高等教育出版社 中國·北京
Higher Education Press, Beijing, China

英漢實用中醫藥大全

趙樸初題

16

DERMATOLOGY
皮膚病學

THE ENGLISH–CHINESE ENCYCLOPEDIA OF PRACTICAL TRADITIONAL CHINESE MEDICINE

Chief Editor   Xu Xiangcai
Assistants   You Ke   Kang Kai
                  Bao Xuequan Lu Yubin

英汉实用中医药大全

主　编　　徐象才
主编助理　尤　可　　康　凯
　　　　　鲍学全　　路玉滨

Higher Education Press
高等教育出版社

16
皮肤病学

	中文	英文
主　编	赵纯修	李　磊
副主编	杜锡贤	王宏理
编　者	杨东海	

DERMATOLOGY

	English	Chinese
Chief Editor	Li Lei	Zhao Chunxiu
Deputy Chief Editor	Wang Hongli	Du Xixian
Editor		Yang Donghai

DERMATOLOGY

The Leading Commission of Compilation and Translation
编译领导委员会

Honorary Director 名誉主任委员	Hu Ximing 胡熙明
Honorary Deputy Directors 名誉副主任委员	Zhang Qiwen　Wang Lei 张奇文　　　王镭
Director 主任委员	Zou Jilong 邹积隆
Deputy Director 副主任委员	Wei Jiwu 隗继武

Members 委员
(以姓氏笔划为序)

Wan Deguang 万德光	Wang Yongyan 王永炎	Wang Maoze 王懋泽
Wei Guikang 韦贵康	Cong Chunyu 丛春雨	Liu Zhongben 刘申本
Sun Guojie 孙国杰	Yan Shiyun 严世芸	Qiu Dewen 邱德文
Shang Chichang 尚炽昌	Xiang Ping 项平	Zhao Yisen 赵以森
Gao Jinliang 高金亮	Cheng Yichun 程益春	Ge Linyi 葛琳仪
Cai Jianqian 蔡剑前	Zhai Weimin 翟维敏	

Advisers 顾问

Dong Jianhua 董建华	Huang Xiaokai 黄孝楷	Geng Jianting 耿鉴庭
Zhou Fengwu 周凤梧	Zhou Ciqing 周次清	Chen Keji 陈可冀

The Commission of Compilation and Translation
编译委员会

Director 主任委员	Xu Xiangcai 徐象才

Deputy Directors 副主任委员	Zhang Zhigang 张志刚	Zhang Wengao 张文高	Jiang Zhaojun 姜兆俊
	Qi Xiuheng 亓秀恒	Xuan Jiasheng 宣家声	Sun Xiangxie 孙祥燮
Members 委员 (以姓氏笔划为序)	Yu Wenping 于文平	Wang Zhengzhong 王正忠	Wang Chenying 王陈应
	Wang Guocai 王国才	Fang Tingyu 方廷钰	Fang Xuwu 方续武
	Tian Jingzhen 田景振	Bi Yongsheng 毕永升	Liu Yutan 刘玉檀
	Liu Chengcai 刘承才	Liu Jiaqi 刘家起	Liu Xiaojuan 刘晓娟
	Zhu Zhongbao 朱忠宝	Zhu Zhenduo 朱振铎	Xun Jianying 寻建英
	Li Lei 李磊	Li Zhulan 李竹兰	Xin Shoupu 辛寿璞
	Shao Nianfang 邵念方	Chen Shaomin 陈绍民	Zou Jilong 邹积隆
	Lu Shengnian 陆胜年	Zhou Xing 周行	Zhou Ciqing 周次清
	Zhang Sufang 张素芳	Yang Chongfeng 杨崇峰	Zhao Chunxiu 赵纯修
	Yu Changzheng 俞昌正	Hu Zunda 胡遵达	Xu Heying 须鹤瑛
	Yuan Jiurong 袁久荣	Huang Naijian 黄乃健	Huang Kuiming 黄奎铭
	Huang Jialing 黄嘉陵	Cao Yixun 曹贻训	Lei Xilian 雷希濂
	Cai Huasong 蔡华松	Cai Jianqian 蔡剑前	

Preface

I am delighted to learn that THE ENGLISH-CHINESE ENCYCLOPEDIA OF PRACTICAL TRADITIONAL CHINESE MEDICINE will soon come into the world.

TCM has experienced many vicissitudes of times but has remained evergreen. It has made great contributions not only to the power and prosperity of our Chinese nation but to the enrichment and improvement of world medicine. Unfortunately, differences in nations, states and languages have slowed down its spreading and flowing outside China. At present, however, an upsurge in learning, researching and applying Traditional Chinese Medicine (TCM) is unfolding. In order to maximize the effect of this upsurge and to lead TCM, one of the brilliant cultural heritages of the Chinese nation, to the world for it to expand and bring benefit to the people of all nations, Mr. Xu Xiangcai called intellectuals of noble aspirations and high intelligence together from Shandong and many other provinces in China and took charge of the work of both compilation and translation of THE ENGLISH-CHINESE ENCYCLOPEDIA OF PRACTICAL TRADITIONAL CHINESE MEDICINE. With great pleasure, the medical staff both at home and abroad will hail the appearance of this encyclopedia.

I believe that the day when the world's medicine is fully

developed will be the day when TCM has spread throughout the world.

I am pleased to give it my preface.

Prof. Dr. Hu Ximing
    Deputy Ministerof the Ministry of Public Health of the People's Republic of China,
    Director General of the State Administrative Bureau of Traditional Chinese Medicine and Pharmacology,
    President of the World Federation of Acupuncture —Moxibustion Societies,
    Member of China Association of Science & Technology,
    Deputy President of All-China Association of Traditional Chinese Medicine,
    President of China Acupuncture & Moxibustion Society.

December, 1989

Preface

The Chinese nation has been through a long, arduous course of struggling against diseases and has developed its own traditional medicine—Traditional Chinese Medicine and Pharmacology (TCMP). TCMP has a unique, comprehensive, scientific system including both theories and clinical practice. Some thousand years since ito—beginnings, not only has it been well preserved but also continuously developed. It has special advantages, such as remarkable curative effects and few side effects. Hence it is an effective means by which people prevent and treat diseases and keep themselves strong and healthy.

All achievements attained by any nation in the development of medicine are the public wealth of all mankind. They should not be confined within a single country. What is more, the need to set them free to flow throughout the world as quickly and precisely as possible is greater than that of any other kind of science. During my more than thirty years of being engaged in Traditional Chinese Medicine(TCM), I have been looking forward to the day when TCMP will have spread all over the world and made its contributions to the elimination of diseases of all mankind. However it is to be deeply regretted that the pace of TCMP in extending outside China has been unsatisfactory due to the major difficulties in expressing its concepts in foreign languages.

Mr. Xu Xiangcai, a teacher of Shandong College of TCM, has sponsored and taken charge of the work of compilation and translation of The English—Chinese Encyclopedia of Practical Traditional Chinese Medicine—an extensive series. This work is a great project, a large—scale scientific research, a courageous effort and a novel creation. I deeply esteem Mr. Xu Xiangcai and his compilers and translators, who have been working day and night for such a long time, for their hard labor and for their firm and indomitable will displayed in overcoming one difficulty after another, and for their great success achieved in this way. As a leader in the circles of TCM, I am duty—bound to do my best to support them.

I believe this encyclopedia will be certain to find its position both in the history of Chinese medicine and in the history of world science and technology.

Mr. Zhang Qiwen
Member of the Standing Committee of
All—China Association of TCM,
Deputy Head of the Health Department
of Shandong Province.
March, 1990

Publisher's Preface

Traditional Chinese Medicine(TCM) is one of China's great cultural heritages. Since the founding of the People's Republic of China in 1949, guided by the farsighted TCM policy of the Chinese Communist Party and the Chinese government, the treasure house of the theories of TCM has been continuously explored and the plentiful literature researched and compiled. As a result, great success has been achieved. Today there has appeared a world-wide upsurge in the studying and researching of TCM. To promote even more vigorous development of this trend in order that TCM may better serve all mankind, efforts are required to further it throughout the world. To bring this about, the language barriers must be overcome as soon as possible in order that TCM can be accurately expressed in foreign languages.

Thus the compilation and translation of a series of English-Chinese books of basic knowledge of TCM has become of great urgency to serve the needs of medical and educational circles both inside and outside China.

In recent years, at the request of the health departments, satisfactory achievements have been made in researching the expression of TCM in English. Based on the investigation into the history and current state of the research work mentioned above, the English-Chinese Encyclopedia of Practical TCM has been published to meet the needs of extending the knowledge of TCM around the world.

The encyclopedia consists of twenty-one volumes, each dealing with a particular branch of TCM. In the process of compilation, the distinguishing features of TCM have been given close attention and great efforts have been made to ensure that the content is scientific, practical, comprehensive and concise. The chief writers of the Chinese manuscripts include professors or associate professors with at least twenty years of practical clinical and / or teaching experience in TCM. The Chinese manuscript of each volume has been checked and approved by a specialist of the relevant branch of TCM. The team of the translators and revisers of the English versions consists of TCM specialists with a good command of English professional medical translators, and teachers of English from TCM colleges or universities. At a symposium to standardize the English versions, scholars from twenty-two colleges or universities, research institutes of TCM or other health institutes probed the question of how to express TCM in English more comprehensively, systematically and accurately, and discussed and deliberated in detail the English versions of some volumes in order to upgrade the English versions of the whole series. The English version of each volume has been re-examined and then given a final checking.

Obviously this encyclopedia will provide extensive reading material of TCM English for senior students in colleges of TCM in China and will also greatly benefit foreigners studying TCM.

The assiduous efforts of compiling and translating this encyclopedia have been supported by the responsible leaders of the State Education Commission of the People's Republic of China, the State Administrative Bureau of TCM and Pharmacy, and the Education Commission and Health Department of Shandong

Province. Under the direction of the Higher Education Department of the State Education Commission, the leading board of compilation and translation of this encyclopedia was set up. The leaders of many colleges of TCM and pharmaceutical factories of TCM have also given assistance.

We hope that this encyclopedia will bring about a good effect on enhancing the teaching of TCM English at the colleges of TCM in China, on cultivating skills in medical circles in exchanging ideas of TCM with patients in English, and on giving an impetus to the study of TCM outside China.

Higher Education Press
March, 1990

Foreword

The English-Chinese Encyclopedia of Practical Traditional Chinese Medicine is an extensive series of twenty-one volumes. Based on the fundamental theories of traditional Chinese medicine(TCM) and with emphasis on the clinical practice of TCM, it is a semi-advanced English-Chinese academic works which is quite comprehensive, systematic, concise, practical and easy to read. It caters mainly to the following readers: senior students of colleges of TCM, young and middle-aged teachers of colleges of TCM, young and middle-aged physicians of hospitals of TCM, personnel of scientific research institutions of TCM, teachers giving correspondence courses in TCM to foreigners, TCM personnel going abroad in the capacity of lecturers or physicians, those trained in Western medicine but wishing to study TCM, and foreigners coming to China to learn TCM or to take refresher courses in TCM.

Because Traditional Chinese Medicine and Pharmacology is unique to our Chinese nation, putting TCM into English has been the crux of the compilation and translation of this encyclopedia. Owing to the fact that no one can be proficient both in the theories of Traditional Chinese Medicine and Pharmacology and the clinical practice of every branch of TCM, as well as in English, to ensure that the English versions express accurately the inherent meanings of TCM, collective translation measures have been taken. That is, teachers of English familiar with TCM, professional medical translators, teachers or physicians of TCM and even teachers of palaeography with a strong command of English were all invited together to co-translate the Chinese manuscripts and, then, to co-deliberate and discuss the English versions. Finally English-speaking foreigners studying TCM or teaching English in China were asked to polish the English versions. In this way, the skills of the above translators and foreigners were merged to ensure the quality of the English versions. However, even using this method, the uncertainty that the English versions will be wholly accepted still remains. As for the Chinese manuscripts, they do reflect the essence, and give a general picture, of traditional Chinese medicine and pharmacology. It is not asserted, though, that they are perfect, I whole-heartedly look forward to any criticisms or opinions from readers in order to make improvements to future editions.

More than 200 people have taken part in the activities of compiling, translating and revising this encyclopedia. They come from twenty-eight institutions in all parts of China. Among these institutions, there are fifteen colleges of TCM:Shandong, Beijing, Shanghai, Tianjin, Nanjing, Zhejiang, Anhui, Henan, Hubei, Guangxi, Guiyang, Gansu, Chengdu, Shanxi and Changchun, and scientific research centers of TCM such as China Academy of TCM and Shandong Scientific Research Institute of TCM.

The Education Commission of Shandong province has included the compilation and translation of this encyclopedia in its scientific research projects and allocated funds accordingly. The Health Department of Shandong Province has also given financial aid together with a number of pharmaceutical factories of TCM. The subsidization from Jinan Pharmaceutical Factory of

TCM provided the impetus for the work of compilation and translation to get under way.

The success of compiling and translating this encyclopedia is not only the fruit of the collective labor of all the compilers, translators and revisers but also the result of the support of the responsible leaders of the relevant leading institutions. As the encyclopedia is going to be published, I express my heartfelt thanks to all the compilers. translators and revisers for their sincere cooperation, and to the specialists, professors, leaders at all levels and pharmaceutical factories of TCM for their warm support.

It is my most profound wish that the publication of this encyclopedia will take its role in cultivating talented persons of TCM having a very good command of TCM English and in extending, rapidly, comprehensive knowledge of TCM to all corners of the globe.

Chief Editor   Xu Xiangcai
Shandong College of TCM
March, 1990

Contents

Notes ·· 1

Part I General Discussions

1 **The Dermapathic Physiology in TCM** ······················· 1
   1.1 The Skin and the Theory of *Wei−Qi*
        (defensive energy)··· 1
   1.2 The Relation between the Skin and Viscera ················ 3
   1.3 The Relation Between the Skin and the Channels
        and Collaterals ·· 5
2 **Traditional Chinese Dermatopathology** ····················· 7
   2.1 Wind−type ··· 7
   2.2 Dampness ·· 8
   2.3 Heat ·· 9
   2.4 Poison ··· 9
   2.5 Dryness ··· 10
   2.6 Blood Stasis ·· 11
   2.7 Deficiency of the Liver and Kidney ··························· 12
3 **Traditional Chinese Medical Differentiation of
    Dermapathic Symptoms and Signs** ···························· 13
   3.1 Subjective Symptoms ·· 13
   3.2 Skin Lesion ·· 16
4 **TCM Treatment of Dermatoses** ································ 19
   4.1 Internal Treatment ·· 20

    4.2   External Treatment ··· 23

Part II Discussions on Individual Dermatoses

1 Viral Dermatoses ··· 28
    1.1   Herpes Simplex ··· 28
    1.2   Herpes Zoster ·· 31
    1.3   Verruca ·· 35

2 Bacterial Dermatoses ··· 42
    2.1   Impetigo Herpetiformis ····································· 42
    2.2   Erysipelas ·· 46

3 Tinea ··· 50
    3.1   Hand−foot Tinea ··· 50
    3.2   Nail Tinea ·· 53
    3.3   Tinea Corporis and Tinea Cruris ····················· 55
    3.4   Tinea Capitis ·· 56
    3.5   Tinea Versicolor ·· 59

4 Insect−borne Dermatoses ······································ 61
    4.1   Scabies ·· 61
    4.2   Insect Dermatitis ··· 64

5 Physicogenic Dermatoses ····································· 67
    5.1   Chilblain ··· 67
    5.2   Rhagades of Hand and Foot ··························· 69
    5.3   Sudamen ·· 70
    5.4   Corns ·· 72

6 Allergic Dermatoses ·· 75
    6.1   Contact Dermatitis ·· 75
    6.2   Eczema ·· 79
    6.3   Urticaria ·· 85

	6.4	Papular Urticaria ···	91
	6.5	Drug-induced Dermatitis ··	95
	6.6	Allergic Purpura ··	103
7	**Dysneuria Dermatoses** ···		111
	7.1	Cutaneous Pruritus ··	111
	7.2	Neurodermatitis ··	116
8	**Erythematous Dermatoses** ···		121
	8.1	Polymorphic Erythema ··	121
	8.2	Erythema Nodusum ···	125
9	**Erythroderma Desquamativum** ··		129
	9.1	Pityriasis Rosea ··	129
	9.2	Psoriasis ··	132
10	**Desmosis** ···		142
	10.1	Lupus Erythematosus ··	142
	10.2	Dermatasclerosis ···	152
	10.3	Dermatomyositis ···	159
11	**Disease of Cutaneous Appendages** ··································		167
	11.1	Acne Vulgaris ···	167
	11.2	Brandy Nose ···	170
	11.3	Seborrhea and Seborrheic Dermatitis ························	175
	11.4	Alopecia Areata ··	179
	11.5	Tragomaschalia ···	183
12	**Pigmentary Dermatoses** ··		186
	12.1	Vitiligo ···	186
	12.2	Chloasma ··	188
	12.3	Freckle ···	192

Formula Index ·· 195
The English-Chinese Encyclopedia of Practical TCM (Booklist) ······ 415

Notes

DERMATOLOGY is the sixteenth of the volumes constituting the English—Chinese Encyclopedia of Practical Traditional Chinese Medicine.

There have long been records of skin diseases in traditional Chinese medical works. As early as the fourteenth century B. C, oracle—bone scriptures were found to contain records of such dermatoses as sarcoptidosis and psoriasis. The Treatise on the Causes and Symptoms of Diseases (by Chao Yuanfang in the Sui Dynasty) includes detailed descriptions of dozens of dermatoses, among which are verrucae, tinea and measles. Two Ancient books, Prescriptions Worth a Thousand Gold for Emergencies and Medical Secrets of an Official, both compiled in the Tang Dynasty, have descriptions of treating skin diseases by using realgar, alumina, sulphur and other traditional Chinese medicines. Over the years, physicians of various historical periods have developed unique therapies for the treatment of dermatoses, and have accumulated a wealth of clinical experience. Traditional Chinese dermatology, with its long history, is an important component of the treasure—house of Traditional Chinese Medicine (TCM). Clinical experience has manifested that many skin diseases for which modern medical remedies do not prove quite effective or have no effect at all may be treated by traditional Chinese medicine and herbs with significant results. Thus, traditional Chinese dermatology is receiving more and more attention both at home and abroad.

The volume consists of two parts, the first of which has four chapters. Contained in these four chapters is a brief introduction to the dermapathic physiology and dermatopathology in terms of traditional Chinese medicine and a brief account of the treatment of skin diseases, as well as the differentiation of their signs and symptoms in TCM. The second part has twelve chapters, in which forty common skin diseases are discussed. Efforts have been made to render this volume concise and practical, by using language that is simple yet popular. This is our first attempt to compile and translate such a book and we would greatly appreciate your opinions and advice concerning our work.

Finally, we wish to express our thanks to Professor Bian Tianyu, Professor Lei Xilian, and Professor Tracey L.Bailey an American scholar, who have made valuable suggestions for the improvement of the book, and, also, to Mr. Zhou Xing, Miss Yang Yang and Miss Li Xiaoman, who have contributed their efforts to our editorial work.

The Editors

Part I General Discussions

1 The Dermapathic Physiology in TCM

1.1 The Skin and the Theory of *Wei–Qi* (defensive energy)

Over 2000 years ago, traditional Chinese medicine (TCM) developed the physiological theories involving *Zang* and *Fu* (viscera), channels and collaterals, *Qi*, blood and body fluid. The so-called *Qi* performs a vital physiological function; it refers, in TCM, to one of the most fundamental elements constituting the body, and that which maintains vital activities of the body. The concept of *Qi* involves many senses, but on the whole, it refers to two different aspects: first, the refined nutritive substance flowing within the body, and second, the function of the internal organs and tissues in general. Since the refined nutritive substance exists in every part of the body, *Qi* derives its different names from different parts of the body, such as *Zong–Qi* (pectoral *Qi*), which gathers in the chest, *Yuan–Qi*, which originates from the kidneys, *Ying–Qi*, which circulates through the blood vessels, and

Wei-Qi, which circulates outside the blood vessels and originates in the striae of skin, muscles, viscera, and sweat pores.

In TCM physiology, the theory of *Wei-Qi* is most closely related to the skin. The Miraculous Pivot says, "*Wei-Qi* warms up the flesh, strengthens the skin, nourishes the striae of skin and muscles, and controls the openning and closing of the skin pores" and ,"If the harmony of *Wei-Qi* is achieved, the muscles will be healthy and strong, the skin smooth and soft, and their striae refined and firm". In short, the *Wei-Qi* has three physiological functions: first, to protect the superfical portion of the body against exogenous pathogenic factors; second, to warm up and nourish the organs both internally and externally (such as skin, hair, muscles, viscera, etc.), and to moisten the skin as well; and third, to open and close sweat pores, regulate the secretion of sweat, and to maintain a relatively constant temperature within the body.

The power of *Wei-Qi* is related to the health of the skin and its susceptibility to exogenous pathogenic factors. An abundance of *Wei-Qi* will make the skin soft, smooth and strong, the muscles plump, and the striae refined and firm so that the exogenous pathogenic factors can be checked. The deficiency of *Wei-Qi* will make the skin dry, the hair drop, the muscles weak, and the pores loose. This in turn will cause sweating due to debility, and the exogenous pathogenic factors will be allowed to take advantage of this condition to affect the body. As the saying goes, "where pathogenic factors take effect, there is a deficiency of *Wei-Qi*". Therefore, the *Wei-Qi* performs a crucial physiological function, namely, defending and strengthening the uperficial proportion of the body.

1.2 The Relation between the Skin and Viscera

The human body is a complete organic system, whose various organs, though performing different functions, are related to each other and influence each other. In other words, the condition of one particular organ may affect other organs. Skin, (including the attached hair and nails), is an important component of the human body, closely related to other organs. For instance, the condition of the heart, which controls blood vessels, is reflected on the face. Whether the heart functions normally or not can easily be judged by the complexion of the face: when the heart is in normal condition, the face has a healthy complexion, but if the heart—Qi is in deficiency and circulation is poor, the complexion of the face may be pale or bluish. The liver controls the tendons, its condition being reflected on the fingers, toes and nails, i.e, it takes charge of the action of the tendons, commanding the movement of all the muscles and joints of the body. Since the nails are the endings of the tendons, the liver is therefore closely related to the nails. When the liver—blood is abundant, the tendons will be stout and powerful, the nails will be strong and show a high complexion; but, if the liver—blood is deficient, the tendons will be weak, and the nails will wither. Hence, the colour and shape of the nails will change, and they are liable to become crisp. The spleen is in charge of digestion, and its condition is reflected on the lips. When the spleen performs normally the function of digesting and transporting, the refined nutritive substance of food and water will nourish the body, the Qi and blood will be abundant, the limbs strong, the muscles and skin sturdy, and the lips rosy. But, if the spleen is weak and the digestive function is abnormal, the muscles and skin will be thin and weak, the limbs feeble, and the lips pale, withered, or yellowish. In the case of the lungs, they control all the *Qi* in the body and influence the skin and hair. Here, the skin and hair refer to the superficial portion of the body, including the pores and some other tissues as well. The external function of the lungs lies in their dispersing action, by which the refined nutritive substance of food and water is spread over the superficial portion of the body, nourishing the tissues of the skin, hair and muscles. Such refined nutritive substance includes *Wei—Qi*, which, when dispersed to the superficial portion of the body, will perform the function of strengthening the surface and resisting the attack of pathogenic factors. As the lungs and skin are so closely related, they influence each other pathologically. For instance, when exogenous pathogenic factors invade the surface portion of the body, they also attack the lungs simultaneously, causing the skin and lungs to show symptoms such as fever, chills, and cough. If the lung—*Qi* is weak, so that it cannot disperse the *Wei—Qi*, it will result in the withering of the skin and hair, and will lessen the function of strengthening the body's surface portion and hency cause vulnerability to exogenous pathogenic factors. As a result, invasion by exogenous factors is made easy. The kidney stores the vital essence and energy, a condition which is reflected in the hair. Whether the hair is growing or shedding, shiny or withered, depends on whether the essential *Qi* of the kidney is abundant or deficient. When the kidney stores plentiful vital essence and energy, the hair is thick, pitch—black and shiny. But, if the essential *Qi* in the kidney is insufficient, the hair will shrivel or turn white and lack luster.

In short, the skin and viscera are closely related. Whether the viscera are performing their functions normally or not is often reflected on the skin and hair. Conversely, the condition of the skin and hair will reflect the state of the actions of the viscera. Such a close relation between the skin and viscera is, in part, due to the connecting and conveying function of the channels and collaterals.

1.3 The Relation Between the Skin and the Channels and Collaterals

In the book Plain Questions, which is part of the Internal Classic, the chapter entitled Discussion on Skin states, " The twelve channels belong to the skin", indicating that the skin is an important area through which the channels move. The meridian system is the general term for channels and collaterals, which are component parts of the tissues and are spread all over the human body. Physiologically, channels and collaterals perform the role of transporting *Qi* and blood, connecting the interior and exterior, resisting exogenous pathogenic factors and safeguarding the functions of the organs.

In the meridian system, the twelve channels are connected directly with the viscera. Each channel runs across a certain area of the superficial portion of the body and is connected with a certain inner organ. The channels themselves are linked to each other by collaterals. Thus, all the organs are joined together as a systematic whole. Since the channels and collaterals connect the viscera inwardly and the body surface outwardly, pathogenic factors can move between the viscera and the body surface through channels and collaterals. For instance, the pathogenic factors in the superficial portion of the body can enter the body, bringing harm to the viscera, while the pathologic change in the viscera can also be conveyed to the surface portion of the body, causing certain skin diseases.

By judging the particular area where a skin disease exists and by examining the route and net-work of channels and collaterals in the body, it is possible to decide which inner organ the diseased area belongs to. This method plays a guiding role in the differentiation of dermapathic symptoms and signs and in the medication for skin diseases. For example, the nose belongs to the Lung Channel and the cheeks belong to the Stomach Channel. Therefore, diseases like brandy nose and acne on the face are considered to be caused by warm and hot pathogens moving upward from the lungs and stomach. In such a case, the therapy of removing heat from the lungs and stomach can be applied. The areas around the ears, the chest and the pudenda belong to the Liver Channel and Gallbladder Channel; therefore, eczema around the ears, herpes zoster on the chest and eczema on the pudenda are believed to be caused by damp-heat in the Liver and Gallbladder Channels. In such a case, the therapy of clearing away dampness and heat from the Liver Channel and Gallbladder Channel is adopted.

2 Traditional Chinese Dermatopathology

Dermatoses are of great variety, and their clinical manifestations are also varying, but in terms of pathological changes, there are mainly seven types: wind, dampness, heat, poison, dryness, blood stasis, and deficiency of the liver—Qi and kidney—Qi. These pathological changes often act together and lead to onset of diseases, showing complex symptoms and causing damage to the skin.

2.1 Wind—type

1. Characteristics of Wind Pathological Changes

(1) Abrupt onset: The attack of disease is sudden or the patient's condition deteriorates rapidly, as in the case of urticaria.

(2) Liability to move and waver as in the case of urticaria.

(3) Tendency to spread outward and upward. Thus, the skin diseases caused by wind appear mostly on the head, face and the superficial portion of the body, such as alopecia areata.

(4) Wind is liable to lodge in the blood and attack the blood, often having a close relation with heat, dryness and deficiency of blood. Therefore, wind is not likely to be suppressed without first treating the blood, just as the Ancients said:"To suppress the wind, it is necessary to treat the blood first; and the wind will vanish itself when the blood becomes fluent and normal."

(5) Wind is the chief pathogenic factor in various diseases,

with a tendency to combine with other pathogenic factors to cause diseases. Consequently, many skin diseases exhibit characteristics of wind pathology.

2. Clinical Manifestations of Wind

Most skin damages take the form of urticaria, papular eruption, and erythema, which are inclined to be on the move and spread over the whole body, characterized by sudden onset, rapid advance, abrupt disapperance, and irregular itching.

2.2 Dampness

1. Characteristics of the Pathological Changes of Dampness

(1) Dampness is a turbid pathogen with a tendency to spread downward and outward. The tendency of downward spreading is manifested by the fact that many pathological changes take place on the lower limbs or spread downward from upper parts of the body, while the tendency of outward spreading is shown by the fact that such pathological changes of dampness are liable to cause hidroa, tumefaction and exudation.

(2) Dampness is inclined to stay and persist, and is difficult to exterminate. This is manifested by the fact that pathological changes of dampness usually linger for a long time, attack repeatedly, and are difficult to cure, as in the case of eczema.

(3) Dampness often mixes with wind and heat to produce various pathological changes, which in turn cause diseases.

2. Clinical Manifestations of Dampness

The skin damage in this case often takes the form of tumefaction, hidroa, erosion, exudation, hypersteatosis and lipoid furfures. The general symptoms include acratia as well as chest distress and loss of appetite. Also there is often local itching.

2.3 Heat

1. Characteristics of Heat Pathological Changes.

(1) Heat is a *Yang* pathogen, whose attack is usually abrupt and sudden, such as the cases of erysipelas, and scald, etc.

(2) Heat tends to rise upward, often affecting the head and face, and causing diseases such as brandy nose and adolescent acne.

(3) Heat is liable to penetrate the skin, causing warm-heat pathogens there. For instance, the damp-heat in the liver and gallbladder may penetrate the skin and cause herpes zoster.

(4) Heat is active and abundant, liable to enter blood and cause a general fever. When the abundant heat scorches the skin, it will turn red and hot, causing a feeling of pain or even the formation of pus.

2. Clinical Manifestations of Heat

The damage to skin by heat is manifested by reddened skin, erosion, pustulae, scorching, itching and pain, accompanied possibly by constipation and dark urine, as well as heat sensation and thirst.

2.4 Poison

Generally there are four common types of poisoning: drug poisoning, food poisoning, insect poisoning, and rhus poisoning.

1. Characteristics of the Pathological Changes of Poison

(1) The pathogenic factors of poison are most likely to cause diseases to those who are of a weak constitution.

(2) Poison is characterized by its great violence, capable of causing serious and dangerous side effects. The pathogens usually

gather on the skin, causing various forms of skin damage. They may attack the viscera, resulting in their dysfunction, or even injuring them. They may also enter the blood, causing general symptoms like fever and shivering, as in the case of serious dermatitis medicamentosa.

2. Clinical Manifestations of Poison

Skin damage by poison may be manifested in the form of red swelling, purple maculae, papular eruption, urticaria, vesicle, erosion, ulcera, epidermal necrolysis and exfoliation. The attack is often abrupt and recurrent, and the advance is rapid, accompanied by local burning heat, itching, or pain. There may also be general fever, fatigue and discomfort.

2.5 Dryness

1. Characteristics of the Pathological Changes of Dryness

(1) Domination of dryness brings about deficiency of fluid, causing impairment of *Yin* and reduction of blood. Consequently, xeroderma, pachylosis and squamae often result.

(2) Deficiency of blood causes dryness, while dryness of blood causes wind. When wind dominates, itch will ensue.

(3) The pathological changes of dryness take place mostly during the anaphase of a skin disease. The process is usually slow and prolonged.

2. Clinical Manifestations of Dryness

The skin damage in the case of dryness is manifested by xerosis cutis, pacchylosis, lichenoid dermatitis, rhagades, squamae, atrophia trichoxerosis, trichomadesis, as well as the nails growing thin and withered. Itching is usually the subjective symptom.

2.6 Blood Stasis

1. Characteristics of the Pathological Changes of Blood Stasis

(1) Being a parenchymatous pathological change, blood stasis may gather in the superficial portion of the body, or block the channels, or form blood clots, causing various kinds of skin damage and disease.

(2) The pathological change process of blood stasis is closely related with *Qi*: The fluency of *Qi* will result in the fluency of blood, while the stagnancy of *Qi* will lead to blood stasis; conversely, blood stasis can also result in stagnancy of *Qi*. Consequently, the method of promoting the flow of *Qi* and circulation of blood is often adopted clinically in the treatment of syndromes of blood stasis.

(3) The area where the pathological changes take place is often invariable, and the course of disease is usually chronic.

2. Clinical Manifestations of Blood Stasis

The skin damage under this category is manifested by the following diseases: Petechia, Ecchymosis, violet red or dark red spots, pigmented spots, nodes, lumps, capillarectasia, varicosity, thickened and hardened skin, verrucous vegetation or cicatrix, etc, which may be accompanied by such pathological changes as purple lip, tongue ecchymosis, and menstrual disorder as well. The subjective symptoms may include pain, numbness, and bradyesthesia.

2.7 Deficiency of the Liver and Kidney

1. Characteristics of the Pathological Changes of Liver / Kidney Deficiency

(1) Deficiency of the liver blood will fail to nourish the nails, which in turn will dry up and wither.

(2) Deficiency of liver blood cannot enrich the tendons, while inadequacy of *Qi* in the tendons will cause warts.

(3) Deficiency of liver—*Yin* and kidney *Yin* will result in the malnutrition of skin, which, in turn, will cause white patches.

(4) Deficiency of liver—kidney essence and blood causes malnutrition of hair, which may result in trichoxerosis and trichomadesis or achromotrichia.

(5) Deficiency of kidney—*Qi* causes the black *Qi* to ascend, effecting chloasma on the face.

2. Clinical Manifestations of Liver—Kidney Deficiency

(1) Pigmentary skin diseases like chloasma and melanosis.

(2) Diseases of hair and nails, such as trichomadesis, grey hair, and malnutrition of nails.

(3) Diseases of the connective tissues like systemic lupus erythematosus and systemic scleroderma.

The subjective symptoms include light—headedness, tinnitus, deafness, pain and weakness in the knee and lumbar regions, sexual impotence, and prospermia. Most of them are of chronic courses.

3 Traditional Chinese Medical Differentiation of Dermapathic Symptoms and Signs

Dermapathic symptoms are classified into two groups: first, the subjective symptoms, which are the patient's sensations of the diseases, and second, the skin damages, ei, the manifastations of dermatopathologic changes on the skin or mucosa, which are objective signs called skin lesion or eruption.

The TCM perception of dermapathic symptoms, or, the TCM differentiation of subjective symptoms and skin lesion, is the theoretical basis for the TCM treatment of dermatoses. To diagnose and treat dermatoses well, it is essential first to identify the dermapathic symptoms and lesion and to grasp the differentiation of them in terms of TCM. In addition, it is also necessary to analyze the patient's state of Qi and blood, any deficiency or excess of the internal viscera and the physical condition of the individual, as well as the changes of the tongue coating and pulse.

3.1 Subjective Symptoms

The main subjective symptom of dermatoses is itching. Other symptoms include burning heat sensation, aching, and numbness etc.

1. Itching

Itching, the most common symptom in dermatoses, is caused mostly by five pathological changes on the skin, namely, wind, dampness, heat, dryness and insect poison. It is differentiated in TCM as follows:

(1) Itching due to Wind Pathogen

This sort of itching is caused mainly by wind pathological changes, often occuring all over the body or itching intensely. It is characterized by sudden attack, quick development, and irregular wandering with involvement of the whole body, as in the case of urticaria.

(2) Itching due to Dampness

This type of itching is chiefly due to the pathological changes of dampness. It is often accompanied by such skin damages as skin swelling, blister, exudation and erosion, as in the case of eczema and foot tinea.

(3) Itching due to Heat

This is mainly caused by the pathological changes of heat, mostly accompanied by inflammation, reddened skin, and burning heat sensation, as in the case of acute dermatitis and eczema.

(4) Itching due to Dryness

This type of itching is also known as blood-deficiency itching caused by deficiency of blood which in turn changes into dryness of blood. This will cause wind pathogen. It is often accompanied by skin dryness, roughness, desquamation and lichenoid changes, such as neurodermatitis and chronic eczema.

(5) Itching due to Insect Poison

This is caused by insect poison affecting the skin or mucosa. The itching area is usually fixed, but it may also spread elsewhere.

The affected area usually itches intensely and it may also be infectious, as in the case of scabies and foot tinea.

2. Ache

Aching results mainly from stagnation of Qi and blood and blockage of the channels as well. It is differentiated in TCM into the following types:

(1) Heat Ache: The affected area shows inflammatory redness, and the ache is alleviated when coming into contact with cold.

(2) Cold Ache: The skin colour of the affected area is unchanged, and the pain is alleviated when coming into contact with warmth.

(3) Ache Caused by Anger: The aching occurs at no fixed place or time. It is alleviated during happy moods but intensified with a bad temper.

(4) Ache Caused by Blood Stasis: The aching area is fixed and the skin colour shows reddish brown or purplish blue.

3. Numbness

This is caused by deficiency of Qi and blood and malnutrition of the skin, which is due to blockage of the skin channels and hindered flow of Qi and blood. In this case, the skin shows normal colour or slightly pale, with a decline in sense of touch and sense of pain. It is differentiated in TCM as deficiency of Qi and blood.

4. Cauma

This is caused by heat pathogenic changes affecting the skin, often accompanied by itching as well as some red skin lesion. It is differentiated in TCM as overabundance of heat.

3.2 Skin Lesion

1. Macular Eruption, a skin lesion with distinct bounds and change of skin colour, the surface of the diseased area being on the same level as the surrounding skin.

Differential Diagnosis: Red maculae are due to heat or blood-heat, purple maculae are due to blood stasis or excess of toxic heat, white maculae are due to stagnation of *Qi* and blood stasis or deficiency of liver-*Yin* and kidney-*Yin*, brown maculae are due to stagnation of *Qi* and blood stasis or deficiency of the liver and kidney, and black maculae are due to deficiency of the kidney. Secondary pigmented spots are mostly due to blood stasis as well as derangement of *Qi* and blood.

2. Papular Eruption, characterized by small solid papulae prominent on the surrounding skin with clear bounds.

Differential Diagnosis: Red papulae are due to blood-heat and wind-heat, purple papulae are due to blood stasis and toxic heat, and skin-coloured papulae are due to stagnation of *Qi* or wind-cold.

3. Blisters, skin lesion containing liquid and being prominent out of the surrounding skin.

Differential Diagnosis: Blisters full of water-like liquid are due to the accumulation of the damp pathogen; blisters surrounded by awla, or blisters growing on red papulae, are due to damp-heat; blisters with bloody liquid are due to blood-heat; and blisters with turbid liquid are due to noxious dampness.

4. Pustulae——a kind of skin lesion, prominent out of the surrounding skin, containing pus.

Differential Diagnosis: Pustulae are caused by noxious heat.

5. Tubercles: Local parenchymatous subcutaneous lesion.

Differential Diagnosis: Red tubercles are due to blood—heat or blood stasis; skin—coloured tubercles are due to accumulation of blood stasis or phlegm—dampness.

6. Urticaria——temporary, local flat edematous prominance usually occurring and vanishing abruptly and repeatedly, leaving no trace after disappearance.

Differential Diagnosis: Red urticaria is due to wind—heat or blood—heat, white urticaria due to wind—cold, wind—dampness or deficiency of blood plus wind pathogen.

7. Squamae——scale—like furfures resulting from skin accumulation and exfoliation of skin.

Differential Diagnosis: Squamae formed at the early stage of a skin disease are due to wind—heat pathogen whereas those at the late stage are due to dryness from deficiency of blood and malnutrition of skin; lipoidal squamae are due to excessive dampness, and dry squamae are due to dryness of blood.

8. Erosion—— wet erosive formation resulting from skin damage of lesions such as blister and pustulae. It leaves no trace after recovery.

Differential Diagnosis: Erosion with seepage is mostly due to damp—heat pathogen; erosion with profuse seepage is due to excess of dampness, and erosion with pus is due to noxious dampness.

9. Ulcer——local tissue lesion of skin or mucoca, caused by inflammatory or non—inflammatory damage, deep in the true skin.

Differential Diagnosis: Acute ulcer, red granulation at the bottom with thick and yellowish pus, accompanied by red swelling and pain with heat-sensation, is due mainly to noxious heat; chronic ulcer is slow in healing, with dusky or reddish granulation at the bottom and scant secretion, due mainly to deficiency of Qi and blood. If edema is found in the granulation on the ulcer's surface, it is due to excessive dampness.

    10. Rhagades——thread-like cracks in the skin, found mostly on hands and feet.

    Differential Diagnoses: Rhagades is due to deficiency of blood, wind-dryness and excessive cold.

    11. Lichenoid changes——skin lesion characterized by local pachydermia, xerosis. Pachylosis and the prominence of deep cleavage lines, or tiny, thin furfures.

    Differential Diagnosis: Lichenoid changes are due to deficiency of blood and wind-dryness.

    12. Cicatrices——connective tissues formed during recovey from ulcer and damage; or lumps of primary neoplastic connective tissues. They are classified into two classes: atrophic cicatrices and hypertrophic cicatrices.

    Differential Diagnosis: Cicatrices are due to blood stasis.

4 TCM Treatment of Dermatoses

Treatment of dermatoses in China has a long history with rich clinical experience, which constitutes an important component of the valuable inheritance of TCM. Chinese traditional dermatology has made valuable contributions to international dermatology. For instance, the cure for leprosy with chaulmoogra seeds, the cure for syphilis with arsenic and mercurial, and the cure for scabies with sulphur were all first developed in China and, later on, introduced to the rest of the world.

The traditional Chinese medical treatment of dermatoses relies, in principle, on '*bianzheng lunzhi*', a term referring to the whole process of grasping the overall condition of the patient's disease and learning about the pathological signs and symptoms through analysis with the TCM theory of differential diagnosis, and lastly, deciding on the correct treatment, selecting the suitable formula, and administering the medicine. As the saying goes, "To treat the exterior, it is essential to base the treatment on the interior factors". The integrative concept of connecting local pathological changes with the overall condition of the body and environment is the basic concept of traditional Chinese therapeutics and is the basic principle in the TCM treatment of dermatosis.

The treatment of dermatosis is divided into two classes: internal treatment and external treatment, both of which have inherited the theories and achievements of TCM-treatment and TCM-pharmacology, with characteristics different from those of modern Western medicine.

4.1 Internal Treatment

There are various internal therapeutic methods for dermatosis. In clinical practice, one particular therapeutic method is usually adopted as the chief method for a case, accompanied by some other methods.

1. Therapy for Dispelling Wind and Removing Heat

This therapy is used to treat skin diseases caused by wind and heat pathogens existing in the skin, among which are urticaria and pityriasis rosea, etc.

Typical Formula: *Xiaofeng San* (Formula 1).

Basic Drugs for Use: Flos Chrysanthemi, Herba Menthae, Periostracum Cicadae, Herba Spirodelae, Folium Mori, Fructus Arctii, Cortex Dictamni Radicis, Fructus Kochiae and Gypsum Fibrosum.

2. Therapy for Expelling Wind and Cold Pathogens

This therapy is used to treat skin diseases caused by wind and cold pathogens invading the skin, such as urticaria and cutaneous pruritus, etc.

Typical Formula: *Jingfang Baidu San* (Formula 2).

Basic Drugs for Use: Schizonepeta, Radix Ledebouriellae, Rhizoma seu Radix Notopterygii, Radix Angelicae Pubescentis, Radix Ephedrae, Ramulus Cinnamomi, Radix Angelicae Dahuricae, Herba Asari and Folium Perillae.

3. Therapy for Promoting Blood Circulation and Removing Wind Pathogen

This method is used to treat diseases caused by long-existing pathogenic wind in the blood system. These diseases have defied medical treatment for a long time and may be accompanied by blood stasis. Such diseases include prurigo nodularis and pigmented purpuric lichenoid dermatitis.

Typical Formula: *Siwu Xiaofeng Yin* (Formula 3).

Basic Drugs for Use: Radix Angelicae Sinensis, Rhizoma Ligustici Chuanxiong, Radix Salviae Miltiorrhizae, Caulis Spatholobi, Herba Schizonepetae, Radix Ledebouriellae, Scorpio, Zaocys and Bombyx Batryticatus.

4. Therapy for Nourishing the Blood to Expel Wind

This therapy is used to treat skin diseases like neurodermatitis and chronic eczema which are due to blood deficiency and wind-dryness or blood dryness.

Typical Formula: *Danggui Yinzi*(Formula 4).

Basic Drugs for Use: Radix Angelicae Sinensis, Radix Paeoniae Alba, Radix Rehmanniae, Radix Rehmanniae Praeparata, Radix Polygoni Multiflori, Fructus Cannabis, Caulis Spatholobi, Radix Salviae Miltiorrhizae, Herba Schizonepetae, Radix Ledebouriellae, Fructus Tribuli, etc.

5. Therapy for Clearing away Heat and Toxic Material

This method is used to treat diseases like impetigo herpetiformis, erysipelas, and furuncle caused by noxious heat.

Typical Formulae: *Wuwei Xiaodu Yin* (Formula 5), and *Huanglian Jiedu Tang* (Formula 6).

Basic Drugs for Use: Flos Lonicerae, Herba Taraxaci, Herba Violae, Fructus Forsythiae, Radix Scutellariae, Rhizoma Coptidis, Capejasmine Fruit, Cortex Phellodendri, Flos Chrysanthemi Indici, Folium Isatidis and Radix Isatidis, etc.

6. Therapy for Removing Pathogenic Heat from Blood

This method is used to treat skin diseases like psoriasis and allergic purpura caused by heat pathogen in the blood.

Typical Formula: *Xij iao Dihuang Tang* (Formula 7).

Basic Drugs for Use: Radix Rehmanniae, Radix Paeoniae Rubra, Cortex Moutan Radicis, Radix Arnebiae seu Lithospermi, Radix Scrophulariae, Radix Cynanchi Atrati, Rhizoma Imperatae, Cortex Lycii Radicis, Gypsum Fibrosum, etc.

7. Therapy for Clearing away Heat and Promoting Diuresis

This method is used to treat skin diseases like herpes zoster and acute eczema caused by the accumulation of noxious damp-heat in the skin.

Typical Formulae: *Longdan Xiegan Tang* (Formula 8), the liver-fire and *Wushen Tang* (Formula 9).

Basic Drugs for Use: Radix Gentianae, Capejasmine Fruit, Radix Scutellariae, Cortex phellodendri, Radix Sophorae Flavescentis, Herba Artemisiae Capillaris, Rhizoma Dioscoreae Septemlobae, Semen Plantaginis, Poria, Rhizoma Alismatis, Caulis Akebiae, Radix Stephaniae Tetrandrae, Semen Phaseoli, etc.

8. Therapy for Activating Blood Flow and Removing Blood Stasis

This method is employed to cure such diseases as erythema nodusum, dermatasclerosis and keloid, which are caused by blood stasis.

Typical Formula: *Taohong Siwu Tang* (Formula 10).

Basic Drugs for Use: Semen Persicae, Flos Carthami, Radix Paeoniae Rubrum, Rhizoma Ligustici Chuanxiong, Radix

Salviae Miltiorrhizae, Squama Manitis, Resina Olibani, Myrrha, Rhizoma Sparganii, Rhizoma Zedoariae, Eupolyphaga Sinensis Walker, Lumbricus.

9. Therapy for Resolving Hard Lumps

This therapy is employed to treat skin diseases like tuberculoderm, verruca vulgar is and acne, belonging to subcutaneous nodule and verrucosis.

Typical Formula: *Taohong Erchen Tang* (Formula 11).

Basic Drugs for Use: Rhizoma Pinelliae, Pericarpium Citri Reticulatae, Bulbus Fritillariae, Semen Citri Reticulatae, Spica Prunellae, Rhizoma Peionis, Concha Ostreae, Fructus Forsythiae, Thallus Laminariae, Thallus Eckloniae and Sargassum.

10. Therapy for Tonifying the Liver and Kidney

This method is employed for treating skin diseases like allopecia areata and chloasma, which are caused by deficiency of the liver—Qi and kidney—Qi.

Typical Formula: *Shenying Yangzhen Dan* (Formula 12)

Basic Drugs for Use: Radix Rehmanniae Praeparata, Radix Polygoni Multiflori, Radix Angelicae Sinensis, Radix Paeoniae Alba, Fructus Corni, Semen Cuscutae, Fructus Lycii, Herba Ecliptae, Fructus Ligustri Lucidi, etc.

4.2 External Treatment

External treatment is a local treatment, based on subjective symptoms and the condition of the skin lesion, using various kinds of drug and dosage forms, it plays an important part in the treatment of dermatoses and, in the case of some skin diseases, may alone yield satisfactory effects. Here are listed as follows the common dosage forms, their uses and actions:

1. Liquor for Steaming or Dressing: It is a water solution obtained through boiling a single drug or compound prescription to a certain concentration and then filtering off the drug remains. It has the following actions: clearing away heat and toxic material, expelling wind, arresting itchings, removing dampness, astringing, promoting blood circulation to remove swelling, destroying parasites and getting rid of verruca. For the use of liquor, there are two therapeutic methods: first, the steaming and washing method and, second, the wet packing method. The first method consists of heating the affected part of the skin with the steam of the hot liquor before soaking and washing it in the liquor, usually once or twice a day for thirty minutes each time. Preparing such a liquor for use requires only ten minutes' boiling. Moreover, in soaking and washing the affected part, the temperature of the liquor should not be too high. This method is employed to treat chronic pruritic dermatoses, such as neurodermatitis and chronic eczema. The wet packing method consists of placing on the lesion six to eight layers of disinfectant gauze or towels soaked with the liquor (squeezing them a little bit before use), and changing the layers every few minutes. This is done two or three times daily, each time lasting 30 to 60 minutes. Cool wet packing is often preferred clinically with the temperature of decoction equal to or slightly lower than the indoor temperature in summer, and in winter 10℃ is usually preferred. This method is used to treat acute or subacute eczema, dermatitis and skin lesion with obvious seepage and swelling.

Basic drugs for choice in making the liquor are as follows: Herba Taraxaci, Flos Chrysanthemi Indici, Herba Portulacae,

Radix Sophorae Flavescentis, Cortex Phellodendri, Radix Sanguisorbae, Fructus Cnidii, etc.

Compound Prescriptions for choice: *Jiedu Xiyao* (Formula 13); *Zhiyang Xiyao* (Formula 14); *Qie feng Xiyao* (Formula 15); *Xiaofan Xiyao* (Formula 16).

(2)Powder: It is a preparation of one or more drugs ground into powder, with the action of protecting the skin, removing heat pathogen and promoting the subsidence of swelling, astringing heat, destroying parasites and relieving itching. Depending on the condition of a particular case, the powder may be applied dry on the diseased part, or mixed with cool boiled water, vinegar and sesame oil into a paste to be applied to the diseased part. However, powder should not be applied to the hairy parts or those parts with much exudation. Generally, powder is used to treat acute or subacute skin lesions having little or no exudation.

Typical Formula: *Huang Bo San* (Formula 17); *Qingha San* (Formula 18); *Diandao San* (Formula 19) and *Dahuang Fen*, etc.

3. Oleo—infusions: This is prepared by frying drugs in oil until they are brown and then removing them from the oil, or by mixing sesame oil, peanut oil, or other plant oil with drug powder or drug oil obtained from oil—containing drugs. It has the action of clearing away heat and toxic material, subduing swelling and pain, astringing dryness and dampness, protecting and nourishing the skin.

Administration and Dosage: Apply the oleo—infusion on the diseased part with a cotton stick or a writing brush, twice or three times daily.

Uses: It is indicated in intermission of wet dressing for skin lesion with erosion and exudation, in pyoderma with erosion and pus, or in chronic dermatitis or eczema.

Typical Oleo—infusions: *Zicao You* (Formula 20); *Huanglian You* (Formula 21); *Heidou Liuyou* (Formula 22) and *Kang Liuyou* (Formula 23), etc.

4. Tincture: This is made by soaking a single drug or a complex prescription in white spirit or ethyle alcohol, with the remains filtered out at the end of the process. It has the actions of detoxicating, parasite—killing, promoting blood circulation and itch—arresting.

Administration and Dosage: It is applied directly to the diseased part with a cotton stick or a brushpen, twice or three times daily.

Uses: It is indicated in localized and chronic dermatitis with no ulceration, such as neurodermatitis, localized cutaneous pruritus, mycosis cutis, alopecia areata and vitiligo, etc.

Typical Tincture: Malaytea Scurfpea Tincture (obtained by infusing for 25 g of malaytea scurfpea in 100 g of 75% alcohol for one week) alcohol, indicated in vitiligo and alopecia areata etc; Radix Stemonae Tincture (obtained through infusing for a week 25 g of Radix Stemonae in 100 g of 75% alcohol), indicated in neurodermatitis, urticaria and head lice; and *Fufang Tujingpi Ding* (Formula 24).

5. Acetum: This is made by soaking drugs in vinegar, with the remains filtered out at the end of the process. It has the actions of killing parasites, arresting itching and softening cutin, indicated mainly in such diseases as hand—foot tinea and nail tinea.

Administration and Dosage: Wash the diseased part clean and then wipe it dry before soaking it in the acetum for 15 to 40 minutes each time, 2 to 3 times daily.

Typical Aceta: *Ezhangfeng Cujinji* (Formula 25) and *Huohuang Jinji* (Formula 26), etc.

6. Ointment: This is made by boiling or mixing the powder of medicinal herbs together with plant oil, animal fat, or with vaseline and beeswax. It has the actions of clearing away heat and toxic material, killing parasites, arresting itching as well as nourishing and astringing the skin. Ointments are indicated in chronic dermatoses with such skin lesions as scab, rhagades, and lichenoid changes, and it is also used in treating acute and infective nonulceration dermatoses.

Administration and dosage: Apply the ointment directly to the diseased part, twice daily, or spread the ointment on a cotton gauze before applying it to the diseased part, changing the dressing once a day or once every other day.

Typical ointment: *Runf u Gao* (Formula 27), *Huanglian Gao* (Formula 28), *Jinhuang Gao* (Formula 29) and *Daqing Gao* (Formula 30).

Part II Discussions on Individual Dermatoses

1 Viral Dermatoses

1.1 Herpes Simplex

Herpes simplex is an acute herpetic dermatosis caused by simplex herpetic virus, characterized by the fact that it is inclined to appear where the dermatomucosae join one another, and takes the form of local, clustered vesicles. It is known as heat sore in TCM, so called because it tends to accompany febrile diseases.

Etiology and Pathogenesis

Herpes simplex results from febrile diseases, gastrointestinal dysfunction, or overfatigue, which lower the body's resistance to illness, i.e, they weaken the vital—Qi and thus allow the pathogenic factors to take effect.

Clinical Manifestations

1. This disease, normally found in adults, usually attacks where the skin and mucous membrane are connected, often occurring in areas around the lips and nostrils, or on cheeks and ex-

ternal genitalia.

2. A sensation of local itching and burning heat first occurs, followed by the appearance of erythema, on which are soon formed vesicles in clusters. The base of the vesicle shows reddish, and the liquid in it is hyaline or slightly turbid. It may also be accompanied by intertrigo, exudation or scab, etc, and after recovery, some temporary pigmentation often remains.

3. If there is secondary infection, it may be accompanied by suppuration and pain; the local lymph node is often tumescent with tenderness.

4. Subjective symptoms include sensation of burning heat, the feeling of itching and slight pain.

5. The course of the disease lasts one or two weeks. It is capable of spontaneous cure, but is likely to recur.

Type and Treatment

1. Internal Treatment

(1) Treatment For Diseases Caused by Damp-heat Symptoms and Signs: Erythema and vesicles appear around the lips and nostrils or on cheeks, with the sensation of itching and burning heat. The tongue proper shows red while the tongue coating thin and yellow. The pulse is mostly floating.

Therapeutic Method: Clear away heat and dampness from the lungs and stomach.

Recipe —— Modified *XinYi Qingfei Yin* (Formula31), a decoction of Flos Magnoliae for clearing away lung-heat:

Flos Magnoliae	9 g
Radix Scutellariae	9 g
Capejasmine Fruit	9 g
Folium Eriobotryae	9 g

Rhizoma Anemarrhenae	9 g
Bulbus Lilii	9 g
Semen Pruni Armeniacae	9 g
Semen Amomum Cardamomun	9 g
Gypsum	15 g
Semen Coicis	15 g
Radix Glycyrrhizae	6 g

(2) For Diseases Caused by Downward Flow of Damp—heat.

Symptoms and Signs: Erythema and vesicles are found on the external genitalia, with the sensation of burning heat and itching. The tongue proper shows red, and the tongue coating yellowish or yellowish and greasy. The pulse in this case feels slippery.

Theraputic Method: Clear away the damp—heat from Liver and Gall—bladder.

Recipe——Modified *Longdan Xiegan Tang* (Formula 8):

Radix Bupleuri	9 g
Radix Scutellariae	9 g
Capejasmine Fruit	9 g
Radix Rehmanniae	9 g
Herba Plantaginis	9 g
Rhizoma Alismatis	9 g
Radix Angelicae Sinensis	9 g
Radix Sophorae Flavescentis	9 g
Rhizoma Dioscoreae Hypoglaucae	9 g
Caulis Aristolochiae Manshuriensis	6 g
Radix Glycyrrhizae	6 g

2. External Treatment

(1) Mix the Powder of Cortex Phellodendri (Formula 17)

with decoction of tea and apply the mixture to the diseased part.

(2) Rinse the diseased part with the solution of 2% Borneolum.

1.2 Herpes Zoster

This is an acute Herpetic dermatosis due to viral infection, characterized by clusters of vesicles usually appearing abruptly, accompanied by neuralgia, and arranged in the shape of a belt along unilateral side with eneurosis; rare recurrence after recovery is also one of the characteristics.

This disease is known in TCM classics as "Pellets of fire spreading round the waist".

Etiology and Pathogenesis

This disease is caused by (1) depression and by the liver−fire moving randomly, which leads to excessive fire in the liver and gall−bladder, or (2) by unrestrained diet resulting in the disorder of the function of the spleen, hence, the formation of spleen−dampness, or (3) by the invasion of toxic material at a time when the vital−*Qi* has been weakened after an illness.

Clinical Manifestations

1. This disease, more popular in spring and autumn than in other seasons, is found mostly on one side of the waist or on the chest, face and neck.

2. Before the onset of the disease, there are often symptoms of mild fever, lassitude, mental inactivity, general discomfort, local stabbing pain on the skin, itching, burning heat sensation and hyperesthesia. An abrubt onset may also be possible.

3. At first, the diseased part exhibits patchy erythema, followed by clusters of red papular eruptions which soon become

grouped in pellet-shaped blisters surrounded by areolae. Each group contains five to seven blisters. The herpes blisters are arranged band-shaped along the unilateral nerve trunk, and normal skin can often be found among the herpes.

4. There are subjective feelings of pain, burning heat, and hyperesthesia. The feeling of pain in the case of infants being milder than in the case of elderly people. The latter may still suffer from neuralgia to a greater or lesser degree even after the skin lesion has disappeared.

5. Herpes, in a serious case, may exhibit bloody bulla and necroses accompanied by general symptoms such as fever. Normal herpes will last a few days before a crust is formed and leave a reddish maculae or pigmentation after decrustation.

6. The course of the disease lasts two or three weeks. But among some elderly and weak patients, the pain of the skin may last several weeks or months.

Type and Treatment

1. Internal Treatment

(1) Treatment for the Type Overabundance of Heat

Symptoms and Signs: The symptoms and signs of this type are found approximately during the early stage of herpes zoster. The diseased part has erythema, clusters of reddish papular eruption, pain, burning heat sensation, and itching, etc. Other symptoms may include restlessness, thirst, bitter taste, red tongue proper, yellowish tongue coating, taut and rapid pulse.

Therapeutic Method: Remove heat from the blood.

Recipe——*Liangxue Qinggan Tang* (Formula 32)

    Radix Rehmanniae   15 g

    Radix Paeoniae Rubrum   15 g

Moutan Bark	12 g
Radix Bupleuri	9 g
Rhizoma Ligustici Chuanxiang	9 g
Radix Scutellariae	9 g
Capejasmine Fruit	9 g
Radix Gentianae	9 g
Radix Arnebiae seu Lithospermi	9 g
Pericarpium Citri Reticulatae Viride	9 g
Flos Lonicerae	15 g
Fructus Forsythiae	15 g
raw Radix Glycyrrhizae	6 g

(2) Treatment for the Type Damp-heat

Symptoms and Signs: The symptoms and signs of this type are found during the metaphase of the disease. The skin of the diseased part is reddish and moist, with clustered blisters surrounded by areola or with diabrosis and exudation. Other symptoms include pain, burning-heat sensation, restlessness, thirst, red tongue proper, yellow tongue coating, and slippery pulse.

Therapeutic Method: Remove damp-heat from the liver and gallbladder.

Recipe——Modified *Longdan Xiegan Tang* (Formula 8).

Flos Lonicerae	15 g
Fructus Forsythiae	15 g
Radix Rehmanniae	12 g
Semen Plantaginis	12 g
Rhizoma Alismatis	12 g
Radix Bupleuri	9 g
Radix Gentianae	9 g
Capejasmine Fruit	9 g

Radix Scutellariae	9 g
Radix Paeoniae Rubrum	9 g
Rhizoma corydalis	9 g
Caulis Akebiae	6 g
raw Radix Glycyrrhizae	6 g

(3) Treatment for the Type Blood Stasis: The symptoms and signs of this type are found during the advanced stage of herpes zoster. The diseased part is covered with herpetic scabs on which there are reddish and brownish maculae or pigmentation, and associated pain.

Therapeutic Method: Disperse the depressed liver-Qi, promote blood circulation, and remove obstruction in the channels to relieve pain.

Recipe——Modified *Chaihu Shugan Tang* (Formula 33)

Radix paeoniae Alba	15 g
Radix Paeoniae Rubra	15 g
Radix Salviae Miltiorrhizae	15 g
Radix Bupleuri	9 g
Rhizoma Cyperi	9 g
Rhizoma Ligustici Chuanxiong	9 g
Fructus Aurantii	9 g
Pericarpium Citri Reticulatae	9 g
Rhizoma Corydalis	9 g
Pericarpium Citri Reticulatae Viride	9 g
Fructus Meliae Toosendan	9 g
Radix Glycyrrhizae	6 g

Modification: When there exists overabundance of heat, Folium Isatidis, Radix Isatidis and larger amount of Radix Scutellariae and Radix Gentianae are to be added.

If the chest and loin area ache intensely with burning heat, add fairly large quantities of Cortex Phellodendri and Radix Achyranthis Bidentatae.

When dysphoria exists, add Concha Margaritifera Usta, Os Draconis, Concha Ostreae, Radix Polygalae and Rhizoma Ziziphi Aurantii. When excessive pain exists, choose some of the following as additional ingredients: Resina Boswelliae Carterii, Radix Curcumae, Radix Angelicae Dahuricae, Herba Asari and Rhizoma Ligustici Chuanxiong.

2. External Treatment

(1) *Wugong San* (Scolopendra Powder):

It is a powder containing 10 g of baked Scolopendra and 1 g of Borneolum, to be mixed with water into a paste before application on the diseased part.

(2) Powder of Radix et Rhizoma Rhei and Cortex Phellodendri: It is a powder of the two drugs, equal in amount, plus a little Borneolum, mixed with water into a paste for application on the diseased part.

(3) Herba portulacae: Wash clean a certain amount of Herba Portulacae and then hammer it into a paste before applying it to the diseased part.

1.3 Verruca

Verruca is a common skin disease caused by virus. it is a vegetative growth underneath the skin surface. Clinically, it can be classified into four groups: verruca vulgaris, flat verruca, soft infectious verruca, and damp pointed verruca.

Etiology and Pathogenesis

Verruca lesion is of great variety, caused by the disharmony between *Qi* and blood, the loosening of skin striae, and the invading pathogens; hence, the resultant accumulation and stasis of *Qi* and blood.

Clinical Manifestations

1. Verruca Vulgaris

(1) It is most liable to occur among teenagers and young adults on the dorsum of hands and on the head and face.

(2) At first, there are only one or two verruca, which are hyperkeratosis each of which is and the size of a mung bean or a soybean. The surface of it is rough and fairly hard, showing light brown or normal skin colour. In the later stage, the size grows and the number increases, while the top becomes nipple-shaped or prickle-shaped huperplasia.

(3) Usually there exhibits no subjective symptoms. A chronic case may last as long as several years, or it may heal by itself without leaving any trace.

Clinically there can be found the following extraordinary types of verruca vulgaris.

(1) periungual Wart, in the form of prickle-shaped hyperplasia, is found on the edge of the nail body, even extending under the nail, with gaps that are prone to develop pyoganic infection.

(2) Verruca Filliformis, afilamentous Protuberance, soft and slender, mostly occuring on the skin of the neck and eye-lid of the aged and the middle-aged.

(3) Digitate Warts, in the shape of uneven digitationes, usually appearing on the scalp.

(4) Plantar Wart, usually appearing on the heel, is in the form of stratum corneum, which is on the same level as the sur-

rounding skin, and is caused by pressure and friction. When the upper layer of the cutin is removed, a cream-coloured cutin core is revealed. Warts usually occur on one side of the heel in varying numbers.

2. Flat Wart

(1) It is usually found on the face, the dorsum of the hand and the forearm, and among young people, especially young women.

(2) It often occurs abruptly as a papular eruption, first the size of a needle-end or a sesame seed, and later the size of a rice grain. The colour is light brown or light grey, and the surface is smooth. They may appear either separate and loose or densely distributed.

(3) It has a chronic process with slight itching or without any subjective symptoms. It may heal itself, but may also recur again.

3. Infectious Soft Wart

(1) Slightly infectious, it is usually found on the torso or limbs among children and youth.

(2) At first it is a small papular eruption the size of a needle-end; gradually it grows larger and the number increases. When it becomes as big as a mung bean or a soybean in the shape of a semiglobe, the surface shows smooth and shiny like wax, with a omphaloid-like center showing greyish white or normal skin colour. If its surface is cut open, a milky-white substance is obtained, which is known as molluscum bodies.

(3) Itching is felt by the patient and the course of disease is slow.

4. Pointed Condyloma

(1) This disease is found among adults, mostly on the exter-

nal genital organs, the perianal region, the arm-pit, and the region under a woman's breasts.

(2) At first, a few nipple-like papular eruptions appear, and then the number and size grow until they overlap each other, with the shape like a warty thorn, a nipple, a fungoid, a flower of a Chinese cabbage or an enormous dermoid cancer, etc. The colour may be dark brown or greyish. It is liable to bleed when pressed. It's surface feels moist, with erosion, fissure, serous fluid or pus, and it usually smells putrid.

(3) There are no subjective symptoms in the early stage, but in the advanced stage, there may be itching and a feeling of pressure.

Type and Treatment

1. Internal Treatment

This treatment applies to cases with warts vastly distributed, such as flat wart, infectious soft wart, and verruca vulgaris. There are varied interpretations concerning pathology, diagnosis and treatment. One theory holds that warts are caused by deficiency of the liver-Qi and blood and by malnutrition of the tendons as well; another theory maintains that warts are caused by stasis of both Qi and blood in the skin; and still another theory is based on the concept of pathogenic and toxic factors attacking the skin, causing multiplication and stasis. Thus the disease is clinically classified into three types: deficiency of the liver-Qi and blood, blood stasis, and accumulation of pathogens.

(1) The Type Deficiency of the Liver-Qi and Blood

Symptoms and Signs: Large amount of verrucae, its surface being dry, rough and withered.

Therapeutic Method: Nourish the blood, calm the liver and

subdue the exuberance of the liver—*Yang*.

Recipe——*Zhiyou Fang* (Recipe for Verruca, a proven prescription).

Radix Angelicae Sinensis	12 g
Radix Paeoniae Alba	12 g
Magnetitum	12 g
Concha Mauritia	12 g
Ochra Haematitum	12 g
Concha Ostreae	12 g
Semen Persicae	9 g
Flos Carthami	9 g
Rhizoma Pleionis	9 g
Cortex Lycii Radicis	9 g
Cortex Phellodendri	9 g

(2) The Type Blood Stasis

Symptoms and Signs: The warts are solid and vastly distributed, showing reddish brown.

Therapeutic Method: Activate blood flow and remove blood stasis.

Recipe—— *Zhihou Fang* (Recipe for verruca vulgaris, a proven prescription).

Radix Rehmanniae Praeparatae	12 g
Radix Polygoni Multiflori	12 g
Cortex Eucommiae	12 g
Radix Paeoniae Alba	12 g
Radix Paeoniae Rubra	12 g
Cortex Moutan Radicis	9 g
Semen Persicae	9 g
Flos Carthami	9 g

Squama Manitis	9 g
Semen Phaseoli	9 g
Rhizoma Atractylodis Macrocephalae	9 g
Radix Achyranthis Bidentatae	9 g

(3) The Type Accumulated pathogens in a Mass

Symptoms and Signs: The size of verrucous hyperplasia is considerable, with exudation or pus.

Recipe——*Zhiyou Tang* (Decoction for Verrucae).

Flos Lonicerae	12 g
Fructus Forsythiae	12 g
Herba Taraxaci	12 g
Folium Isatidis	12 g
Radix Isatidis	12 g
Cortex Dictamni Radicis	12 g
Radix Bupleuri	9 g
Semen Persicae	9 g
Flos Carthami	9 g
Radix Paeoniae Rubra	9 g
Cortex Moutan Radicis	9 g
Radix Arnebiae seu Lithospermi	9 g
Spica Prunellae	15 g

2. External Treatment

(1) Steaming and Washing Method

a. Decoct 30 g of Radix Isatidis and wash the diseased part with the decoction once or twice daily.

b. *Xiyou Fang* (Recipe for Washing Verrucae): Decoct Radix Isatidis 30 g, Radix Arnebiae seu Lithospermi 15 g, Rhizoma Cyperi 15 g, Semen Persicae 15 g and wash the diseased part with the decoction once or twice daily.

c. *Cayou Fang* (Recipe for Rubbing Verrucae): make 300 ml of a condensed decoction by boiling thoroughly the following ingredients: Cortex Dictamni Radicis 60 g, Alumen 20 g, Rhizoma Cyperi 30 g, Herba Equiseti Hiemalis 30 g, water 1000 ml; and rub the condensed decoction into the diseased part three times daily, each time lasting five minutes.

(2) Dressing Method

a. Dressing with mashed Fructus Bruceae: Soak the Fructus Bruceae in water before peeling them to obtain the nuts, which are to be mashed. Apply the mashed material to the diseased part and fix it with adhesive plaster. Change the dressing every three or four days.

b. Dressing with Powder of Fructus Mume:

Grind the Fructus Mume into Powder, make a mash by mixing the powder with water, and then apply the mash onto the diseased part. Fix the dressing with adhesive plaster.

2 Bacterial Dermatoses

2.1 Impetigo Herpetiformis

Impetigo herpetiformis is a kind of superficial impetigo, the onset of which usually occurs in children in summer and autumn. It is capable of contact infection and autoinfection, and liable to become an epidemic among children.

Etiology and Pathogenesis

This disease attacks, in most cases, children whose physical constitution is weak. Since a child has tender skin, he / she is easily affected by toxic material, especially in summer when the skin is exposed to sweat and dirt. The toxicant will turn into pathogenic heat, which will accumulate in the skin, causing the kind of skin lesion characteristic of impetigo herpetiformis.

Clinical Manifestation

Clinically, impetigo herpetiformis vulgaris is the most common type. There is also infantile impetigo herpetiformis, ecthuma herpetiformis, as well as large-size impetigo herpetifomis.

1. Impetigo Herpetiformis Vulgaris

At first, it appears as enthema or papular eruption, but soon develops into soybean-sized vesicles surrounded by areola, which then become impetigo herpetiformis in a day or two. Impetigo herpetiformis will spread separately on the skin, its wall being thin and tight and easy to break. Once the wall is broken, a red erosive surface will be revealed, and pus and exudation will flow out, causing the pathogen to spread about. This in turn leads to the growth of new impetigo herpetiformis. When the pus dries up, a yellow wax—like crust will form. There is a sensation of itching and, in serious cases, it is accompanied by fever and swelling of the lymph nodes.

2. Large—size Impetigo Herpetiformis

The pustule is comparatively large, the size of a broad bean, or even bigger, with no apparent aula surrounding it. The pustule wall is tight at first, but loose afterwards. Owing to the body position, the pus usually stays in the lower part of the pustule, hanging in the shape of a crescent. When the pustule breaks, the pus will dry up and a yellowish crust will form. As soon as it heals the crust drops off, leaving some temporary pigmentation.

3. Infantile Impetigo Herpetiformis

The onset usually takes place some time after birth, mostly among infants with a poor physical constitution. The pustule is as big as a Juglans regia, and its wall is thin and liable to break. Erosion appears upon diabrosis and a pus scab is formed afterwards. This disease is characterized by abrupt onset, high infectivity, quick development, and it is capable of spreading over large areas swiftly. The disease exhibits general symptoms of fever, weariness, vomiting and eccoprotic, etc. It may cause death from complications like hematosepsis or toxemia if it is not properly treated.

4. Ecthuma Herpetiformis

This disease occurs mainly on the lower limbs, first in the form of erythema or big induration, then turning into a pustule surrounded by aula. It expands gradually into the deep—layer tissues. Ulcers will form after it breaks up, and a pus scab will appear that is thick and clings firmly. When it heals, it leaves a scar and a feeling of pain.

Type and Treatment

1. Internal Treatment

Symptoms and Signs: The skin lesion is mainly in the form of pustule circled by aula. When the pustule breaks, a scab will form, the local lymph nodes will swell and there is a sensation of burning heat, itching, or pain. In a serious case, it may be accompanied by fever, anxiety, thirst, constipation or yellow urine, etc. It is a disease due to noxious heat.

Therapeutic Method: Clearing away heat and toxic material.

Recipe——*Huanglian Jiedu Tang* (Formula 6), plus *Wuwei Xiaodu Yin* ,(Formula 5).

Flos Lonicerae	15 g
Herba Taraxaci	15 g
Herba Violae	15 g
Flos Chrysanthemi Indici	15 g
Rhizoma Coptidis	9 g
Cortex Phellodendri	9 g
Capejasmine Fruit	9 g
Radix Scutellariae	9 g
Radix Semiaquilegiae	9 g

In treating a serious case of infantile impetigo herpetiformis, modern therapeutic method should also be employed.

2. External Treatment

Ordinary mild cases can be treated by mere external treatment.

(1) Remove the pus—pocket before clearing away the pus and crust with Detoxicating Decoction (Formula 13) or with the decoction of the following drugs:

Flos Lonicerae	15 g
Flos Chrysanthemi Indici	15 g
Radix Sophorae Flavescentis	15 g
Cortex Phellodendri	15 g
Alumen	6 g

Then spread on the pustule *Huangbai San* (Formula17), or *Huanglian Fen* , the powder of Rhizoma Coptidis. The application is done once a day.

(2) Make an ointment by mixing 45 g of vaseline with a powder made of the following drugs:

Rhizoma Coptidis	6 g
Cortex Phellodendri	9 g
Alumen exsiccatum	3 g
borneol	1 g
zinc oxide	24 g

Apply the ointment onto the affected part, twice or three times daily.

Prevention and Nursing

1. Pay attention to hygiene and give timely treatment to itchy skin diseases.

2. Once a child affected with this desease is discovered, he / she should be isolated and treated. The clothes and objects the child has used should be sterilized.

3. Moisten the diseased part for a few moments with sesame oil so as to remove the previous ointment before applying the new.

2.2 Erysipelas

This is an acute phlegmonosis of the skin or subcutaneous tissues caused by Hemolysis Streptococcus, most likely occuring on the lower limbs and face, and characterized by localized and clear-bounded swelling. It is accompanied by some general symptoms like fever and aversion to cold. The onset is swift, and only a few cases have suppuration.

Etiology and Pathogenesis

Erysipelas is caused mostly by pathogenic heat and other intruding pathogenic factors, or by toxic materials penetrating a wound. Such toxic material turns into pathogenic heat which accumulates in the skin tissues causing swelling, burning-heat sensation, and pain. When it is found on the head and face, wind is often part of the cause; When found on the lower limbs, dampness may be one of the factors. When toxic heat is in excess, it may invade the blood, causing serious complicaions.

Clinical Manifestation

1. At the beginning of the onset, there are some general symptoms like fever, aversion to cold, and general discomfort.

2. The diseased part shows red papulae which swiftly expand. The surface is smooth and shining, the colour bright red and the boundary extinct. When the onset occurs on the areas with loose skin (such as lips and eyelids) there is apparent swelling accompanied by local swollen lymph nodes.

3. An exact sensation of burning heat and pain is felt in the affected part.

4. In serious cases, there may be vesicles, huge blisters and necrosis, which may expand elsewhere.

5. Symptoms like high fever, anxiety, restlessness, coma, delirium, sickness and vomiting may also be found.

6. In the case of repeated attacks, the diseased part may have secondary lymphoid hydrops.

7. During the attack, there may appear a rise in the white blood cell count, blood sedimentation and antistreptolysin.

Type and Treatment

1. Internal Treatment

(1) Treatment for the Type Noxious Heat plus Wind

Symptoms and Signs: Swelling is found on the head and face. There is also fever, aversion to cold, inflammatory pain or itching.

Therapeutic Method: Clear away heat and toxic material, and reduce swelling by dispersing pathogenic wind.

Recipe——Modified *Puj i Xiaodu Yin* (Formula 34).

Radix Isatidis	18 g
Flos Lonicerae	18 g
Fructus Forsythiae	18 g
Rhizoma Coptidis	9 g
Radix Scutellariae	9 g
Lasiosphaera seu Calvatia	9 g
Fructus Arctii	9 g
Herba Menthae	9 g
Bombyx Batryticatus	
Radix Bupleuri	
Radix Platycodi	
Radix Glycyrrhizae	

(2) Treatment for the Type Noxious Heat

Symptoms and Signs: Localized swel

lower legs and there is fever, sickness, burning—heat sensation, and pain as well.

Therapeutic Method: Clear away heat and toxic material, and remove dampness by diuresis.

Recipe—— *Yinchen Chixiaodou Tang* (Decoction of Herba Artemisiae Capillar and Semen Phaseoli, a proven prescription)

Radix Isatidis	30 g
Caulis Lonicerae	30 g
Cortex Phellodendri	9 g
Radix Sophorae Flavescentis	9 g
Herba Artemisiae Capillaris	9 g
Radix Stephaniae Tetrandrae	9 g
Rhizoma Alismatis	9 g
Cortex Moutan Radicis	9 g
Radix Paeoniae Rubra	9 g
Radix Achyranthis Bidentatae	9 g
Rhizoma Atractylodis	9 g
Semen Phaseoli	15 g
Semen Coicis	15 g

(3) Treatment for the Type Excessive Noxious Heat

Symptoms and Signs: Red swelling is found on the affected part accompanied by inflammatory burning heat and pain, high fever, aversion to cold, coma and delirium.

Therapeutic Method: Clear up the *Ying* system and remove pathogenic heat from blood and toxic material from the body.

Recipe——*Xijiao Dihuang Tang* (Formula 7), plus *Huanglian Jiedu Tang* (Formula 6), with some modification.

Flos Lonicerae	30 g
Fructus Forsythiae	30 g

Gypsum Fibrosum	30 g
Radix Rehmanniae	15 g
Radix Paeoniae Rubra	15 g
Moutan Bark	15 g
Rhizoma Coptidis	9 g
Radix Scutellariae	9 g
Cortex Phellodendri	9 g
Capejasmine Fruit	9 g
Rhizoma Anemarrhenae	9 g
Cornu Rhinoceri	6 g

The decoction may be taken together with *Zixue Dan* (Formula 35), or *Angong Nuihuang Wan* (Formula 36), dosage, one bolus a time, twice daily.

2. External Treatment

(1) Apply *Jinhuang Gao* (Formula 29) or *Daqing Gao* (Formula 30) onto the diseased part, once a day.

(2) Make a paste by mixing water with the powder of Cortex Phellodendri or with the powder of Radix et Rhizoma Rhei. Apply the paste to the affected part twice a day.

(3) Make a paste by grinding fresh and clean Herba Portulacae. Apply it to the diseased part twice daily.

Prevention and Nursing

1. When there is rupture of the skin, it should be treated timely lest it should get infected.

2. Give timely treatment to primary focus, such as Hongkong foot.

3. During the onset, the patient should be confined to bed and should drink sufficient water. If the disease is on the lower leg, the diseased leg should be raised when the patient is in a lying position.

3 Tinea

Tinea is an infectious mycosis of the skin, due to a fungus intrusion of the skin, hair, or nails. Common cases include hand-foot, tinea, tinea corporis, tinea cruris, tinea unguium, tinea capitis and tinea versicolor. In TCM, hand tinea is known as tinea unguium, foot tinea as tinea pedis, tinea corporis as tinea circinata or coin-like tinea, tinea cruris as tinea inguinalis, nail tinea as grey nail, tinea capitis as white acomous sore or tinea favosa, and tinea versicolor as sweat patch or pityriasis simplex on the face. Since tinea appears on various parts of the body, the clinical manifestations vary with different cases. Moreover, this infectious disease has a high incidence rate in warm seasons and areas.

Etiology and Pathogenesis

It is held in traditional Chinese medicine that the pathogenic factor in tinea is insect (referring to fungus). When fungus intrudes into the skin, it gives rise to heat, wind dryness, and dampness, which in turn, cause various respective clinical symptoms.

3.1 Hand-foot Tinea

Clinical Manifestation

This is found mainly among adults and rarely among children. The onset, exacerbation and recurrence of the disease usually takes place in the summer and autumn, while in the winter, the case may show abatement. The skin lesion is in most cases limited to the palm, sole, and between the toes. Clinically, the cases may be classified into three types:

1. Vesicle Type: At first, vesicles, the size of a millet grain, appear either separately or in clusters on palmaris et plantaris and between the toes. The vesicle wall is quite thick, and not easily broken. It may cause severe itching.

2. Erosive Type: This type is found mostly between the toes. When the vesicle breaks, it leaves localized wetting, with white skin due to soaking. With the denudation of the white decayed skin, a red erodible surface with exudation is revealed, accompanied by itching. This disease is often found among people with hyperhidrosis on the hands and feet.

3. Keratotic-scale Type: Vesicles no longer exist, or only appear occasionally. The skin becomes dry and thick, producing scales continuously. It then becomes coarse or even takes on rhagadates. This type is often found on the palmaris et plantaris, or on the edge of hands and feet, accompanied by itching.

Erosive type is likely to have a secondary bacterial infection, incurring lymphangitis, lymphnoditis and erysipelas on the lower legs.

Type and Treatment

1. External Treatment

(1) Use of Lotion and Fumigant. Decoct one of the following drugs: *Zhiyang Xiyao* (Formula 14) or *Qufeng Xiyao* (Formula 15) or *Xiaofan Xiyao* (Formual 16), then steam and cleanse the affected part while the decoction is warm. If there is a secondary bacterial infection, *Jiedu Xiyao* (Formula 13), should be added.

(2) Use of Tincture: Apply the complex prescription *Fufan Tuqingpi Ding* (Formula 24) to the affected part three times daily.

(3) Use of Acetum: Soak the affected part twice a day in *Huoxiang Cuqin Ji* (Formula 26), or in Acetum of Tinea Unguium (Formula 25)

(4) Apply on the diseased part *Jiaoqi Fen* (Formula 37).

2. Internal Treatment (Suitable for cases with erosion, exudation, or combined acute bacterial infections.)

(1) Treatment for the Excessive Dampness Type

Symptoms and Signs: The diseased part has erosion and exudation, or blisters which appear repeatedly in clusters.

Therapeutic Method: Induce diuresis; remove heat to expel wind.

Recipe —— Modified *Bixie Shenshi Tang* (Formula 53)

Cortex Dictamni Radicis	15 g
Talcum	15 g
Semen Coicis	15 g
Rhizoma Dioscoreae Hypoglaucae	9 g
Poria	9 g
Rhizoma Alismatis	9 g
Cortex Phellodendri	9 g
Cortex Moutan Radicis	9 g
Radix Sophorae Flavescentis	9 g
Caulis Akebiae	6 g
Radix Glycyrrhizae	6 g

(2) Treatment for the Moist Heat Type

Symptoms and Signs: The skin lesion includes blisters, erosion, exudation and some mild swelling on the affected part.

Therapeutic Method: Clear away heat and promote diuresis.

Recipe —— Decoction of Herba Atemisiae Capillaris (a proven prescription, see 'Erysipelas' in part II)

(3) Treatment for the Toxic Heat Type

Symptoms and Signs: There is exudation, swelling and pain in the affected part, or there may be secondary erysipelas in the lower legs. The lymph nodes in the groin are swollen with tenderness. It may also be accompanied by fever.

Therapeutic Method: Clear away heat and toxic material and remove dampness by diuresis.

Recipe: Modified *Huanglian Jiedu Tang* (Formula 6) and *Wushen Tang* (Formula 9).

Flos Lonicerae	30 g
Herba Violae	30 g
Rhizoma Coptidis	9 g
Cortex Phellodendri	9 g
Radix Scutellariae	9 g
Capejasmine Fruit	9 g
Radix Sophorae Flavescentis	9 g
Cortex Moutan Radicis	9 g
Poria	9 g
Semen Plantaginis	9 g
Radix Achyranthis Bidentatae	9 g
Herba Lycopi	9 g

3.2 Nail Tinea

Clinical Manifestation

Nail tinea results mainly from the spreading of hand-foot tinea, which invades only a few nails at the beginning, but gradually involves many more as time goes by. Without proper treatment it usually becomes incurable throughout one's life. Its clinical manifestations include thick growth of the nail edge or the whole nail, with rough and uneven surface, loss of luster, opaqueness of the nail and the colour turning greyish brown, greyish yellow, or greyish white. It is also manifested by crispness of the diseased nail, which is often incomplete or misshaped, with no feeling of discomfort in the main.

Type and Treatment

External Treatment

1. Soak the diseased part in *Huoxiang Cujingji* (Formula 26), or in *Ezhangfeng Cujingji* (Formula 25), Acetum—infusion of Tinea Unguium.

2. Soak for seven days in 1 500 g of acetum the following drugs:

Herba Schizonepetae	18 g
Radix Ledebouriellae	18 g
Semen Hydoocapi (Hydnocarpi)	18 g
Spina Gleditsiae	15 g
Flos Persicae	15 g
Cortex Lycii Radicis	15 g
Alumen	12 g

The residue should be removed afterwards. Then soak the diseased part in the infusion twice a day, each time lasting 20–30 minutes. This treatment may also be applied to hand–foot tinea

3. Grind the following drugs into grains before soaking them in colourless vinegar (250 ml) for seven days:

Spina Gleditsiae	30 g
Flos Impatiens Balsamina	30 g
Pericarpium Zanthoxyli	15 g

Apply a proper quantity of the infusion to the diseased part with degreased absorbent cotton, bind it up with gauze, and change it every twelve hours until recovery.

During the treatment, the softened portion of the diseased nail should be gently scraped regularly with a clean blade.

3.3 Tinea Corporis and Tinea Cruris

Clinical Menifestation

Tinea on the face, neck, torso or limbs is classified as tinea corporis, while tinea cruris refers to those on the inside surface of the upper end of the thigh, including those which spread to the genital organs or buttocks. It is manifested by ring—shaped or multi—ring—shaped erythemas with clear and prominent boundaries, papular eruptions, vesicles, squamae or scab, which are mostly near the boundaries. The tinea center tends to be capable of a natural cure and gives a feeling of itching. Without proper treatment it may show centrifugal expansion. Besides, skin lesion of the eczema type or lichenification type may result from too much scratching.

Type and Treatment

External treatment is the main treatment employed in this case, with the following therapies for choice:

1. *Fufang Tuqinpi Ding* (Formula 24) or *Pifu Ruangao* (Formula 85), for external application, twice or three times daily.

2. Soak 60 g of Radix et Rhizoma Rhei in 250 g of alcohol (density: 75%) for three days before being filtered for external application, twice or three times daily.

3. *Xiaofan Xiyao* (Formula 16), Washing Medicament of Nitrified Alum, for external application, twice daily, 30 minutes each time.

3.4 Tinea Capitis

This is a kind of surface mycosis on the scalp and hair, found mainly among children. A highly infectious disease, it is clinically divided into three classes: yellow ringworm, white ringworm and black—dotted ringworm.

1. Yellow Ringworm

(1) At first there is mild inflammation around the hair follicles, with a few scales forming tiny yellowish red spots which expand gradually into yellowish dish—shaped tinea scabs, through which hair grows. The scabs may join together without regular shape, spread separately, or cover the whole scalp.

(2) The diseased hair is dry and crisp; gradually it begins scaling off unevenly. Later, the hair follicles become damaged, resulting in permanent trichomadesis and, possibly, leaving atropic scars.

(3) The scalp itches and smells.

(4) It is a chronic disease, which may become less severe during adolescence, but does not have a natural cure.

2. White Ringworm

(1) At first there appear papular eruptions on the hair follicles. These are covered with greyish white scales, which later expand gradually into spots of greyish white scales. These spots may exist singly or in great numbers.

(2) The diseased hair is dry and crisp, and locks luster. The section of the hair near the scalp becomes dry with a greyish white bacterial sheath, and is likely to break at 2—4 mm from the scalp. Therefore, the diseased hair is uneven.

(3) There is a feeling of itching.

(4) The course is a chronic one and it is capable of a natural cure when the patient reaches adolescence. No scar will be left after recovery. Those who have a secondary purulent infection will have a scar left after recovery, and on the scar there will be permanent baldness.

3. Black—dotted Ringworm

(1) At first there appears separate local erythema, which gradually develop into white round scale squama with clear boundaries.

(2) The diseased hair is liable to break near the scalp, leaving a black dot.

(3) There is a feeling of itching. The course is a chronic one, and after recovery a small scar is left.

Type and Treatment

External Treatment

(1) have a hair—cut once a week

(2) Wash the head everyday with 10 g of Alumen or 30 g of Fructus Cnidii

(3) Apply ointment onto the diseased part every morning and evening. Below are different kinds of ointment for choice:

——Sulphur Ointment (5% sulphur by weight)

——Realgar Ointment (Containing 30 g of Realgar, 30 g of Zinc Oxide, and 300 g of vaseline)

——*Yi Shaoguan Ointment,* which is made of powder of the following drugs:

Radix Sophorae Flavescentis	500 g
Cortex Phellodendri	500 g
Cattle Skin Oily Liquid (obtained by smoking)	500 g
Aumen Exsiccatum	90 g

Momordicae Cochinchinensis	90 g
Chaulmoogra Seed	90 g
Fructus Cnidii	90 g
red cayenne pepper	90 g
Camphora	90 g
Sulfur	90 g
Alumen	90 g
Hydrargyrum	90 g
Calomelas	90 g
while arsenic	15 g

Mix the powder of the above drugs with 1 120 g of melted pig fat.

(4) In the course of applying the ointments mentioned above, dissolve the hair once every week with *Xiong Hui Hu* (Paste of Realgar and Calx). Here is the method of making and using the Paste of Realgar and Calx: Put into a container Realgar and Calx in a ratio of 1:4, pour cool water in it to make a thin paste for use after keeping it in the container for a whole day.

Administration: Apply the *xiong Hui Hu* onto the scalp evenly and twenty minutes later wash the head; the hair will then drop off. This medical paste has a dissolving function with no side effects so that the hair will grow up again without destroying the hair follicles.

The above treatment should continue until the examination of fungus confirms a cure.

3.5 Tinea Versicolor

Clinical Manifestations

1. Tinea Versicolor is liable to be found among adults on the chest, back, and upper end of the arm or neck. It usually becomes severe in summer and milder in winter.

2. The lesion takes the form of small dots the size of a soy bean, in white, yellowish brown or greyish white. The boundaries are distinct, and the surface is smooth and covered with tiny scales.

3. Normally there are no subjective symptoms, but possibly some mild itching.

4. It is a chronic course, possibly lasting many years without cure.

Type and Treatment

External Treatment

1. Acetum—infusion of Sulphur: Infuse 30 g of sulphur in 100 ml of Acetum for a week before applying it to the diseased part. The medicine is administered two or three times daily.

2. Use Sulphur—emulsion (5–10% sulphur by weight) or Compound Tincture of Cortex Pseudolaricis for external application, two or three times daily.

3. Grind the following drugs into a fine powder: 30 g of Lithargyrum, 15 g of sulphur, 30 g of Os Sepeilla seu Sepiae, 15 g of pericarpium Zanthoxyli. Then before application, cut at a slant a lump of ginger, and dip the section of the ginger into the powder so that the powder clings to the ginger section. Rub the powder covered ginger section over the diseased part until the lesion

turns light red. This should be repeated twice a day, morning and evening. After each application, the rubbed part should not be washed with water. In most cases, the disease can be cured in one or two weeks. The application should be continued for another 3—6 days in order to prevent recurrence.

Prevention

1. Prevention of Tinea Capitis

Any articles for daily use usch as hats, pillows, and combs that have been used by the patient must be sterilized before use again. Tools and devices for hair—cutting must be strictly sterilized. The disease should be treated as early as possible after discovery and a child with such a disease should not be permitted to enter school or kindergarten until recovery.

2. Prevention of Foot Tinea

Keep the feet clean and dry; basins and towels for foot washing and slipperies, etc. should not be exchanged; the shoes, socks, and stockings of the patient should be frequently washed and dried in the blazing sun.

4 Insect-borne Dermatoses

4.1 Scabies

Scabies is a highly infectious skin disease, liable to be epidemic among family members and those in close contact. It is termed *Jie Chuang* or *Chongje* (Insect—sarcoptidosis) in TCM works.

Etiology and Pathogenesis

This disease is due to invasion by sarcoptic mites parasitized in the body after contact with a scabies—patient or use of his / her clothing.

Clinical Manifestation

1. The patient has a record of contact with a scabies—patient or has used the clothes and articles of such a patient so that the sarcoptic mites have invaded the skin, causing the disease.

2. This disease may attack people of any age, often occurring on those parts of the body where the skin is thinner and softer, such as the grooves under the nail—edge, the surface of the wrist, the cubital fossa, the area around the naval, the abdomen, the bend of the upper thigh, and the external genital organs, etc. Normally, it is not found on the head, face or the ball of the foot.

3. The skin lesions appear mainly in the form of tiny pimples, vesicles, and tunnels. The pimples are usually as big as the end of a needle or a grain of rice. Tunnels are characteristic of this disease. They are caused by sarcopic mites working their way under the skin, thus resulting in tunnels, about 3—15mm long. They are

usually twisted, slightly prominent, grey or skin—coloured, and often have tiny vesicles at their ends. Skin lesions in the form of nodular may appear on the scrotum, penis, groin, or arm—pits.

4. There is severe itching, mainly in the night, often affecting sleep.

5. As a result of constant scratching, the following forms of lesion will ensue: scratched scar, thickened skin, pigmentation, and pyogenic infection.

6. Microscopic observation of the liquid from the vesicles will show the existence of sarcoptic mites.

Type and Treatment

1. External Treatment

In most cases, this disease does not require internal treatment, but relies on the external application of medicine for destroying sarcoptic mites. Clinically, sulfur ointment is often employed (with children use ointment containing 5—10% sulphur; with adults use ointment containing 10—15% sulphur. The patient should take a bath using warm water and soap, and then dry the body before applying the ointment to the whole body except the head and face. The ointment should be applied with some force, and on those parts with skin lesion more ointment should be applied. The application is repeated every morning and night for three days in succession, during which time no bath should be taken and no clothes changed until the fourth day. When the patient should take a second bath and change to disinfected clothes, quilts, and bedding. This is then followed by observation for a week. If there appears no skin rash during the observation period, it means a recovery. If it has not yet been cured, the above treatment should be repeated once more.

2. Internal Treatment

When there is secondary pyogenic infection, the modified *Wuwei Xiaodu Yin* (Formula 5), may be administered.

Radix Rehmanniae	15 g
Radix Paeoniae Rubra	15 g
Flos Lonicerae	30 g
Herba Taraxaci	30 g
Cortex Dictamni Radicis	30 g
Flos Chrysanthemi Indici	15 g
Herba Violae	15 g
Fructus Forsythiae	15 g
Radix Glycyrrhizae	9 g

Nursing and Prevention

1. During the treatment, efforts should be made to exterminate sarcoptic mites, since only by doing this can the scabies be cured. In order to prevent recurrence, attention should be paid to substituting clean and sterilized clothes, quilts, and bedding in between courses of treatment. The changed clothing and beddings must be sterilized through boiling, sunning, or ironing, and if necessary, using pharmacal means so that further contact of infection may be avoided.

2. In order to prevent infection, those who share the same room with the patient in a family or in a dormitory, should also be treated at the same time.

3. Personal hygiene and hygienic control in services should be enhanced so that transmission of scabies may be prevented.

4.2 Insect Dermatitis

Insect dermatitis is an inflammatory skin disease caused by insect bites or stings which leaves poison, poisonous stings or poison seta irritating the skin. The common insects likely to cause this disease include midges, mosquitoes, ants, fleas, bugs, bees, scorpions, catepillars, leeches, centipedes, and snakes. In TCMclassic works, it is termed biting by vicious insects or wound caused by poisonous insect–bite.

Etiology and Pathogenesis

The disease is caused by a poisonous insect–bite leaving poison which intrudes and stagnates in the skin and flesh.

Clinical Manifestation

1. Insect dermatitis is found mostly in summer and autumn when destructive insects are prevalent. It is liable to attack the exposed parts of the body.

2. Petechia, papular erruption, and wheal are commonly found on the skin. Sometimes, there may occur vesicles, bullae, or running sore, in the center of which there is usually a tiny petechia, the size of a needle end. These spread on the skin separately or in small groups. The area bitten by a bee, scorpion, or centipede usually shows red swelling; but if it is bitten by a leech, it is manifested by bleeding.

3. The affected area has, more or less, a local feeling of itching, numbness, burning heat or pain. In some severe cases, it may be accompanied by such systemic toxic symptoms as aversion to cold, fever, dizziness, chest distress, sickness vomiting, or even convulsion and coma.

Type and Treatment

1. External Treatment

Since insect dermatitis is usually a mild case with only some local symptoms, external treatment is employed in most cases.

(1) If a poisonous stinger has lodged in the skin, it should be pulled out with great care; and if it is a poison seta, it can be pulled out by means of an adhesive plaster or a *Goupi Gao* (Formula 38). If the opening of the wound is big and obvious, the poison can be sucked out by a breast pump or a cupping glass.

(2) Wash thoroughly the affected area with soap and water (wounds caused by a wasp, centipede, or scorpion should be washed in vinegar), then apply onto the affected part one of the following selectively: *Bisu Gao* (Formula 39), *Fengyou Jin* (Formula 40), and *Zhiyang Ding* (Formula 41), Antipruritic Tincture.

(3) Soak in cool boiled water a certain amount of *Nantong Sheyao Pian* (Formula 42), so that it becomes a paste—like stuff, and then apply it to the area surrounding the wound (the center of the wound should get no medicine).

(4) Mash up a certain amount of purslane for application to the affected area.

2. Internal Treatment

Since severe cases often show some systemic toxic symptoms, the following internal treatment is to be employed in addition to local external treatment: Take the Nantong Snake Tablets, three times daily, 10 tablets each time. At the same time, the *Wuwei Xiaodu Yin* (Formula 5) and *Huanglian Jiedu Tang* (Formula 6), may be administered with some modifications:

Flos Lonicerae	30 g
Herba Taraxaci	30 g

Flos Chrysanthemi Indici	15 g
Herba Violae	30 g
Radix Scutellariae	9 g
Rhizoma Coptidis	9 g
Capejasmine	12 g
Herba Plantaginis	30 g
Radix Glycyrrhizae	9 g

Nursing and Prevention

1. When dermatitis appears, it should never be irritated by scratching or by washing it with hot water.

2. Attention should be paid to the improvement of environmental hygiene; the breeding ground of insects should be sprayed with insecticides.

3. Protective articles such as mosquito-nets and mosquito-repellent incense should be used in summer.

5 Physicogenic Dermatoses

5.1 Chilblain

Chilblain is a blood—stasis type of dermatosis occurring in cold seasons, often on such parts of the body as hands, feet, external ears and faces. A light—coloured purple tumor is found among mild cases, but in severe cases, ulceration develops and becomes a sore.

Etiology and Pathogenesis

This disease is caused by insufficiency of *Yang*, allowing the invasion of pathogenic cold, which in turn stagnates in the skin and flesh, leading to stagnancy of *Qi* and blood stasis.

Clinical Manifestation

It is manifested by onset in cold seasons, usually appearing on hands, feet, external ears and face, and often in symmetry. Moreover, in the early stage, the affected area exhibits puffy erythema, which gradually turns dull purple, and, in severe cases, the surface of the dull purple erythema will grow vesicles and bulla which will ulcerate after breaking. There is a sensation of swelling. Itching will occur with warmth and a feeling of pain is felt as it ulcerates. The ulcerating wound does not heal easily, but it will get a spontaneous cure when the weather turns warmer.

Type and Treatment

1. Internal Treatment

It is advisable to adopt the therapeutic method of warming up the channels to expel pathogenic cold, and promoting blood circulation to regulate channels. The Modified *Danggui Sini Tang* (Formula 43), to be administered:

Radix Angelicae Sinensis	15 g
Radix Paeoniae Alba	15 g
Ramulus Cinnamomi	15 g
baked ginger	9 g
Radix Aconiti Praeparata	9 g
Herba Asari	3 g
Medulla Tetrapanacis	9 g
Fructus Ziziphi Jujubae	5 paice
Radix Aconiti Kusnezoffii	9 g
Radix Aconiti	9 g
Radix Glycyrrhizae	9 g

2. External Treatment

(1) Make a decoction by boiling the *Huoxue Zhitong San* (Formula 44) or dried Fructus Capsici, then wash the affected part with the hot decoction, once or twice daily; or, it may also be rinsed with the hot decoction made from 120 g of Fructus Crataegi

(2) External application of ginger tincture, capsicum tincture or *Dongchuang Gao* (Formula 45).

(3) The ulcerated part may be treated with fresh Fructus Crataegi, the cores of which are to be removed before the fructus crataegi is ground to a paste for application, or the ready-made Fructus Crataegi Onitment may be directly used for application.

Nursing and Prevention

1. Careful attention should be paid to keeping warm and protection against cold, especially for those parts already inflicted with chilblain. When going outside in cold weather, one should be

dressed with more clothes, wear masks and gloves; the shoes and socks should be loose, big enough and warm so that the body may not be exposed to cold for a long time.

2. Keep hands and feet dry; damp masks, gloves, shoes and socks should be changed or dried.

5.2 Rhagades of Hand and Foot

This disease occurs in the filiform fissures on the palms and soles. It is a common skin disease in winter, which is known as *Junlie* or *Junlie* Sore in TCM works.

Etiology and Pathogenesis

This disease is caused by the invasion of pathogenic wind, cold and dryness which stay in the skin and flesh causing the stagnation of *Qi* and blood, and hence the malnutrition of the skin.

Clinical Manifestation

1. This disease occurs mainly in cold weather, and on those parts of the body where the skin is thick and subject to frequent brushing, like the fingers, the edge of the palm, the heel, and the edge of the ball of a foot, etc.

2. At first, the skin becomes dry, tight, and hard, and later, it turns rough, thick, and lusterless, followed by the appearance of gaps with different depths and lengths.

3. Those with gaps may suffer from unbearable pain. The gaps may bleed, hinder the twisting movement, or even affect one's work and life.

Type and Treatment

This disease does not require internal treatment in most cases, and some drugs for external application will suffice for the treatment.

1. Wash the affected part with a hot decoction obtained by boiling *Huoxue Zhitong Shang* (Formula 44), Powder for Promoting Blood Circulation to Stop Pain, once or twice a day, each time lasting 30 minutes, or wash it with a decoction obtained from Cortex Lycii Radicis 30 g and Alumen 15 g.

2. Use of *Waiyong Runji Gao* (Formula 46), *Hali You* (Formula 47) or *Runfu Gao* (Formula 27), for external application, two to four times a day.

Nursing and Prevention

When doing one's work, one should keep warm, protect against cold weather, avoid the stimulation of brushing and shaking, and avoid the contamination by grease and dirt. Hands should not be washed with over-basic soap, and in winter they should be rubbed with skin-protecting grease.

5.3 Sudamen

This is a dermatosis occurring in hot summer characterized by skin covered with papular eruption. In TCM works it is also termed heat-caused pimples or sweat pimples.

Etiology and Pathogenesis

This disease is caused by summer-heat and dampness blocking the pores and hindering the release of sweat.

Clinical Manifestation

1. It occurs mostly in hot summer.

2. It is often found among fat children and women, on their foreheads, necks, chests, backs, folds under the breasts, arm-pits and groins, where sweat is profuse.

3. The onset is abrupt; with densely clustered pimples, the

size of a needle end, and occupying large areas, each pimple surrounded by areola. The pimples usually appear in large numbers and are coarse to the touch and feel prickly.

4. There is a feeling of itching and burning—heat.

5. When the weather gets cooler, the pimples may disappear naturally and have a spontaneous cure with some desquamation.

6. It may also have secondary infections called sudamen poison in TCM works due to scratching, thus leading to diseases such as folliculitis, pus—pocket and furuncle.

Type and Treatment

1. Internal Treatment

If the skin lesion involves vast areas, the *Qingshu Tang* (Formula 48) with some modification is used, which has the effect of removing summer—heat and resolving dampness.

Modified *Qingshu Tang*.

Radix Paeoniae Rubra	9 g
Rhizoma Imperatae	30 g
Flos Lonicerae	12 g
Fructus Forsythiae	9 g
Herba Plantaginis	15 g
Rhizoma Alismatis	9 g
Herba Lophatheri	9 g
Talcum	18 g
Fructus Arctie	9 g
Radix Glycyrrhizae	3 g

If it has changed into 'sudamen poison', the modified *Wuwei Xiaodu Yin* (Formula 5), may be administered.

Radix Rehmanniae	12 g
Flos Lonicerae	15 g

Herba Taraxaci	15 g
Flos Chrysanthemi Indici	15 g
Herba Violae	15 g
Fructus Forsythiae	9 g
Herba Plantaginis	15 g
Radix Glycyrrhizae	9 g

2. External Treatment

Bathe in the decoction made by boiling 250 g of Semen Allii Tuberosi or of Herba Portulacae, and, after drying the body, spread on one of the following powders: *Liuyi San* (Formula 49), *Zhiyang Fen* (Formula 50) and *Feizi Fen* (Formula 51).

Nursing and Prevention

1. The affected part should not be bathed with hot water, rubbed heavily with a towel, or scratched.

2. Living accommodations should be well ventilated; and in hot seasons, attention should be paid to the lowering of temperature, too. When sweating profusely, one should not take a cold shower.

3. One should not wear too much, and the clothes should be big enough, clean and dry.

4. Bathe regularly in the case of babies, and *Feizhi Fen* can be applied after the bath.

5.4 Corns

Corns are caused by prolonged pressing. They are rod-shaped hyperkeratosis growing in the affected part, which looks like a chicken's eye. It is also termed as clavus in TCM works.

Etiology and Pathogenesis

Constant pressure and friction upon the crus cerebri and areas between toes cause hindrance for the circulation of *Qi* and blood, hence, the malnutrition of the skin, which in turn results in corns.

Clinical Manifestation

This disease is found mostly among young men who do too much standing and walking. The skin lesion usually occurs in the center of the end section of a toe, the bending side of the great toe, the stretching side of the small toe, the back of the toes, and the heel, etc. In some rare cases, it can be found on the hands. It may either occur singly or in several places simultaneously, but usually a patient has only one or two corns. The skin rash is yellowish, the size of a mung bean or a pea. At the early stage, the skin of the affected area turns thickened, and gradually it grows into a cone-shaped solid mass which is slightly prominent with a concave center. When it is pressed longitudinally, a pain is keenly felt.

Type and Treatment

This disease is treated mainly with external therapeutic method.

1. Bathe the affected part with a decoction obtained by boiling *Huoxue Zhitong San* (Formula 44).

2. Apply *Jiyang Gao* (Formula 52), onto the affected part, or alternatively, make a paste of Fructus Bruceae nuts, removing their shells, and apply it to the affected part and fasten it there with adhesive plaster. Change the dressing every two or three days until the corns have completely disappeared. Better results can be obtained if, before the application of corn plaster or paste, the affected part is bathed with hot decoction obtained by boiling

Huoxue Zhitong San or with hot water, and then chip the corn to make it thinner.

Nursing and Prevention

1. prevent the local parts from being pressed or rubbed. The size of shoes and socks should fit the feet well, and the heel of shoes should be soft.

2. Those people with abnormal foot bones should receive corrective therapy as soon as possible.

3. Refrain from using powerful errosive drugs.

4. Never use unclean knives and scissors for chipping the corns lest secondary infection could result.

6 Allergic Dermatoses

6.1 Contact Dermatitis

This is an acute latent and inflammatary dermatosis in a certain local part, caused by the contact of skin or mucosa with a certain substance. It is manifested by the existence of erythema, swelling, papular eruption, vesicles or even necroses. There are two types of contact dermatitis: the primary and the allergic, the latter being the majority. In TCM works, there are different names for the disease, which vary according to the different contact objects, for instance, lacquer sores, pollen sores, plaster sores and closetstool sores.

Etiology and Pathogenesis

This disease is caused by the following factors: weak congenital resistance, loose striae of skin and muscles, invasion of exogenous pathogenic factors and the accumulation of pathogenic heat in the skin and muscles.

Clinical Manifestation

1. Primary contact dermatitis usually attacks the patient abrubtly without an incubation period, while allergic contact dermatitis has an incubation period of between five and twenty−one days.

2. The part with skin lesion is just the part of contact, with a clear edge. It may also attack the surrounding areas of a contact part or attack other parts of the body. This is due to scratching or the rubbing of clothing. There are also cases in which the

dermatitis spreads through the whole body due to high sensitivity.

3. In mild cases, it is manifested by erythema, papular eruption and swelling, but severe cases may involve vesicles, large blisters, erosion, scab, or even ulcer and necrosis.

4. There is a feeling of itching and burning heat in varying degrees. A severe case may involve burning pain accompanied by general discomfort.

5. It is a self-limited disease. When the pathogenic factors have been removed, or when proper treatment has been given, the skin lesion will soon disappear in a few days. Otherwise, the course will develop into a chronic one like chronic eczema with lichenoid changes on the affected part.

Type and Treatment

1. Internal Treatment

(1) Treatment for the Damp-heat Type

The Main Symptoms and Signs of this type are as follows: abrupt onset, short course, flush local skin lesion, swelling, papular eruption, vesicles, erosion, exudation, painful itching, reddened tongue with white or sticky yellow fur, floating or slow pulse.

Therapeutic Method: Remove heat and dampness factors.

Recipe——Modified *Bixie Shenshi Tang* (Formula 53)

Rhizoma Dioscoreae Septemlobae	15 g
Rhizoma Alismatis	15 g
Semen Coicis	30 g
Poria	15 g
Herba Plantaginis	30 g
Radix Rehmanniae	15 g
Cortex Moutan Radicis	15 g

Radix Scutellariae	12 g
Cortex Phellodendri	12 g
Caulis Aristolochiae Manshuriensis	9 g
Fructus Kochiae	30 g
Radix Glycyrrhizae	9 g

Modification: For cases accompanied by high fever, Gypsum Fibrosum 30 g and Rhizoma Anemarrhenae 12 g are to be added; for cases with severe dampness, add Herba Artemisiae Capillaris 15 g and Exocarpium Benincasae 15 g; for those with severe itching, add Cortex Dictamni Radicis 30 g and Periostracum Cicadae 9 g.

Proprietaries: *Longdan Xiegan Wan* (Formula 8) or *Fangfeng Tongsheng Wen* (Formula 54).

(2) Treatment for the Blood—dryness Type

Main Symptoms and Signs: The course is a protracted one, the skin lesion is thick, coarse, with the surface covered with scratching marks, blood scab, pigmantation or showing lichenoid changes. There exists severe itching. The tongue is pale, covered with white fur. The pulse feels deep or slow.

Therapentic Method: Promote blood circulation and expel wind—evil to arrest itching.

Recipe——Modified *Dangui Yinzi* (Formula 4).

Radix Angelicae Sinensis	15 g
Radix Rehmanniae	15 g
Radix Paeoniae Rurae	15 g
Radix Paeoniae Alba	15 g
Radix Salviae Miltiorrhizae	15 g
Radix Polygoni Multiflori	15 g
Radix Astragali Seu Hedysari	24 g

    Fructus Xanthii   15 g
    Radix Glycyrrhizae   9 g

Modifications: In case of severe itching add Scorpio 9 g, Zaocys 9 g, Cortex Albiziae 15 g and parched Semen Ziziphi Spinosae 15 g. For those with dry excrement, add Folium Cassia angustifolia 6 g.

Proprietaries: *Qinjiu Wan* (Formula 55) or *Runfu Wan* (Formula 56)

2. External Treatment

(1) For the acute attack, make a decoction by boiling the *Jiedu Xiyao* (Formula 13) and *Zhiyang Xiyao* (Formula 14), and apply it on the affected part after the decoction has cooled down, and then put *Huangbai San* (Formula 17) or *Shizhen San* (Formula 57), on the affected part (those powders may be mixed with sesame iol before application). The application is repeated twice or three times daily

(2) Chronic dermatitis may be treated by applying *Heidou Liuyou Ruangao* (Formula 58), twice to 4 times daily.

Nursing and Prevention

1. Find out the cause of the disease, eliminate pathogenic substance and avoid further contact.

2. Avoid such stimulations as scratching, rubbing, bathing with hot or soap water, etc.

3. Fish, shrimps and irritating food with bitter or hot tastes should not be eaten.

4. Avoid constipation and dyschesia

6.2 Eczema

Eczema is a common hypersensitive and inflammatory dermatosis which may attack people of all ages, either occurring all over the body or being confined in certain parts. Clinically, it is classified into three groups: acute eczema, subacute eczema and chronic eczema.

In TCM works, there are various names for this disease, according to the different parts it attacks and different manifestations; for instance, the eczema that attacks the whole body is termed *JinYin Chuang* (acute eczema), or *Shi Chuang*, and the eczema that attacks some local parts gets its names like *Xuan Er Chuang*, *Siwan Feng* and *Shennang Feng* (scrotal eczema) according to the particular parts.

Etiology and pathogenesis

This disease is basically due to congenital defect, and the pathogenic factors of wind dampness, heat and dryness.

Acute and subacute eczema are mostly due to pathogenic wind and damp-heat staying in the skin and flesh so that blood circulation is hindered and the harmony between *Ying* and *Wei* is disturbed. Chronic eczema is usually recurrent, caused by prolonged accumulation of pathogens, the impairment of *Yin* and blood, and by malnutrition of the skin.

Clinical Manifestation

1. Acute Eczema

(1) The onset is abrupt, capable of attacking any part of the skin, mostly the face, head, limbs and perineum.

(2) The skin lesion appears symmetrically.

(3) The skin lesion is polymorph.

At first the affected part shows flush, later it is followed by the appearance of papular eruption, vesicles, erosions, exudation, crust, etc. The skin rush is ofter clustered over a large area, without distinct edges. Usually, several different kinds of lesion exist, but may also be just one or two kinds of skin rash.

(4) There is severe itching and a burning—heat sensation. Those with general skin rash may have slight feverr.

(5) It may be healed after two or three weeks of proper treatment. But it is liable to relapse and tends to be chronic.

2. Subacute Eczema

(1) This is a stage in between acute eczema and chronic eczema; it is often turned into a protracted case when acute eczema has not received timely treatment or has been treated imroperly.

(2) The skin lesion is less severe than that of acute eczema, with inflammation gradually disappearing, exudation reduced, itching lessened, and with the appearance of scales, crust and skin rash.

3. Chronic Eczema

(1) Chronic Eczema originates mainly from acute and subacute eczema, although some cases are chronic from the beginning.

(2) The skin of the affected part is thick, coarse and hard, dark red or brown, possibly with scales or lichenoid changes. The dege is more distinct than in acute and subacute cases. Occasionally, some skin lesion may contain a little erosion, exudation and crust with a limited amount of papular eruptionsor vesicles, and, if the eczema occurrs on hands and feet, it is often accompanied by rhagadia.

(3) There exists a severe paroxysmal itching, and it becomes more serious when the skin gets into contact with heat or before the patient is going to bed.

(4) A chronic course may last for days or even years, sometimes severe and sometimes mild, relapsing alternatively in acute and subacute forms, especially when the patient is in the state of mental stress.

The three types of eczema mentioned above are not fixed forms, they may change into each other. On the whole, eczema has four characteristics as follows:

(1) The skin lesion is characterized by polymorphism and a tendancy towards exudation.

(2) The affected areas are arranged symmetrically.

(3) There exists intense itching.

(4) The course tends to become chronic, and it is liable to relapse.

Type and treatment

1. Internal Treatment

(1) Treatment for the Damp—heat Type

Symptoms and Signs: The skin lesion shows flush and swelling, accompanied by erosion, exudation or scabs, with intense itching and burning heat sensation. The patient feels anxious and thirsty, with his tongue red and covered with white or yellow thin fur, his pulse being slippery or taut and rapid.

Therapeutic Method: Clear away heat and remove dampness, expel pathogenic wind to stop itching.

Recipe——Modified *Longdan Xiegan Tang* (Formula 8).

Radix Gentianae	9 g
Capejasmine Fruit	9 g

Radix Scutellariae	12 g
Fresh Radix Rehmanniae	15 g
Radix Scrophulariae	15 g
Herba Plantaginis (and Semen Plantaginis)	30 g
Rhizoma Alismatis	15 g
Caulis Akebiae	9 g
Cortex Dictamni Radicis	30 g
Fructus Kochiae	30 g
Periostracum Cicadae	9 g
Radix Glycyrrhizae	9 g

Modifications: For cases with excessive heat, add Gypsum 30 g and Rhizoma Imperatae 30 g, for those with excessive dampness add Poria peal 15 g and Exocarpium Benincasae 15 g; for those with intense itching, add Scorpio 9 g and Zaocys 9 g; for cases with dry stool, add Radix et Rhizoma Rhei 9 g (to be added some time after the boiling of other drugs); if it attacks the upper part of the body, add Rhizoma Cimicifugae 9 g, and if it attacks the lower part of the body, add Radix Achyranthis Bidentatae 9 g

Proprietaries: *Longdan Xiegan Wan* (Formula 8) or *Fangfen Tongsheng Wan* (Formula 54).

(2) Treatment for the Wind—heat Type

Symptoms and Signs: The skin lesion is mainly in the forms of erythema, papular eruption, scab and scales. Swelling is lessened and exudation reduced. The patient feels itching, his tongue shows red covered with white fur, and his pulse is floating or rapid.

Therapentic Method: Expel wind, clear away heat and remove dampness.

Recipe——*Xiaofen San* (Formula 1).

Fructus Arctii	9 g
Radix Rehmanniae	15 g
Radix Sophorae Flavescentis	9 g
Rhizoma Atractylodis	15 g
Radix Angelicae Sinensis	15 g
Rhizoma Anemarrhenae	12 g
Gypsum Fibrosum	30 g
Caulis Aristolochiae Manshuriensis	9 g
Fructus Rochiae	30 g
Cortex Dictamni Radicis	15 g
Periostracum Cicadae	9 g
Radix Glycyrrhizae	9 g

Modifications: For cases with intense itching, add Scorpio 9g and Zaocys 9 g; for cases with obvious exudation, add Rhizoma Alismatis 15 g and Herba Plantaginis 30 g; for those with poor appetite, omit Radix Sophorae Flavescentis, Caulis Aristolochiae, but add Pericarpium Citri Reticulatae 9 g and Alpiniae Katsumadai 9 g; for cases with the skin lesion on the chest, flanks, external ears and the pudendum, add Radix Bupleuri 12 g and Radix Gentianae 9 g

Proprietaties: *Longdan Xiegan Wan* (Formula 8) or *Fangfeng Tongsheng Wan* (Formula 54)

(3) Treatment for the wind—dryness Type

Symptoms and Signs: The course is protracted and recurrent, with skin—pachynsis or lichenoid changes and with paroxysmal intense itching. The tongue is red covered with while fur; the pulse is weak or slow.

Therapentic Method: Nourish the blood to ease dryness; expel pathogenic wind to stop itching.

Recipe——Modified *Danggui Yinzi* (Formula 4)

Radix Angelicae Sinensis	15 g
Radix Salviae Miltiorrhizae	15 g
Radix Paeoniae Alba	15 g
Radix Polygoni Multiflori	15 g
Rhizom Ligustici Chuangxiong	9 g
Radix Astragali seu Hedysari	24 g
Radix Ledebouriellae	15 g
Fructus Tribuli	15 g
Fructus Xanthii	15 g
Radix Cynanchi Paniculati	30 g
Radix Glycyrrhizae	9 g

Modifications: For cases with red skin rash and heat symptoms add Radix Rehmanniae 15 g and Rhizoma Imperatae 30 g; for cases with intense itching, add Scorpio 9 g and Zaocys 9 g

Proprietaries: *Qinjiu Wan* (Formula 55) or *Runfu Wan* (Formula 56).

2. External Treatent

(1) If there are obvious erosions and exudation, *Zhiyang Xiyao* (Formula 14), or *Zaoshi Xiyao* (Formula 59) may be boiled into a decoction for wet packing after cooling dowm. The wet packing has to be repeated twice or three times daily, each time lasting thirty minutes.

(2) When there is little exudation, Antieczema Powder or Powder of Phellodendri may be applied onto the affected part or can be mixed with sesame oil into a paste before application. The application has to be repeated twice or three times daily.

(3) When there exists skin pachynsis or lichenoid changes, *Zhiyang Pufeng* (Formula 50) or *Qufeng Xiyao* (Formula 15) may

be boiled into a decoction for bathing the affected part while it is still hot, twice or three times daily, each time lasting thirty minutes. Besides, the Unguentum Picis Fabae Nigrae or Borneolum Powder may also be selected for external application.

Nursing and Prevention

1. Scratching should be avoided; during acute onset, the affected part should not be bathed in hot water or with alkali or soap.

2. Refrain from eating such foods as fish, sea-animals, eggs, beef, mutton, chicken, duck and goose, which are likely to induce or intensify eczema; besides, pungent food and alcohol should also be avoided.

3. Take enough rest and refrain from overwork and too much mental stress.

4. Preventive injection should not be offered to patient during the acute stage.

5. Trace the inducing factors and reduce relapsing.

6.3 Urticaria

Urticaria is a commonly-found itching dermatosis, characterized mainly by wheal on the skin. In TCM classics, this disease is termed *Yinzhen, Fengbei Liu,* etc.

Etiology and Pathogenesis

1. The patient has some congenital defects and has eaten irritative food such as fish and shrimps.

2. Loose striae of skin and muscles results in the failure of superficial-*Qi* to protect the body while the body has come under the attack of pathogenic factors of wind-heat and wind-cold.

3. Improper diet results in disharmony of stomack and intes-

tines, causing the growth of pathogenic damp—heat; besdies, pathogenic wind has invaded the bady.

4. The patient is of weak constitution or has become weak through protracted illness, with deficiency of Qi and blood, which makes easier the invasion by pathogenic wind.

Clinical Manifestation

1. This disease may attack people of all ages and of both sexes in any season.

2. The onset is usually abrupt. At first, the skin feels itching, later wheals appear either because of scratching or as a natural course. The wheals are of varying shapes and sizes, sometimes merged into each other in bright red, or pink or milkly white. The skin lesions appear and disappear alternately and rapidly without leaving trace, possibly several times a day. The urticaria does not appear on a fixed position, often disappearing from one place but appearing soon in another. In severe casses, it may appear all over the body.

3. During the onset, it is accompanied by intense itching, and possibly by a burning—hest sensation or stabbing pain. In some severe cases, it may be accompanied by fever (usually below 38.5°C), nausea, vomiting, stomachache, diarrhea and other symptoms of digestive tract, or by symptoms of respiratory tract such as chest distress, sensations of throat of throat and difficulty in breathing.

4. The course varies in different cases. Mostly, an acute case recovers in a few days or a fortnight. If the disease continues in a recurrent manner for over three months, it is chronic urticaria, which may last several months or years, with a continuous attack or with some remission stages.

Type and Treatment

1. Internal Treatment

(1) Treatment for the Wind—heat Type

Symptoms and Signs: Red in colour, the wheals emerge or become intensified when heated, but abate when cooled down. The skin rash gives a burning—heat sensation and intense itching. It may be accompanied by thirst and restlessness. The tongue is red, covered with thin, white or yellow fur. The pulse feels floating and rapid.

Therapeutic Method: Remove heat to expel wind and remove dampness.

Recipe——Modified *Xiaofeng San* (Formula 1).

Fructus Arctii	9 g
Radix Rehmanniae	15 g
Radix Sophorae Flavescentis	9 g
Rhizoma Atractylodis	15 g
Radix Angelicae Sinensis	15 g
Rhizoma Anemarrhenae	12 g
Gypsum Fibrosum	30 g
Caulis Akebiae	9 g
Semen Sesamum Indicum	15 g
Fructus Kochiae	30 g
Cortex Dictamni Radicis	15 g
Periostracum Cicadae	9 g
Scorpio	9 g
Radix Glycyrrhizae	9 g

Modifications: For cases with intense heat, add Rhizoma Imperatae 30 g and Flos Lonicerae 15 g; for those with insomnia, add Cortex Albiziae 15 g and Semen Ziziphi Spinosae 15 g; for cases with thirst, add Radix Scrophulariae 15 g; and for those with restlessness, add Plumula Nelumbinis (4.5 g).

(2) Treatment for the Wind—cold Type

Symptoms and Signs: The wheals are red or milky—white, liable to attack the patient when it is cold. The patient tends to hate wind and cold. The case will abate when it is warmer, and it is inclined to be severe in winter but milder in summer. The tongue is pale, covered with thin, white fur, and the pulse is floating and slow.

Therapeutic Method: Expel pathogenic wind and cold to harmonize *Yin* and *Wei*.

Recipe——Modified *Magui Ge Ban Tang* (Formula 60).

Herba Ephedrae	9 g
Ramulus Cinnamomi	9 g
Radix Paeoniae Alba	15 g
Parched Semen Armeniacae Amarum	9 g
Rhizoma Zigiber is Recens	3 chips
Fructus Ziziphi Jujubae	5 dates
Herba schizonepetae	9 g
Radix Ledebouriellae	15 g
Fructus Cnidii	12 g
Fructus Xanthii	15 g
Radix Glycyrrhizae	9 g

Modifications: For those with weak constitution and profuse sweat, omit Herba Ephedrae and add Radix Astragali seu Hedysari 30 g; for recurrent cases add Radix Astragali seu Hedysari 30 g, parched Rhizoma Atractylodis Macrocephalae 30g, Scorpio 9 g and Lumbricus 9 g.

(3) Treatment for Gastrointestinal Damp—heat Type

Symptoms and Signs: When wheals appear, they are accompanied by abdominal pain or nausea and vomiting, and by dry stool or hypercatharsis. The tongue is yellow and stickly, and pulse floating and rapid.

Therapeutic Method: Expel pathogenic wind, relieve exterior syndrome, and remove pathogenic heat from the stomach and intestines.

Recipe——Modified *Fangfeng Tongsheng San* (Formula 54).

Radix Ledebouriellae	15 g
Radix Platycodi	9 g
Gypsum Fibrosum	30 g
Talcum	18 g
Radix et Rhizoma Rhei (to be put into the boiling fluid)	9 g
Natrii Sulfas	9 g
Rhizoma Atractylodis Macrocephalae	15 g
Cortex Dictamni Radicis	30 g
Herba Menthae	9 g
Fructus Forsythiae	12 g
Radix Scutellariae	12 g
Capejasmine Fruit	12 g
Radix Glycyrrhizae	9 g

Modifications: For cases with abdominal pain, add Rhizoma Corydalis 12 g, and Pericarpium Papaveris 12 g, for cases with diarrhea, omit Radix et Rhizoma Rhei and Natrii Sulfas, but add Semen Dolichoris Album 15 g and Flos Lonicerae 15 g; for cases with nausea and vomiting, add Caulis Bambusae 9 g and Haematitum 30 g.

Proprietary: *Fangfeng Tongsheng Wan* (54)

(4)Treatment for the Type of Deficiency of Both *Qi* and Blood

Symptoms and Signs: The patient is of weak constitution or has suffered from a protracted illness; wheals relapse frequently, usually intensified when the patient is tired or suffering from cold. Other Symtoms include listleness, colourless complexion, pale tongue, thin and white tongue-coating, weak and deep pulse, etc.

Therapentic Method: Nourish the blood to expel wind, strengthen *Qi* to enhance the superficial power of resistance.

Recipe— — Modified *Dangui Yinzi* (Formula 4) plus *Yupingfeng San* (Formula 61).

Radix Angelicae Sinensis	15 g
Radix Paeoniae Alba	15 g
Radix Salviae Miltiorrhizae	30 g
Rhizoma Ligustici Chuanxiong	9 g
Radix Polygoni Multiflori	15 g
Herba Schizonepetae	9 g
Radix Ledebouriellae	15 g
Radix Astragali seu Hedysari	30 g
Parched Semen Armeniacae Amarum	15 g
Raidx Cynanchi Paniculati	30 g
Fructus Xanthii	15 g
Fructus Cnidii	12 g
Radix Glycyrrhizae	9 g
Scorpio	9 g

Modifications: For cases with poor appetite, add Fructus Crataegi 9 g and Endothelium Corneum Gigeriae Galli 9 g; for those with insomnia, add parched Semen Ziziphi Spinosae 15 g and Caulis Polygoni Multiflori 15 g; for those with listleness and drowsiness, and Radix Aconiti Praeparata 9 g and Herba Epimedii 12 g.

Proprietaries for Choice: *Shiquan Dabu Wan* (Formula 62), *Yupingfeng San* (Formula 61) and *Guipi Wan* (Formula 63).

2. External Treatment

(1) Cases with fast skin lesion bathe in the decoction made by boiling *ZhiYang Xiyao* (Formula 14) and *Zaoshi Xiyao* (Formula 59), once or twice daily.

(2) For external application: *Zhiyang Ding* (Formula 41) and *Baibu Ding* (Tincture of Radix Stemonae) (Please refer to Chapt.4, Paer I: Internal Treatment).

(3) Rub the affected part with *Zhiyang Feng* (Formula 64).

Nursing and Prevention

1. Refrain from eating marine-products like fish, lobsters, crabs, and pungent, irritating food as well. Alcohol Should not be drunk either. When a certain food has be found to be the cause of the onset, it should not be eaten again.

2. Avoid various kinds of irritating factors, such as wearing chemical fibre clothing, cold, scratching and mental stress.

3. Those patients who are hypersensitive to pollen, should not keep flowers in their rooms.

6.4 Papular Urticaria

Papular Urticaria is an allergic dermatosis found mostly among children, characterized by red wheal-like lesions with small vesicles or papular eruptions in the center, and accompanied by severe itching. In TCM works it is termed *Xipi Fengzhen* (thin-skinned Wind-rash) or *Shui Jie* etc.

Etiology and Pathogenesis

1. The patient, being of weak constitution, has been bitten by mosquitoes or other insects, with poison left inside and then spreading through skin and flesh.

2. Intake of improper food. such as irritating heavy food, has caused the growth of damp—heat inside the body, or exogenous pathogenic Pactors of wind, dampness and heat have intruded into the body and stagnate in skin and flesh.

Clinical Manifestations

1. The disease is liable to attack children under the age of eight, mostly in summer and autumn.

2. The skin rash tends to appear on the limbs and the flanks of the torso, spreading either seperately or in clusters.

3. Skin rash appears abruptly like red wheals, in the shape of a ring or similar to a spindle, the size of a mung—bean or of an earth—nut. Its long axis mostly runs parallel to skin—wrinkles. It feels a bit hard, with pseudopods on the deges and small vesicles or pimples on its top, Some vesicles may be just as big as the skin rash, the liquid in the vesicle being clear, without areola around.

4. Skin rash often appears in lage amount, and both old and new rash may exist together. The skin rash of the same group will disappear in a couple of days or in a fortnight at most, leaving some temporary, light pigmentation. This disease may relapse, lasting for several days or even several years.

5. Usually there are no general symptoms. The patient feels intense itching, and scratches may give rise to erosion and infestation.

Type and Treatment

1. Internal Treatment

(1) Treatment for the Wind—heat Type

Symptoms and Signs: The skin-rash is mainly in the form of wheal-like papular eruptions or erythema, but rarely in the form of vesicles. It is red in colour, with intense itching. The tongue is red, covered with thin, yellow coating.

Therapeutic Method: Expel wind and clear away heat.

Recipe—— *Shengdi Fang* (Decoction of Radix Paeoniae Rurae, a proved prescription).

Radix Rehmanniae	9 g
Rhizomaa Imperatae	30 g
Flos Lonicerae	15 g
Herba Taraxaci	15 g
Fructus Kochiae	30 g
Periostracum Cicadae	6 g
Herba Schizonepetae Spica	6 g
Radix Ledebouriellae	9 g
Semen Phaseoli	30 g
Radix Glycyrrhizae	9 g

Modifications: For cases with severe heat, add Gypsum Fibrosum 30 g and Fructus Arctii 9 g; for cases with intense itching add Cortex Dictamni Radicis 12 g and Fructus Xanthii 9 g

Proprietaries: *Xij iao Huadu Wan* (Formula 65) or *Fangfeng Tongsheng Wan* (Formula 54).

(2) Treatment for the Damp-heat Type

Symptoms and Signs: Skin-rash mainly appears on the limbs in various sizes. Erosions, exudation, scab and intense itching will possibly follow the rupture of vesicles. The tongue is red, covered with sticky yellow fur.

Therapeutic Method: Strengthen the spleen to remove dampness, and remove pathogenic heat and wind.

Recipe——Modified *Xiaoer Huasi Tang* (a proven prescription).

Rhizoma Atractylodis	9 g
Pericarpium Citri Reticulatae	6 g
Poria	9 g
Rhizoma Alismatis	9 g
parched Fructus Hordei Germinatus	9 g
Talcum	15 g
Fructus Kochiae	30 g
Periostracum Cicadae	9 g
Radix Ledebouriella	9 g
Radix Glycyrrhizae	6 g

Modifications: For cases with severe dampness add Herba Plantaginis 15 g and Exocarpium Benincasae 9 g; for those with intense heat add Radix Rehmanniae 9 g and Gypsum Fibrosum 30 g; for those with secondary infection add Flos Lonicerae 15 g and Fructus Forsythiae 9 g.

Proprietaries: *Xijiao Huadu Wan* (Formula 65) or *Fangfeng Tongsheng Wan* (Formula 54).

2. External Treatment

(1) When the skin lesion shows no ulceration, use either *Fengyou Jin* (Formula 40) or *Ziyang Ding* (Formula 41) for external application three or four times daily. Alternatively, dissolve 150 pills of *Houzhen Wan* (Formula 66), in 3 ml of vinegar, and then apply the mixture onto the affected part; repeat the application twice or three times daily.

(2) If there exist erosion, exudation or secondary infections, apply to the diseased part a paste made by mixing *Huangbai San* (Formula 17) or *Shizhen San* (Formula 57), with sesame oil, twice

or three times a day.

Nursing and Prevention:

1. Avoid scratching as much as possible, and use antipruritic drugs for timely application.

2. Enough attention should be paid to home hygiene, preventing mosquitobites by spraying insecticides' and hanging mosquito-nets; children should not play in places with thick growth of weeds so as to avoid insect-biting.

3. Refrain from eating irritative heavy food like fish.

6.5 Drug-induced Dermatitis

This disease is also termed drug rash; it is an inflammatory reaction on the skin mucous membrane, a manifestation of drug reaction, caused by the entrance of drugs through varying access. In classic TCM works, it is termed drug poisoning reaction.

Etiology and Pathogensis

This disease is due to a weak constitution and the invasion of drug poison which enters the blood, stagnates in the skin and flesh, and spreads through the channels and *ZangFu* organs.

Clinical Manifestation

1. Patients of this disease have a definite record of medication.

2. There is an incubation period usually 20-40 days between the first dose of the medicine and the re-appearance of the skin lesion. If the medicine is taken repeatedly, the incubation period will be greatly shortened, usually to one day or even two hours.

3. The shape of the skin rash is varied, the colour bright, the involved area vast and often symmetric.

4. There is a feeling of itching and burning heat; in severe

cases, it is often accompanied by some general symptoms.

5. Except for a few severe cases, the course is usually short. It can heal fairly soon if the patient ceases to take the dermatitis—inducing drug or receives proper treatment.

Clinically, the common types of drug—induced dermatitis are as follows:

(1) Urticaria—like Type: This type consists of urticaria of various sizes occuring over vast areas. It is redder than the common urticaria, and lasts a comparatively long time. There is a feeling of itching, accompanied possibly by stabbing pain and tenderness.

(2) Scarlet—fever—like and Measle—like Type: This is manifested by extensive bright red macula, papular eruptions, and maculopapule ranging in size from a grain of millet to a soybean, densely spread over the skin in symmetry. There is a feeling of itching. Although the skin rash is obvious, there are no general symptoms. This is the main point that makes it differ from measles and scarlet fever.

(3) Erythema—multiforme—like Type: The skin rash is in the form of edematous purple macula, the size ranging from a soybean to a coin, the center of which is in darker colour and possibly having some vesicles. It occurs in symmetry on the torso and limbs, and sometimes involves the mouth, eyes, lips and pudendum, often accompanied by erosion, exudation, itching, fever, arthralgia and abdominal pain.

(4) Fixed Erythematous Type: This is also a common type. The skin rash appears in the form of edematous bright red or purple macula which are circumscribed, in round or oval shapes, and the center may have some vesicles. It is found mostly in the eyes, anus, glans penis and areas around the mouth where the

skin mucous membranes meet, though it may also be found on the torso and limbs. The time required for the skin rash to vanish varies from one to ten days, but it may take longer if there is ulceration on the pudendum. There exists a feeling of itching, and long-lasting pigmentation will be left after recovery.

When the same dermatitis-inducing drug is used again, the disease will occur in the same place where the previous skin lesion existed.

(5) The Purpuric Type: This type consists of petechia or ecchymosis the size ranging from a needleend to a soybean or even bigger. It feels flat or a little prominent. In mild cases, it is found mostly on the legs, while in severe cases, it may involve the whole body.

(6) Exfoliative-Dermatitis Type: This is a severe drug rash with an incubation period of over twenty days. The onset is often abrupt, with measle-like papular eruption and macula eruption appearing first, then merging into each other and becoming a general diffusive flush. The hands, feet and face may have edema and erosion, followed by repeated scaling, and possibly by exfoliation of hair and nails. There is a general itching and burning-heat sensation, often accompanied by aversion to cold, nausea, vomiting and other general symptoms; the course often lasts for over one month.

(7) Epidermolytic, Big-vesicle-like Type: This is the most severe type among all types of drug rash. The onset is abrupt, with a continuous fever. The skin rash at first shows bright red or purple, with various sizes of macular spots soon covering the whole body. The skin lesion then takes on some folds, followed by loose, dark purple vesicles which are liable to ulcerate. If there

is concurrent infection, hematosepsis often results. It is usually accompanied by exfoliation of mucous membranes in the mouth cavity, esophagus and trachea and by damage to the liver and spleen.

Type and Treatment

First and foremost, the patient must immediately stop taking sensitizing drugs or drugs suspected of being sensitizing before receiving corresponding treatment based on the particular type and condition of the case.

1. Internal Treatment

(1) Treatment for the Wind-heat Type

Symptoms and Signs: Erythra is the main manifestation. The skin takes on erythema, papular eruption and wheals, accompanied by itching, mild fever, and thirst. The tongue is red, and covered with thin yellow fur. The pulse is floating and rapid.

Therapeutic Method: Clear away heat and toxic material; Expel wind and arrest itching.

Recipe——Modified *Xiaofeng San* (Formula 1)

Radix Rehmanniae	15 g
Radix Paeoniae Rubra	15 g
Radix Sophorae Flavescentis	9 g
Flos Lonicerae	30 g
Folium Isatidis	15 g
Fructus Forsythiae	15 g
Fructus Arctii	9 g
Periostracum Cicadae	9 g
Semen Sesami	15 g
Gypsum Fibrosum	30 g
Rhizoma Anemarrhenae	12 g

Radix Glycyrrhizae 9 g

Modifications: For cases with intense heat pathogen, add Rhizoma Imperatae 30 g and Radix Arnebiae seu Lithospermi 12g; for cases with intense itching, add Cortex Dictamni Radicis 30 g and Scorpio 9 g; for cases with dry stool, add Radix et Rhizoma Rhei 9 g, but this is to be added after other drugs have been boiled for some time.

Proprietary: *Xilin Jiedu Wan* (Formula 67).

(2) Treatment for the Damp-heat Type

Symptoms and Signs: This type is manifested mainly by erythra, together with swelling, erosion and exudation, and accompanied by itching. The tongue is red, covered with thin white or yellow fur, and the pulse is floating and rapid.

Therapeutic Method: Clear away heat and toxic material, remove wind and dampness pathogens.

Recipe——*Longdang Xiegan Tang* (Formula 8) with modification.

Radix Gentianae	9 g
Radix Scutellariae	9 g
Capejasmine Fruit	9 g
Flos Lonicerae	30 g
Fructus Forsythiae	15 g
Radix Rehmanniae	30 g
Rhizoma Imperatae	30 g
Semen Plantaginis	15 g
Rhizoma Alismatis	15 g
Caulis Aristolochiae Manshuriensis	9 g
Cortex Dictamni Radicis	15 g
Fructus Kochiae	30 g

Radix Glycyrrhizae 9 g

Modifications: For cases of intense heat, add Gypsum Fibrosum 30 g and Rhizoma Anemarrhenae 12 g; for cases with intense dampness add Poria peel 15 g and Exocarpium Benincasae 15 g; for those with intense itching, add Scorpio 9 g and Radix Sophorae Flavescentis 9 g.

Proprietary: *Longdang Xiegan Wan* (Formula 8).

(3) Treatment for the Noxious—heat Type

Symptoms and Signs: There exist general diffuse flush, skin denudation, or vast violet red macula. There also exist big vesicles, erosion and concurrent infection, accompanied by coma due to high fever, restlessness and thirst. The tongue is dark red, and coated with yellow, dry fur. The pulse is full and rapid.

Therapeutic Method: Clear away heat and toxic material; remove heat from the blood.

Recipe——*Xijiao Dihuang Tang* (Formula 7) plus *Huanglian Jiedu Tang* (Formula 6), with modification.

Cornu Bubali	30 g
Radix Rehmanniae	30 g
Cortex Moutan Radicis	15 g
Radix Paeoniae Rubra	30 g
Rhizoma Coptidis	9 g
Radix Scutellariae	12 g
Capejasmine Fruit	12 g
Flos Lonicerae	30 g
Radix Scrophulariae	15 g
Gypsum Fibrosum	30 g
Rhizoma Anemarrhenae	12 g
Radix Glycyrrhizae	9 g

Modifications: For cases with coma and delirium, add *Zixuedan* (Formula 35) 0.9 g, and the decoction should be taken twice; for cases with thirst, add Herba Dendrobii 12 g and Radix Trichosanthis 12 g.

Proprietaries: *Angong Niuhuang Wan* (Formula 36) or *Zhibao Dan* (Formula 68).

(4) Treatment for the Type Deficiency of *Yin* and Domination of Evil Dryness in Blood.

Symptoms and Signs: As it occurs in the later stage of severe drug-induced dermatitis and convalescence, the high fever has abated, and the skin lesion has healed and become dry with scales. The patient has pale complerion, lassitude and hypodynamia. The Tongue is pale. coated with thin white, scanty fur; the pulse is thready and rapid.

Therapeutic Method: Nourish Yin, supplement blood, invigorate *Qi* and expel wind.

Recipe—— *Danggui Yinzi* (Formula 4) plus *Zengye Tang* (Formula 69) with some modification.

Radix Angelicae Sinensis	15 g
Radix Rehmanniae	15 g
Rhizoma Rehmanniae Praeparatae	15 g
Rhizoma Ligustici Chuanxiong	9 g
Radix Paeoniae Alba	15 g
Radix Scrophulariae	30 g
Radix Ophiopogonis	9 g
Radix Astragali seu Hedysari	30 g
parched Rhizoma Atractylodis Macrocephalae	15 g
Fructus Kochiae	30 g

| Cortex Dictamni Radicis | 15 g |
| Radix Glycyrrhizae | 9 g |

Modifications: For cases with dysphoria and heat, add Radix Adenophorae strictae 15 g, plumula Nelumbinis 4.5 g and Herba Dendrobii 15 g; for cases with severe itching, add Periostracum Cicadae 9 g and Scorpio 9 g.

Proprietaries: *Shiquan Dabu Wan* (Formula 62) or *ZhiBai Dihuang Wan* (Formula 70).

2. External Treatment

External treatment should vary with the different kinds of skin lesion. For particular instructions on such treatment, please refer to Chapter 6.2, Eczema.

3. Other Treatment for Choice

For severe cases of drug-induced dermatitis, in addition to the above mentioned internal and external treatments, some modern medical treatments, such as the administration of hormones and antibiotics, transfusion and hematometachysis may also be employed if the particular condition of a case requires.

Nursing and Prevention

1. One should be very cautious in administering drugs, making a detailed inquiry about the patient's drug allergy record, and strickly following indications and avoiding any abusive use of drugs.

2. In the course of administering drugs, if there occurs signs of a drug allergy like erythema or skin itching, the administration of the suspectable drug must be immediately suspended.

3. To avoid a disease becoming worse or any secondary infections, the skin rash should not be bathed with hot water or

scratched.

4. Drink plenty of water to accelerate the excretion of drugs.

6.6 Allergic Purpura

This is a hemorrhagic disease of the skin and mucous membrane caused by allergic reactions. In TCM classic works, it is also termed *Putao Yi*, *Zidian*, etc.

Etiology and Pathogenesis

This disease is due to constitutional weakness, failure to control one's diet, intake of improper food, the growth of dampness and heat inside the body (which in turn causes blood—heat, harms superficial venules and results in the stagnation of blood in the skin); or due to deficiency of *Yin* of the liver and spleen, and the injury of superficial venules done by fire of deficiency type; or due to deficiency of *Qi*, and the failure of the spleen to govern the blood, leading to the escape of blood from vessels and channels.

Clinical Manifestation

This disease is found mostly among adolescents. There may be a record of exopathic diseases like sore—throat, fever, and aversion to cold, etc. It may also be classified into the following four types according to various affected parts and different manifestations:

1. Purpura Simplex

It is manifested usually by a skin rash which tend to appear on the legs especially on the anterior portion of the lower legs, and occasionally on the upper legs and torso. The skin rash often occur abruptly and relapse repeatedly in large amounts. The eruption is in the form of petechia or an ecchymosis the size of a needle—end or soy bean, bright red at first, then turning dark purple a few days later, and finally yellowish—brown. They disappear in two or three weeks without any general symptoms, Some patients may have some mild itching. The disease is liable to relapse.

2. Arthro—purpura

In addition to skin rash, there exists arthroncus, especially on knee joints, and also on elbow and ankle joints. The skin rash is pleomorphic. There may occur urticaria, vesicles, and bloody vesicles, possibly accompanied by fever tiredness, and other general symptoms as well. The course lasts several weeks or months and it tends to relapse.

3. Purpura Abduminalis

In addition to pleomorphic skin rash, it may be accompanied by nausea, vomiting, abdominal pain, diarrhea or even hematochezia. And, in severe cases, there may even be intussusception, intestinal necrosis, and perforation, etc. There may also exist fever, arthroncus, tiredness, or other general symptoms. The course lasts three or four weeks, and it tends to relapse.

4. Renal Purpura

The skin rash is pleomorphic. It is accompanied by hematuria, proteiunria or cylindruria, and, in a few cases, there may be some nephritic symptoms like edema and oliguria.

The classification mentioned above is not absolute, and the patient may have symptoms of two or more types simultaneously.

Type and Treatment

1. Internal Treatment

(1) Treatment for the Wind—heat Type

Symptoms and Signs: The appearance of maculae on the skin is abrupt, bright red or purple, and does not vanish when the skin is pressed. There may exist mild itching or low fever. The tongue is red, covered with thin yellow fur, and the pluse is floating and rapid.

Therapeutic Method: Remove heat from the blood to stop bleeding, dispel wind and remove heat.

Recipe—— *Xijiao Dihuang Tang* (Formula 7) plus *Sang Ju Yin* (Formula 71), with some modification.

Cornmu Bubali	30 g
Cortex Moutan Radicis	15 g
Parched Radix Rehmanniae	15 g
Radix Paeoniae Rubra	15 g
Folium Mori	9 g
Flos Chrysanthemi	9 g
Parched Flos Carthami	9 g
Fructus Forsythiae	15 g
Parched Nodus Nelumbinis Rhizomatis	9 g
Cacumen Biotae	9 g
Herba Menthae	9 g
Radix Glycyrrhizae	9 g

Modifications: For cases with obvious itching, add Fructus Kochiae 30 g and Periostracum Cicadae 9 g; for those with restlessness, add Medulla Junci 3 g and Herba Lophatheri 9 g.

Proprietaries: *Shihui San* (Formula 72), *Qingwen Baidu Wan* (Formula 73) and *Xiling Jiedu Wan* (Formula 67).

(2) Treatment for the Wind—dampness Type

Symptoms and Signs: The skin rash is polymorphic, with prominent red ecchymosis, accompanied by arthroncus, arthralgia, acratia, or, possibly, fever and edema on the lower limbs. The tongue is red, covered with sticky yellow or white fur and the pulse feels floating and rapid.

Therapeutic Method: Remove heat from the blood, expel wind and clear away dampness.

Recipe——Modified *Xij iao Dihuang Tang* (Formula 7) plus *Duhuo Jisheng Tang* (Formula 74).

Cornu Bubali (powder)	3 g
(to be added to the boiling decoction of other ingredients.)	
Parched Radix Rehmanniae	15 g
Cortex Moutan Radicis	15 g
Radix Paeoniae Rubra	30 g
Radix Angelicae Pubescentis	12 g
Ramulus Loranthi	9 g
Radix Clematidis	15 g
Radix Gentianae Macrophyllae	15 g
Radix Stephaniae Tetrandrae	15 g
Radix Cyathulae	12 g
Semen Coicis	30 g
Caulis Piperis Futokadsurae	15 g
Radix Glycyrrhizae	9 g

Modifications: For cases with edema on the lower limbs, add Poria peel 15 g and Herba Plantaginis 30 g

Proprietaries: *Xiaoluo Tong* (Formula 75) or *Simiao Wan* (Formula 76).

(3) Treatment for the Type Damp-heat in the Spleen and Stomach

Symptoms and Sign: In addition to polymorphic skin rash, there are such symptoms as nausea, vomiting, abdominal pain, diarrhea and hematochezia. The tongue is red, covered with sticky yellow fur, and the pulse is soft, floating and rapid.

Therapeutic Method: Remove heat from the spleen to promote diuresis, and remove heat from the blood to stop bleeding.

Recipe——Modified *Qingpi Chushi Yin* (Formula 77).

Poria	15 g
Parched Rhizoma Atractylodis Macrocephalae	15 g
Radix Scutellariae	12 g
Capejasmine Fruit	15 g
Herba Artemisiae Scopariae	15 g
Radix Rehmanniae (ash)	15 g
Radix Sanguisorbae (ash)	15 g
Rhizoma Alismatis	15 g
Herba Lophatheri	9 g
Caulis Bambusae	9 g
Cortex Magnoliae Officinalis	9 g
Rhizoma Corydalis	9 g
Radix Glycyrrhizae	9 g

Modification: For cases with nausea and vomiting, add Rhizoma Pinelliae 9 g and Rhizoma Zingiber is Recens 6 g; for those with diarrhea add Radix Aucklandiae 9 g and Rhizoma Coptidis 9 g.

Proprietaries: *Fangfeng Tongsheng Wan* (Formula 54) or *Xianglian Wan* (Formula 78).

(4) Treatment for the Type Deficiency of Liver—*Yin* and Kidney—*Yin*

Symptoms and Signs: There is polymorphic skin rash accompanied by symptoms like hematuria, proteinuria, oliguria, edema, low fever, restlessness, tinnitus, loss of weight, lumbago, red tongue with scanty coating, and weak, rapid pulse.

Therapeutic Method: Replenish the vital essence and remove

heat from the blood to cure the macula eruption.

Recipe——Modified *Liuwei Dihuang Wang* (Formula 79).

Radix Rehmanniae	15 g
Cortex Moutan Radicis	15 g
Radix Scrophulariae	24 g
Radix Ophiopogonis	9 g
Radix Paeoniae Rubra	30 g
Rhizoma Alismatis	15 g
Poria	12 g
Fructus Corni	9 g
Herba seu Radix Cirsii Japonici	12 g
Herba Cephalanoploris	12 g
Plastrum Testudinis	12 g
Carapax Trionycis	12 g
Radix Glycyrrhizae	9 g

Modification: For cases with restlessness, add Herba Lophatheri 6 g and Medulla Junci 3 g; for those with edema, add Semen Plantaginis 12 g and Exocarpium Benincasae 15 g; for those with lumbago, add Rhizoma Cibotii 15 g and Radix Achyranthis Bidentatae 15 g.

Proprietaries: *Liuwei Dihuang Wan* (Formula 79) or *Zhi Bai Dihuang Wan* (Formula 70).

(5) Treatment for the Type *Qi*—Failing to Command the Blood

Symptoms and Signs: The course is a protracted one with a tendency to relapse. The skin lesion is dark purple which does not fade away under pressure. Other accompanying symptoms include withering and yellowish complexion, mental exhaustion, tiredness, headache, dizziness, loss of appetite, pale tongue with scanty fur, and weak and rapid pulse.

Therapeutic Method: Invigorate *Qi*, regulate the stomach and reinforce the spleen to command the blood.

Recipe——Modified *Gui Pi Tang* (Formula 63).

Radix Astragali seu Hedysari	30 g
Radix Codonopsis Pilosulae	15 g
Rhizoma Atractylodis Macrocephalae	15 g
Poria	15 g
Radix Rehmanniae Praeparata	15 g
Radix Angelicae Sinensis	15 g
Crinis Carbonisatus	9 g
Herba Agrimoniae	15 g
Radix Polygalae	9 g
Radix Aucklandiae	9 g
parched Semen Ziziphi Spinosae	15 g
Arillus Longan	9 g
Pericarpium Citri Reticulatae	9 g
Radix Glycyrrhizae	9 g

Modifications: For cases with arthralgia, add Herba Siegesbeckiae 15 g and Caulis Trachelospermi 15 g; for those with stomach ache, add Rhizoma Corydalis 9 g and Faeces Trogopterorum 9 g; for those with hematuria, add Herba Cephalanoploris 15 g and parched Nodus Nelumbinis Rhizomatis 9 g.

Proprietaries: *Guipi Tang* (Formula 63) or *Renshen Jianpi Wan* (Formula 113).

2. External Treatment

Please turn to the External Treatment for Eczema (Chapter 6.2) for reference in treating purpura.

Nursing and Prevention

1. During the course of the illness, the patient should rest in bed with the affected limbs placed on a higher level than the torso.

2. Refrain from eating foods liable to invite wind and fire pathogens, foods like sea products (including fish), milk, eggs and those with pungent tastes.

7 Dysneuria Dermatoses

7.1 Cutaneous Pruritus

It is an itching skin disease without primary skin lesion. There often exist scratch marks, bloody scabs, pigmentation, lichenoid changes and some other secondary lesions. This disease is clinically classified into two groups: universal and localized. In TCM classics, universal itching is termed itching wind or wind of itching, while localized itching is termed variably according to the particular itching part of the body, such as pudendum itching, or anal itching etc.

Etiology and Pathogenesis

This disease is mostly due to stagnation of pathogenic wind, cold, dampness and heat in the skin or due to dryness resulting from blood deficiency. This in turn leads to the growth of wind pathogen and the malnutrition of the skin. Pudendum itching and anal itching are often connected with dampness and heat in the liver and kidney.

Clinical Manifestations

1. This disease is found mostly among grown-ups and the elderly.

2. Universal itching occurs on various parts of the body. These parts may itch at the same time or at intervals. In the early stage, the itching is mild and lasts only for a short time, gradually, the intensity will grow and the duration increases. Localized itching mostly attacks such parts as the anus, pudendum and

scrotum.

3. The itching is invariably paroxysmal, usually intense and irregular in daily frequency, each time lasting a period of a few minutes to a few hours. It can be evoked and intensified by excited mood, changed temperature, fatigue, alcoholic drink and intake of pungent food, etc. During sleep at night, the onset is more likely to happen, often affecting one's sleep.

4. Skin examination shows no signs of primary skin rash.

5. Secondary scratch marks, bloody scab and pigmentation may be found on the skin due to seratching Cases with a long course may have thickened skin or lichenoid changes, insomnia, listlessness, or loss of appetite, etc.

6. The course is a long one, varying from weeks to months or years.

Type and Treatment

1. Internal Treatment

(1) Treatment for the Wind—heat Type

Symptoms and Signs: This type occurs in the early stage of the disease. The itching may occur either in various places or in one local place, and it may be worsened by warmth. There exist symptoms such as a burning—heat sensation, scratch marks, bloody scabs, reddened tongue with white or thin yellow fur, and taut and rapid pulse.

Therapeutic Method: Remove heat from the blood, expel wind to arrest itching.

Recipe——Modified *Baixianpi Yin* (Formula 80).

Flos Lonicerae	15 g
Cortex Dictamni Radicis	30 g
Radix Angelicae Sinensis	12 g

Radix Rehmanniae	15 g
Periostracum Cicadae	9 g
Fructus Tribuli	15 g
Radix Scutellariae	9 g
Radix Arnebiae seu Lithospermi	9 g
Radix Ledebouriellae	15 g
Fructus Kochiae	30 g
Radix Glycyrrhizae	9 g

Modifications: For severe cases, add Gypsum Fibrosum 30 g; for those with intense itching add Scorpio 9 g and Zaocys 9 g; for cases with insomnia, add Cortex Albiziae 15 g and Caulis Polygoni Multiflori 15 g, for cases with dry feces, add Radix et Rhizoma Rhei (to be added after other drugs have been boiled for some time).

Proprietary: *Fangfeng Tongsheng Wan* (Formula 54).

(2) Treatment for the Type Blood Deficiency Due to Wind and Dryness

Symptoms and Signs: The course is a protracted one with the following symptoms: dry and thickened skin lesion, or lesion in the form of lichenoid changes, paroxysmal intense itching, pale-looking tongue with thin white fur. The pulse feels deep and weak, or taut and slippery.

Therapeutic Method: Enrich the blood and moisten dryness; expel wind to arrest itching.

Recipe——Modified *Danggui Yinzi* (Formula 4).

Radix Angellcae Sinensis	15 g
Radix Rehmanniae	15 g
Radix Rehmanniae Praeparata	15 g
Radix Paeoniae Alba	15 g

Rhizoma Ligustici ChuanXiong	9 g
Radix Polygoni Multiflori	15 g
Radix Astragali seu Hedysari	30 g
Parched Rhizoma Atractylodis Macrocephalae	15 g
Radix Ledebouriellae	15 g
Fructus Xanthii	15 g
Cortex Albiziae	15 g
Cortex Dictamni Radicis	15 g
Radix Glycyrrhizae	9 g

Modifications: For cases with heat syndrome, subtract Radix Rehmanniae Praeparata and add Gypsum Fibrosum 30 g and Fructus Arctii 9 g; for those with restlessness and insomnia, add Plumula Nelumbinis 4.5 g and Semen Ziziphi Spinosae 15 g; for those with persistent itching, add Zaocys 9 g and Scorpio 9 g.

Proprietaries: *Yangxue Ansheng Wan* (Formula 81), *Sichong Pian* (Formula 82) and *Qinj iu Wan* (Formula 55).

(3) Treatment for the Type Dampness and Heat in the Liver and Gallbladder

Symptoms and Signs: Intense itching on the Scrotum and pudendum, local swelling, flush, reddened tongue with yellow fur, and slippery and rapid pulse.

Therapeutic Method: Remove dampness and heat from the liver and gallbladder, expel wind to arrest itching.

Recipe——Modified *Longdang Xiegang Tang* (Formula 8).

Radix Gentianae	9 g
Radix Bupleuri	12 g
Radix Scutellariae	9 g
Capejasmine Fruit	12 g

Radix Rehmanniae	15 g
Herba Plantaginis	30 g
Rhizoma Alismatis	15 g
Caulis Akebiae	9 g
Fructus Kochiae	30 g
Cortex Dictamni Radicis	15 g
Radix Glycyrrhizae	9 g

Modifications: For cases with intense itching, add Scorpio 9g and Zaocys 9 g; for those with erosion and exudation, add Poria peel 15 g and Herba Artemisiae Capillar is 15 g.

Proprietary: *Longdang Xiegang Wan* (Formula 8).

2. External Treatment

(1) Bathe the affected part once or twice a day in a warm decoction made from either *Zhiyang Xiyao* (Formula 14) or *Quefeng Xiyao* (Formula 15).

(2) The following drugs are offered for choice for external application (usually three or four times daily): *Zhiyang Ding* (Formula 41), Antipruritic Tincture; *Shenjingxing Piyan Yaoshui* Liquid—drug for Neurodermatis (Formula 83), Camphol Powder (2% camphol by weight), Unguentum Picis Fabae Nigrae (Formula 58).

Nursing and Prevention

1. The affected part must not be bathed in hot water or washed with highly basic soap.

2. Keep the affected part clean, but do not wash or rub it too frequently; and in winter, bathing should be limited to once a week. Scratching should be avoided or reduced to a minimum.

3. The quilt, bedding and clothing should be clean and comfortable; clothing made of chemical fiber and woolen material is

not suitable for the patient.

4. Refrain from eating irritative food and drink, such as pepper, alcohol, coffee, or aquatic products like fish, shrimp, and crabs.

5. Keep defecation fluent.

6. Avoid fatigue and mental stress.

7.2 Neurodermatitis

Neurodermatitis is a skin disease characterized by paroxysmal itching and licheonoid changes in the skin. In TCM works, it is termed persistent tinea because of its steadfastness and difficulty in curing; it is also termed cowskin tinea (psoriasis) due to its appearance like the skin of a cow neck, thick and hard.

Etiology and Pathogenesis

At first, it is caused by an emotional disorder and the invasion of wind and heat pathogens into the skin where stagnation results. It gradually worsens as the wind and heat grow more intense, the blood and body fluid become depleted, and blood deficiency brings about dryness and wind, which leads to malnutrition of the skin.

Clinical Manifestations

This disease is clinically classified into two types: the localized and the universal, with the later being the majority.

1. It is found mostly among the young and the old.

2. It tends to occur on the back of the neck and its lateral sides, other possible parts include the lateral side of the elbow, the sacrococygeal region, the popliteal fossa, the ankle, and the eyelid.

3. At first, the skin has paroxysmal itching but no lesion. As

a result of scratching, there appear patches of pimples which are flat and round or multiangled and firm, in normal skin colour, pink, or reddish brown. Gradually, the local skin gets dry and thick, forming lichenoid patches with dermal ridges and deepened stripes, in brownish, yellowish brown, or normal skin colour. These patches have clear edges with a smooth surface or a surface covered with a limited amount of furfuraceous scale surrounded by flat papular eruption. Scratch marks, bloody scabs, erosion, exudation, and even pyogenic infection may result from scratching.

4. The patient has intense paroxysmal itching, especially at night. It is also accompanied by universal neuradermatitis, which often itches so intensely and unbearably that the itching will not cease unless sufficient scratching has caused a pain in the affected local area.

5. The course is a protracted one, with the condition being mild and severe alternately.

Type and Treatment

1. Internal Treatment

(1) Treatment for the Wind—heat Type

Symptoms and Signs: The main symptoms include clusters of red flat pimples, severe itching, palecoloured tongue with thin yellowish or thin white fur, floating and rapid pulse.

Therapeutic Method: Remove heat from the blood; expel wind to arrest itching.

Recipe——Modified *Baixianpi Yin* (Formula 80).

Flos Lonicerae	15 g
Cortex Dictamni Radicis	30 g
Radix Rehmanniae	15 g

Radix Salviae Miltiorrhizae	15 g
Radix Paeoniae Rubra	15 g
Periostracum Cicadae	9 g
Radix Scutellariae	9 g
Radix Arnebiae seu Lithospermi	9 g
Radix Ledebouriellae	15 g
Fructus Kochiae	30 g
Fructus Tribuli	15 g
Radix Glycyrrhizae	9 g

Modifications: For cases with intense itching, add Scorpio 9 g and Zaocys 9 g; for those with insomnia, add Cortex Albiziae 15 g and parched Semen Ziziphi Spinosae 15 g; for those with the neck affected, add Radix Bupleuri 12 g.

Proprietaries: *Fangfeng Tongsheng Wan* (Formula 54) and *Danzhi Xiaoyao Wan* (Formula 84).

(2) Treatment for the Type Blood Deficiency due to Wind-dryness

Symptoms and Signs: As the course continues, the skin lesion takes the form of lichenoid changes or locally thickened skin, possibly with scaling, scratch marks, or a bloody scab. The tongue shows pink, covered with thin white fur, and the pulse is deep and thready.

Therapeutic Methods: Enrich the blood and moisten dryness; expel wind to arrest itching.

Recipe——Modified *Danggui Yinzi* (Formula 4).

Radix Angelicae Sinensis	15 g
Radix Rehmanniae Praeparata	15 g
Rhizoma Ligustici Chuanxiong	9 g
Radix Paeoniae Alba	15 g

Radix Polygoni Multiflori	15 g
Radix Astragali seu Hedysari	30 g
Fructus Tribuli	15 g
Radix Cynanchi Paniculati	30 g
Fructus Xanthii	15 g
Scorpio	9 g
Zaocys	9 g
Radix Ledebouriella	15 g
Radix Glycyrrhizae	9 g

Modifications: For cases with insomnia, add Plumula Nelumbinis 4.5 g and parched Semen Ziziphi Spinosae 15 g; for those with anorexia and abdominal distention, add parched Fructus Hordei Germinatus 15 g, Semen Alpiniae Katsumadai 9 g and parched Semen Raphani 15 g; for those with red skin lesion which gives a burning-heat sensation, subtract Rhizoma Rehmanniae Praeparata and Radix Paeoniae Alba, but add Radix Rehmanniae 15 g, Radix Paeoniae Rubra 15 g and Gypsum Fibrosum 30 g.

Proprietaries: *Qingjiu Wan* (Formula 55), or *Runfu Wan* (Formula 56).

2. External Treatment

(1) For the wind-heat type, *Zhiyang Xiyao* (Formula 14), or *Quefeng Xiyao* (Formula 15) can be used to make a decoction for wet dressing after it gets cool. It is applied once or twice a day, each time lasting 30 minutes. For the type, blood deficiency due to wind-dryness, the same drugs mentioned above may be used to make decoctions, and the affected part is bathed once or twice daily in warm decoctions, each time lasting 30 minutes.

(2) For external application, the following drugs are offered

for choice: *Zhiyang Ding* (Formula 41), *Shenjingxing Piyan Yaoshui* (Formula 83), *Heidou Liuyou Rangao* (Formula 58) and *Huangshen Pifu Rangao* (Formula 85). Three to four applications a day are necessary.

(3) Put a little camphor on either a dogskin plaster (Formula 38) or *Shenj ing Gao* (Formula 86) after the plaster has been heated, and then place the plaster on the affected part. Change the plaster once every three days.

Nursing and Prevention

1. Avoid as much as possible any pessimal stimulations, such as scratching, bathing in hot water, collar-brushing, alcoholic drinks, irritative food, and the application of highly irritative drugs.

2. Avoid mental stress and irritable moods, as well as overwork. If neurosism exists in a certain case, it should be treated at the same time.

8 Erythematous Dermatoses

8.1 Polymorphic Erythema

Polymorphic erythema is a kind of acute inflammatory dermatosis with polymorphic lesion consisting of erythema mainly, together with papular eruption, and vesicles, etc. The typical erythema is in the shape of a cat's eye, hence in TCM works called cat-eye sore; sometimes it is called cold sore, a term based on its characteristics.

Etiology and Pathogenesis

This disease is due to weak constitution or disharmony between *Ying* and *Wei* caused by the invasion of exogenous pathogenic wind-cold. This results in the stagmation of *Qi* and blood, due to exopathic wind-heat affection and stagnation of damp-heat in the skin, or due to uncontrolled diet and the intake of irritating drugs or food, such as fish, shrimp and crabs.

Clinical Manifestation

1. This disease is liable to attack the young and middle-aged, mostly females. It is usually found in the spring, autumn or winter, though there are some cases found in summer.

2. The skin lesion often appears symmetrically on the dorsum manus, palms, finger edge, insteps, heels, face, neck, and also on the mucous membrane of the mouth and genitals as well.

3. The skin eruption appears polymorphic, first in the form of erythema, and later there may appear wheals, papular erruption, vasicles, erosion and purpura. Often, several different

types of skin rash exist together. The erythema is bright red, dark red, or purple, and capable of merging into one another. The edge of some erythema is prominent and in the shape of a ridge while the erythema is umbilicate. A typical erythema usually has over lapping vesicles in the shape of a cat's eye. The lesion on mucous membrane tends to turn into erosion after ulceration.

4. The patient has a feeling of burning—heat and itching. Usually there are no general symptoms. A severe case may have vast skin lesion or even secondary pathologic changes in the viscera. For instance, when it affects the kidneys, there may occur general symptoms such as proteinuria hematuria, loss of appetite, and hypodynamia, etc.

5. The course lasts for two or three weeks, but it is liable to relapse after recovery.

Type and Treatment

1. Internal Treatment

(1) Treatment for the Damp—heat Type

Symptoms and Signs: The macula are bright red, with vesicles, which, after breaking up, or if involving mucous membrane, may have erosion and exudation. There are also such symptoms as burning heat sensation, itching, fever, aversion to cold, restlessness, thirst, arthralgia, yellow urine, dry stool, reddened tongue with yellow sticky coating and rapid and slippery pulse.

Therapeutic Method: Remove heat and dampness, and expel wind.

Recipe——Modified *Bixie Shenshi Tang* (Formula 53).

Herba Taraxaci	30 g
Fructus Forsythiae	12 g

Capejasmine Fruit	9 g
Cortex Phellodendri	9 g
Rhizoma Dioscoreae Septemlobae	9 g
Semen Coicis	15 g
Rhizoma Alismatis	12 g
Caulis Akebiae	6 g
Semen Plantaginis	15 g
Gypsum Fibrosum	15 g
Radix Rehmanniae	15 g
Cortex Moutan Radicis	9 g
Fructus Arctii	9 g
Herba Spirodelae	9 g

(for making a decoction)

Modification: For cases with constipation add Radix et Rhizoma Rhei 9 g (to be added after other drugs have been boiled for some time); for those with arthralgia, add Radix Stephaniae Tetrandrae 12 g and Radix Gentianae Macrophyllae 9 g

(2) Treatment for the Wind—cold Type

Symptoms and Signs: The case relapses or grows more severe when it is cold, and it becomes mild or gradually cures itself when it is warm. The macula is dark purple. Near the end of the limbs, the skin temperature is lower, and the fingers and toes may be swollen. It may also be accompanied by aversion to cold. cool limbs, abdominal pain, loose stool, etc. The tongue fur is thin and white and the pulse is slow and soft.

Therapeutic Method: Expel wind and cold; promote blood circulation to remove blood stasis.

Recipe——modified *Danggui Sini Tang* (Formula 43).

Ramulus Cinnamomi	9 g

Radix Paeoniae Rubra	9 g
Radix Angelicae Sinensis	9 g
Caulis Spatholobi	15 g
Rhizoma Ligustici Chuanxiong	9 g
Radix Salviae Miltiorrhizae	15 g
Herba Asari	3 g
Radix Aconiti Praeparata	6 g
Rhizoma Zingiberis	6 g
Rhizoma seu Radix Notopterygii	9 g
Radix Ledebouriellae	9 g
Radix Glycyrrhizae	6 g

(for making a decoction)

Modification: For cases with abdominal pain, add Rhizoma Corydalis 9 g and Radix Linderae 9 g; and in the case of loose stool, add Poria 12 g and Polyporus Umbellatus 12 g.

2. External Treatment

(1) Treatment for the Damp-heat Type

For cases with erythema and papular eruption as the main symptoms, *Luganshi xiji* (Formula 87) or *Sanshi Shui* (Formula 88) may be chosen for external application; for those with vesicles, erosion or exudation, use *Saoshi Xiyao* (Formula 59) to make a decoction for cool wet dressing. This should be applied with *Huanglian You* (Formula 89). For those with a lesion of the mucous membrane of the mouth, soak Flos Chrysanthemi and Flos Lonicerae (15 g each) in 500 ml. of boiling water and, with the medicated liquid, rinse the mouth several times a day.

(2) Treatment for the Wind-Cold Type

Make a decoction with Lotion No.2 (Formula 90) and bathe the affected part with the decoction twice a day, each time for 20 to 40 minutes.

8.2 Erythema Nodusum

This disease is an acute inflammatory dermatosis, often attacking the anterior side of the lower limbs. It occurs mostly in spring and autumn, often among young females. It is similar to the description of Gourd—vine—like dermatosis and Noxious Dampness Flow recorded in some TCM classics.

Etiology and Pathology

This disease is due to stagnation of *Qi* and blood as well as blockage of channels and vessels, resulting from persistent dampness which turns into heat, causing the retention of damp—heat in the interior, or due to blockage of the vessels resulting from retention of cold—dampness caused by persistent dampness in the weak spleen and by an invasion of cold pathogen.

Clinical Manifestations

1. This disease is liable to attack young females, mostly in spring and autumn.

2. The skin lesion usually occurs symetrically on the lateral side of the lower legs, and in a few cases, may be found on the medial side of the lower legs, and buttocks, etc.

3. The onset is usually abrupt. There may also be, more or less, symptoms such as aversion to cold, fever, headache, throat pain, arthralgia, loss of appetite, listlessness, and acratia, etc.

4. The skin rash takes the form of round subcutaneous nodules, with a diameter of one to five centimeters, slightly prominent or hidden under the surface. The nodule is solid; it will not merge into one another or ulcerate. At first, the nodule is bright red, then gradually turns dark red, reddish purple or tawny, with

the center darker in colour. The number of nodules varies from one to several dozens. The patient feels burning heat, itching, and tenderness. A severe case may have edema on the lower limbs.

5. The course lasts about six weeks in most cases, but a few may continue for several months. It may relapse repeatedly, especially when the patient gets fatigued or during menstruation.

Type and Treatment

1. Internal Treatment

(1) Treatment for the Damp—heat Type

Symptoms and Signs: The onset is abrupt, often accompanied by headache, sore throat, arthralgia or fever. The skin rash shows red, with a burning—heat sensation, and a swelling pain. Other symptoms include thirst, dry stool, yellow urine, reddened tongue with yellowish fur, and a slippery and rapid pulse.

Therapeutic Method: Clear away heat to promote diuresis, and remove obstruction by promoting blood circulation.

Recipe——Modified *Simiao Yongan Tang* (Formula 91).

Flos Lonicerae	30 g
Herba Taraxaci	30 g
Fructus Forsythiae	15 g
Herba Violae	15 g
Capejasmine Fruit	8 g
Cortex Phellodendri	9 g
Radix Stephaniae Tetrandrae	9 g
Radix Scrophulariae	30 g
Radix Salviae Miltiorrhizae	15 g
Radix Paeoniae Rubra	15 g
Radix Angelicae Sinensis	12 g
Radix Cyathulae	9 g

    Radix Glycyrrhizae   6 g
    (for making a decoction)

Modifications: For cases with fever, add Gypsum Fibrosum 30 g, Radix Bupleuri 9 g; for those with throat pain add Fructus Arctii 9 g and Radix Sophorae Subprostratae 9 g; for those with arthralgia, add Radix Clematidis 9 g and Radix Angelicae Pubescentis 9 g.

(2) Treatment for the Cold—dampness Type

Symptoms and Signs: The nodule, coloured purple, is persistent and accompanied by arthralgia. It tends to become worse when the weather is cold, and in some severe cases, it may cause edema on the lower legs. The tongue is pale and covered with white greasy fur. The pulse is deep, weak or slow.

Therapeutic Method: Expel pathogenic cold from channels and clear away dampness to regulate channels.

Recipe——Modified *Danggui Shini Tang* (Formula 43).

Radix Angelicae Sinensis	15 g
Ramulus Cinnamomi	9 g
Herba Asari	3 g
Radix Cyathulae	15 g
Caulis Spatholobi	15 g
Rhizoma Ligustici Chuanxiong	9 g
Radix Salviae Miltiorrhizae	15 g
Radix Clematidis	9 g
Poria	12 g
Rhizoma Atractylodis	12 g
Rhizoma Atractylodis Macrocephalae	9 g
Fructus Chaenomelis	9 g
Semen Coicis	15 g

2. External Treatment

(1) Treatment for the Damp—heat Type:

Use *Daqing Gao* (Formula 30) or *Furong Gao* (Formula 92) for external application. Change the dressing once a day.

(2) Treatment for the Cold—dampress Type:

Bathe the affected part with a hot decoction made by boiling the *Huoxue Zhitong San* (Formula 44), twice a day; or apply *Huiyang Yulong Gao* (Formula 93), changing the dressing once every other day.

9 Erythroderma Desquamativum

9.1 Pityriasis Rosea

Pityriasis rosea is a commonly found erythroderma desquamativum, liable to attack the torso and areas near the end of the limbs. It is purple in colour and covered with white scales, the long axis of the macular eruption being parallel to that of the skin. The above characteristics are similar to those of so-called wind-heat sore described in some TCM works.

Etiology and Pathogensis

This disease is due to the following factors: stagnation of heat in the blood, the invasion of pathogenic wind, and conjoint invasion of pathogenic wind-heat which persists in the skin, blocks the striae of skin, burns the essential fluid of *Ying* and causes dryness in the blood.

Clinical Manifestations

1. It tends to attack the young and middle-aged, mostly in spring and autumn. The skin lesion is usually found on the torso and areas mear the end of limbs, or even the whole body except for the head an face.

2. At first, an erythema, which is termed mother erythema, appears at a certain place on the torso or limbs. It expands gradually into a round or oval shape, the size of a finger-nail or a coin, the edge being a little prominent, and the center comparatively flat and covered with tiny white scales. Its existence is often neglected when there is no itching. The mother erythema tends to

fade away and disappears in about ten days. But in other places, the same macula eruptions, smaller than the mother erythema and of different sizes, called child erythema, appear in groups one after another. They are usually arranged in a symmetrical manner. The long axis of eruption runs parallel to the skin wrinkles, and in the center of the skin rash can be seen some thin fine wrinkles. The eruptions have clear edges, and rarely merge into one another.

3. The patient has, more or less, a sensation of itching. There are no general symptoms in most cases. At the beginning of the course, the patient may have such accompanying symptoms as low fever, headache, throat pain, restlessness, thirst, arthralgia, and general discomfort.

4. The course is self–limited, usually lasting four to six weeks before a natural cure. Some cases may persist for two to three months, or even more, before its cure. On the whole, it is not likely to relapse after it is cured.

Type and Treatment

1. Internal Treatment

At first, the skin eruptions are bright reddish purple in colour, involve vast areas, and are accompanied by low fever, headache, throat pain, restlessness, thirst, and scanty dark urine, etc. Other symptoms include a reddened tongue with thin white or thin yellowish fur, and a pulse which is taut, slippery and slow, due to heat in the blood and excessive pathogenic wind.

Therapeutic Method: Clear away heat from the blood, and expel wind to arrest itching.

Recipe——Modified *Baixianpi Yin* (Formula 80).

Flos Lonicerae   15 g

Folium Isatidis	15 g
Radix Arnebiae Seu Lithospermi	9 g
Radix Scutellaria	9 g
Cortex Dictamni Radicis	15 g
Radix Ledebouriellae	9 g
Periostracum Cicadae	6 g
Fructus Tribuli	12 g
Cortex Moutan Radicis	12 g
Radix Rehmanniae	15 g
Radix Paeoniae Rubra	15 g
Gypsum Fibrosum	15 g
Radix Glycyrrhizae	6 g

Modifications: For cases with severe itching, add Cortex Dictamni Radicis 30 g and Radix Sophorae Flavescentis 9 g; for patients who have suffered from this disease for a long time due to blood deficiency and wind-dryness, subtract Flos Lonicerae, Folium Isatidis, Radix Arnebiae seu Lithospermi, Radix Scutellariae, and add Radix Angelicae Sinensis, Caulis Spatholobi, Radix Polygoni Multiflori and Radix Salviae Miltiorrhizae (each weighing 15 g)

2. External Treatment

(1) Use Calamina Lotion (Formula 87) or Sulfur Emulsion (Sulfur 5%) for external application.

(2) Bathe the affected part once or twice a day with a warm decoction made by boiling in 2000 ml. of water the following drugs: Radix Sophorae Flavescentis 30 g, Fructus Cnidii 30 g, Pericarpium Zanthoxyli 12 g and Alumen 12 g, each time lasting twenty to thirty minutes.

(3) Acupuncture: Puncture the following acupoints: Hegu

(LI4), Quchi (LI11), Dazhui (DU14), Jianyu (LI15), Jianjing (GB21), Xuehai (SP10), Zusanli (ST36), etc, using the reinforcing method once a day, leaving the needle in the skin for ten to fifteen minutes each time.

Nursing and Prevention

1. Refrain from bathing in hot water during acute stage and from using irritating drugs for external applicaton.

2. Refrain from eating pungent foods, fish and other aquatic products.

9.2 Psoriasis

Psoriasis is a common kind of erythroderma desquamativum. Similar descriptions of it can be found in some TCM classics, which term the disease white sore or loose—skin tinea. It is characterized by multi—layer silvery scales which appear repeatedly on the erythema.

Etiology and Pathology

This disease is caused by the invasion of pathogenic wind into the skin, where it stays and later turns into heat, thus causing heat in the blood, dryness in the blood, or blood stasis. It may also be caused by deficiency of both liver—*Yin* and kidney—*Yin*, or by the disharmony between the *Chong* and *Ren* channels, the *Ying—Qi* and blood, or the *Yin* and *Yang* in the *Zang Fu* organs as well.

Clinical Manifestations

This disease is clinically classified into four types: the common type, the articular type, the pus—pocket type, and the erythroderma type, of which the common type is the majority.

1. The Common Type of Psoriasis

(1) The skin eruptions may appear on any part of the body, but most likely on the scalp, the outer side of the limbs, and the lumbosacral portion.

(2) At first, the skin eruption is in the form of red papular eruption or maculopapule, and the size of a grain of rice or a soybean. It gradually grows bigger and merges into one another, covering an area with an extinct edge which may appear in the form of dots. The affected area is shaped like a coin or a map covered with a multi—layer of scales like pine bark. When the scales are removed, a thin translucent membrane can be seen, which is referred to as membrane phenomenon. When the membrane is scraped, some bleeding in the form of dots is seen ,which is called dew--drop phenomenon. The skin eruption on the scalp is dark red, and covered with thick greyish white scales. The hair is often bundled up due to the adhesion of the scales but does not shed thereupon. When the nails are affected, there may appear some tiny concave dots on the nails.

(3) The onset is acute in most cases, and the course is a protracted one, liable to relapse. It is clearly a seasonal disease, attacking the patients or becoming more savere in winter but having a natural cure or becoming less severe in summer. Among some patients, the seasonal condition may just be the reverse. However, this seasonal change is not so obvious among protracted cases. In terms of the changing of the skin eruption, it can be divided into the following stages: active stage, resting stage, and extinctive stage. During the active stage, new skin eruptions emerge continuously while the old ones keep growing bigger, and the scales thicker. There is clear inflamation with areola surrounding the skin eruption. At this stage, isomorphic reactions

frequently take place, ie, psoriasis eruptions occur on a skin wound or around a sty. During the resting stage, the condition stays unchanged with no new eruptions appearing and no old eruptions vanishing. During the extinctive stage, the skin eruptions become flat and smaller until they gradually disappear, leaving some temporary pigmentation or deposit patches.

(4) The patient feels itching to varying degreees.

2. The articular—type of Psoriasis

Apart from the skin eruptions of the common type, it is accompanied by symptoms similar to those of rheumatoid arthritis, such as fever and arthralgia, etc. The severity of these symptoms varies with the change of the condition of the skin eruptions. Articular pathologic changes often involve the small joints of the fingers and toes, sometimes the big joints as well, causing them, in a protracted case, to stiffen and deform, hampering their movements.

3. The Pus—pocket Type of Psoriasis

This type of psoriasis tends to attack the palmaris et plantaris, or in some severe cases, any part of the skin. It is manifested by tiny pus—pockets on the surface of erythema. Cases with pus—pockets covering vast areas often have such symptoms as aversion to cold, fever, and arthralgia.

4. The Erythroderma—type Psoriasis

This type usually stems from the common type of psoriasis, with symptoms as follows: the skin of the whole body is flush or purplish red, moist and with a large amount of desquamation. There is only a small proportion of the skin that remains normal, in the form of patches. It is also accompanied by fever, cornification of palmaris et plantaris and the thickening of nails.

Type and Treatment

1. Internal Treatment

(1) Treatment for the Heat–in –the –Blood Type

Symptoms and Signs: The occurence and growth of the skin rash is considerably rapid, involving large areas, red in colour, and with a great deal of desquamation. There is distinct itching with insomorphic reaction, accompanied by aversion to heat, restlessness, irritability, sensation of dryness in the throat, bitterness in the mouth, constipation and yellow urine. The tongue is reddened or dark red with thin yellow coating. The pulse is rapid and taut or slippery.

Therapeutic Method: Remove heat from the blood, promote circulation of blood and expel pathogenic wind.

Recipe——Modified *Shuanghua Tulin Yin* (Formula 94).

Poria	30 g
Flos Lonicerae	30 g
Flos Sophorae Immaturus (parched)	15 g
Radix Scutellariae	9 g
Rhizoma Anemarrhenae	9 g
Radix Arnebiae seu Lithospermi	9 g
Radix Rehmanniae	15 g
Radix Paeoniae Rubra	15 g
Cortex Moutan Radicis	12 g
Radix Salviae Miltiorrhizae	15 g
Radix Angelicae Sinensis	9 g
Radix Bupleuri	9 g
Periostracum Cicadae	6 g
Cortex Dictamni Radicis	15 g
(for making a decoction)	

(2) Treatment for the Blood—dryness Type

Symptoms and Signs: The course is a protracted one. The skin rash has ceased to grow at this stage and, in some parts, has disappeared. The skin eruption is dry, its colour has faded and scales reduced. The tongue is pink, covered with scanty or thin white fur. The pulse is weak, taut or deep.

Therapeutic Method: Enrich the blood, expel wind and moisten dryness.

Recipe——Modified *Yangsue Runfu Ying* (Formula 95).

Radix Angelicae Sinensis	15 g
Radix Paeoniae Alba	9 g
Radix Paeoniae Rubra	9 g
Radix Rehmanniae	15 g
Radix Rehmanniae Praeparatae	15 g
Caulis spatholobi	30 g
Radix Scrophulariae	15 g
Radix Polygoni Multiflori	15 g
Radix Asparagi	9 g
Radix Ophiopogonis	9 g
Fructus Leonuri	9 g
Cortex Dictamni Radicis	9 g
Fructus Tribuli	9 g
Bombyx Batryticatus	9 g

(3) Treatment for the Blood—stasis Type

Symptoms and Signs: The skin eruption persists for a long time, dark red in colour, or with pigmentation. The scale is thick and in the shape of psoriasis. In some cases, the joints do not function properly. The tongue is dark purple with ecchymosis, and the pulse is weak and uneven.

Therapeutic Method: promote blood circulation to remove blood stasis.

Recipe——Modified *Taohong Siwu Tang* (Formula 10).

Rhizoma Ligustici Chuang Xiong	9 g
Radix Angelicae Sinensis	9 g
Radix Paeoniae Rubra	15 g
Semen Persicae	9 g
Flos Carthami	9 g
Rhizoma Sparganii	9 g
Rhizoma Zedoariae	9 g
Radix Salviae Miltiorrhizae	15 g
Caulis Spatholobi	30 g
Eupolyphaga Sinensis Walker	9 g
Herba Oldenlandiae Diffusae	15 g

(For making a decoction)

(4) Treatment for the Type Disharmony between *Chong* and *Ren* Channels

Symptoms and Signs: This type is found mainly among females. The skin eruption vanishes or abates during pregnancy but will relapse or become exacerbated after delivery. Normally, it is accompanied by irregular menstruation, lumbago, weak limbs, headache, and tinnitus.

Therapeutic Method: Regulate *Chong* and *Ren* channels.

Recipe——Modified *Erxian Tang* (Formula 96) plus *Siwu Tang* (Formula 97).

Radix Rehmanniae Praeparatae	15 g
Radix Angelicae Sinensis	9 g
Radix Paeoniae Rubra	12 g
Radix Paeoniae Alba	12 g

Herba Leonuri	12 g
Radix Polygoni Multiflori	15 g
Rhizoma Polygonati	15 g
Rhizoma Curculiginis	9 g
Herba Epimedii	15 g
Semen Cuscutae	12 g
Radix Morindae Officinalis	9 g
Fructus Xanthii	9 g

(5) Treatment for the Type of Channel-blockage by Wind-dampness

Symptoms and Signs: The symptoms and signs are those of the articular type of psoriasis, such as arthralgia, articular swelling or even stiffness, deformation of joints, and hinderance of articular movement as well.

Therapeutic Method: Expel wind and dampness, promote blood circulation and regulate channels.

Recipe——modified *Duhuo Jisheng Tang* (Formula 74)

Radix Gentianae Macrophyllae	9 g
Radix Ledebouriellae	9 g
Ramulus Mori	30 g
Radix Angelicae Pubescentis	9 g
Radix Clematidis	9 g
Radix Cyathulae	9 g
Radix Angelicae Sinensis	9 g
Rhizoma Ligustici Chuanxiong	9 g
Radix Paeoniae Alba	9 g
Caulis Spatholobi	15 g
Cortex Dictamni Radicis	15 g
Poria	15 g

Radix Glycyrrhizae 6 g

(6) Treatment for the Type of Toxic Heat and Dampness

Symptoms and Signs: Most of the symptoms are similar to those of the pus—pocket type of psoriasis. It may also have flush, erosion, exudation, or other skin lesion. In some severe cases, it may be accompanied by thirst, fever, constipation. yellow urine, and some other general symptoms. The tongue is reddened, covered with yellow or yellow greasy fur. The pulse is taut or slippery.

Therapeutic Method: Clear away heat and toxic material and remove dampness.

Recipe——Modified *Longdan Xiegan Tang* (Formula 8) plus *Wuwei Xiaodu Yin* (Formula 5).

Radix Gentianae	9 g
Radix Scutellariae	9 g
Cortex Phellodendri	9 g
Fructus Capejasmine	9 g
Flos Lonicerae	30 g
Herba Violae	15 g
Herba Taraxaci	30 g
Flos Chrysanthemi Indici	15 g
Fructus Forsythiae	9 g
Poria	15 g
Semen Plantaginis	9 g
Rhizoma Alismatis	9 g
Caulis Akebiae	6 g

(7) Treatment for the Type Excessive Fire—toxin

Symptoms and Signs: The symptoms are those of the erythroderma—type psoriasis. The skin all over the body is diffuse, flushed or dark red, with vast amounts of desquamation and a burning-heat sensation. Protracted cases have moist and thick skin lesions, often accompanied by fever, aversion to cold, restlessness, thirst, constipation, frequent urination, and yellow urine, etc. The tongue is dark red, with scanty or no coating; The pulse is slippery and rapid.

Therapeutic Method: Clear away heat and toxin from the blood.

Recipe——modified *Qingying Tang* (Formula 98).

Cornu Bubali	15 g
Radix Rehmanniae	30 g
Radix Scrophulariae	15 g
Cortex Moutan Radicis	9 g
Radix Paeoniae Rubra	15 g
Flos Lonicerae	30 g
Herba Taraxaci	15 g
Fructus Forsythiae	15 g
Rhizoma Coptidis	6 g
Gypsum Fibrosum	30 g
Herba Lophatheri	6 g
Radix Glycyrrhizae	6 g

Proprietaries: For the common type of psoriasis, administer *Xiaoyin Pian* (Formula 94), to be taken three times daily, ten pills at a time, or *Keyin Wan* (Formula 99) three times daily, one pill at a time, or *Fangfeng Tongsheng Wan* (Formula 54), three times daily, six pills at a time.

2. External Treatment

(1) During the progressive stage, use mild, low-concentration ointment, such as the 5% boric acid ointment, or the 5%

sulphur ointment, etc.

(2) During the resting stage, use the sulphur ointment (5–10% sulphur) or *Heidou Liuyou Gao* (Formula 58) and *Pifu Ruangao* (Formula 85), etc.

(3) Cases with vast skin lesion may receive the following additional treatment: bathing once a day in potassium sulfide solution, or in a hot spring or in a decoction made from the following ingredients: Alumen Exsiccatum 120 g, pericarpium Zanthoxyli 120 g, Flos Chrysanthemi Indici 240 g and Natrii Sulfas 500 g, each time lasting twenty to sixty minutes.

(4) Make an ointment by mixing Pericarpium Granati (in powder form, 10 g) and sesame oil 20 ml. for external application. The application is repeated twice daily.

10 Desmosis

10.1 Lupus Erythematosus

This disease comes within the category of desmosis. As there is autoimmunity against it, this disease also belongs to the category of autoimmune diseases. Clinically, it is classified into two kinds: lupus erythematosus discoides and systemic lupus erythematosus. The former is characterized by skin eruption; it is, in most cases, chronic and circumscribed. In addition to skin eruptions, the latter is also manifested by its effect on internal organs; the pathologic change is usually a progressive one. In TCM classics, there are no exact corresponding names of these diseases. But according to clinical manifestations, it is generally considered that systemic lupus erythematosus corresponds approximately to the terms in TCM as maculae due to *Yang* toxin or *Yin—Yang* toxin, while lupus erythematosus corresponds approximately to ghost—face sore and butter—fly erysipelas. Some classifications are based on symptoms: Cases with arthralgia as the main symptom are grouped under arthralgia—syndrome, those with dropsy as the main symptom are grouped under hydrops, those with dropsy in the chest are termed pleural effusion, those with lesion of cardiac muscles and acute endocarditis are grouped under cardiopalmus or severe palpitation, and those showing syndrome of consumption after a protracted course are grouped under consumptive diseases. As the symptoms of erythematous lupus are very complicated and vary greatly, it is almost impossible to group them under one single category of syndrome.

Etiology and Pathogenesis

This disease is, in most cases, due to a weak constitution, or deficiency of liver—*Yin* and kidney—*Yin*, or damage to *Qi*, blood, and *Zang—Fu* organs by the excessive seven emotions and overwork. These in turn lead to the disharmony between *Yin* and *Yang*, *Qi* and blood, and to the blockage of channels from stagnation of *Qi* and blood stasis; or this is due to severe sun—burning with invasion of noxious heat and blockage of channels, which in turn impair *Zang—Fu* organs internally and the skin externally.

Clinical Manifestions

1. Lupus Erythematosus Discoides

(1) The skin lesion tends to occur on the face, especially on the nose bridge, paranasal sinuses and cheeks, often merging into each other forming a butterfly—like shape. It may also involve lips, external ears, dorsum manus, and scalp, etc. The skin lesion which does not expand beyond the base of the mandible is the topical type, or else it is a dissemination type.

(2) The skin lesion is typified by lifiltrative prominent erythema, with clear edges, the center being convex and atrophic in the shape of a dish. At first, it is bright red, but gradually turns dark red, the surface being covered with adherent greyish yellow or greyish white scales, under which can be found expanded sweat pores in the shape of ethmoidal foramen. On the back of the fallen scale can be seen cuticular pegs in the shape of a board full of pins. Some atrophic scars / or pigmentation or dispigmentation are left after recovery, and some atrophic psilotic maculae are also formed thereafter. The lesion of the mucous

membrane occurs mostly on the lower lip, often showing some greyish white erosion or superficial ulceration.

(3) Mostly, there is no general discomfort. In a few cases, it may be accompanied by low fever, acratia, and arthralgia, etc. Usually, there are no local subjective symptoms, but there may be some mild itching or burning—heat sensation.

(4) The course is a chronic one. A few cases may turn into systemic lupus erythematosus.

2. Systemic Lupus Erythematosus

(1) This disease attacks mostly females between ages 15 to 40.

(2) The skin lesion is often massive and extensive, arranged in symmetry and liable to occur on exposed parts such as face, dorsum manus, and torso. The lesion is polymorphic. The common type of skin lesion is edematous erythema with voilet red macula of various shapes and sizes. The lesion on the face may take the shape of a butterfly. The lesion on the finger ends and toe ends are mostly violet red macula, vesicles, and ulceration. The lesion on the mucous membrane of the mouth is often in the form of bleeding dots, erosion, superficial ulceration, and gingivitis, etc. In other cases, the lesion may take a form similar to polymorphic erythema, livido reticularis, nodular erythema like eruption, or sarcoidosis, wheals, or baldness, etc. About 15% of the cases have no skin lesion during the whole course.

(3) This disease often begins with fever. headache, and arthralgia; later, it may affect some internal organs resulting in various other symptoms. In most cases, it affects the kidneys, causing nephritis or nephrotic syndrome and renal failure. In the anaphase there is often urinaemia and hypertension. 50% of the

cases have pathological changes in the cardiovascular system, such as pericarditis, myocarditis, endocarditis, cardiectasis, and heart—failure, etc. In some cases, it is manifested by thrombotic phlebitis, thromboangiitis obliterans or Raynaud's phenomenon. The respiratory system and digestive system are often involved too, with manifestations of chronic cough, chest pain, hemopysis, dyspneic respiration, or even respiratory failure There may also be symptoms like loss of appetite, nausea, vomiting, abdominal pain, diarrhea, hematochezia and so on. About one third of the patients have their nervous system affected, with symptoms such as irritability, confusion, fantasy, dementia, delirium, hemiparalysis, and periphera paralysis, etc. Other possible symptoms include menstrual disorder, hepato—lienal lymphadenectasis, eyeground bleeding, and pathological changes in the retina, etc.

(4) Laboratory Examination

 a. There is a certain degree of anemia, a reduction of erythrocytes, and, in some cases, a reduction of blood platelets.

 b. Blood sedimentation is quickened in most cases.

 c. The electrophoretic analysis of protein shows some increase in gamma globulin but some decrease in albumin.

 d. The cells of lupus erythematosis can be found in the peripheral Blood or bone marrow. The positive rate is relatively high during the acute stage.

 e. Indirect fluorescent test of immune antinuclear antibody shows, in most cases, positive reaction, with peripheral type or, occasionally, nucleoloid type, as its specificity.

 f. In some cases, the test for rheumatoid factor shows positive.

Type and Treatment

1. Internal Treatment

(1) Treatment for the Type Qi-stagnation and Blood stasis

Symptoms and Signs: This type of symptom is found mostly among cases of lupus erythematosus discoides and systemic lupus erythematosus, which is characterized mainly by hepatic injury. On the face and some other places there is dark red macula, or there may be Raynaud's phenomenon, hepatosplenomegaly, muscle soreness, ness arthralgia pain in the sternocostal region, abdominal distension, and menstrual disorder, etc. the tongue is dark red, or shows some ecchymosis; the fur is thin and white, and the pulse taut and weak.

Therapeutic Method: Relieve the depressed liver, promote blood circulation and remove blood stasis.

Recipe——modified *Chaihu Shugan Tang* (Formula 33) plus *Tongqiao Huoxue Tang* (Formula 100).

Radix Bupleuri	9 g
Radix Paeoniae Rubra	12 g
Radix Paeoniae Alba	12 g
Rhizoma Ligustici Chuanxiong	9 g
Semen Persicae	9 g
Flos Carthami	9 g
Radix Salviae Miltiorrhizae	15 g
Fructus Aurantii	9 g
Radix Curcumae	9 g
Fructus Meliae Toosendan	9 g
Pericarpium Citri Reticulatae	9 g
Herba Oldenlandiae Diffusae	15 g

(For making a decoction)

Proprietaries: (a)*Huoxue Quyu Pian* (Formula 101), to be taken five pills at a time, three times daily. (b) For protracted cases with deficiency of *Yin* and pathogenic heat, administer *Liuwei Dihuang Wan* (Formula 79), to be taken one or two pills each time, twice daily. (c) *Qinggao Mi Wan* (a bolus of Herba Artemisiae powder and honey), each bolus weighing 10 g, to be taken one or two boluses each time, three times daily.

(2) Treatment for the Noxious Heat Type

Symptoms and Signs: This type is found at the acute stage of systemic lupus erythematosus. The main symptoms include fever, arthralgia, restlessness, thirst, an inclination to take cold drinks, dark urine, constipation, trance, and even confusion, delirium and convulsion. The skin lesion takes the form of edematous erythema; other possible symptoms include ecchymosis, spitting blood, hematochezia, and nasal hemorrhage, etc. The tongue is reddened or dark reddish purple, covered with yellow coating; the pulse is taut and rapid or full.

Therapeutic Method: Clear away heat and toxic material; remove heat from the blood to protect *Yin*

Recipe—— modified *Xijiao Dihuang Tang* (Formula 7), or *Huaban Tang* (Formula 102).

Cornu Bubali	6 g
(to be put into the boiling decoction before taking it)	
Radix Rehmanniae	30 g
Cortex Moutan Radicis	9 g
Radix Paeoniae Rubra	15 g
Capejasmine Fruit	12 g
Gypsum Fibrosum	30 g
Rhizoma Anemarrhenae	9 g

Flos Lonicerae	15 g
Fructus Forsythiae	9 g
Radix Scrophulariae	15 g
Radix Ophiopogonis	15 g
Rhizoma Imperatae	30 g

Modifications: For cases with confusion and delirium, add *Angong Niuhuang Wan* (Formula 36), one or two boluses each time, to be dissolved before taking it, or add *Zixue Dan* (Formula 35), 0.9 g each time, to be put into the boiling decoction and soaked before taking it; for cases with persistent high fever, add Cornu Saigae Tataricae Powder (0.3 to 0.6 g each time, to be put into the boiling decoction before taking it)

(3) Treatment for the Type Hyperactivity of Fire due to *Yin* Deficiency

Symptoms and Signs: This type is mostly found in the remission stage of systemic lupus erythematosus, where high fever has receded, turning into persistent low fever. Other symptoms include dysphoria with feverish sensation in the chest, palms and soles, thirst, dry lips, headache, acratia, tinnitus, asthenopia, lassitude in the loin and legs, arthralgia, night sweat, baldness, menstrual disorder, reddened tongue with thin yellow coating or without any coating, and weak rapid pulse.

Therapeutic Method: Replenish the vital essence and remove heat.

Recipe——modified *Zhi Bai Dihuang Tang* (Formula 70).

Radix Rehmanniae	30 g
Radix Scrophulariae	15 g
Radix Asparagi	12 g
Radix Ophiopogonis	12 g

Rhizoma Anemarrhenae	9 g
Cortex Phellodendri	9 g
Herba Artemisiae Chinghao	9 g
Cortex Lycii Radicis	15 g
Cortex Moutan Radicis	9 g
Poria	9 g
Fructus Corni	12 g
Herba Ecliptae	12 g
Fructus Ligustri Lucidi	12 g

(4) Treatment for the Type Deficiency of Both *Yin* and *Qi*

Symptoms and Signs: This type is also mostly found in the remission stage of systemic lupus erythematosus. There are symptoms as follows: general acratia, loss of appetite, listlessness, cardio palmus, shortness of breath; or low fever, thirst but with no desire to drink, constipation, reddened tongue, thready, deep and weak pulse, etc.

Therapeutic Method: Supplement *Qi* and nourish *Yin*.

Recipe——modified *Shengmai San* (Formula 103).

Radix Pseudostellariae	15 g
Radix Ophiopogonis	15 g
Fructus Schisandrae	9 g
Radix Glehniae	15 g
Radix Adenophorae	15 g
Radix Scrophulariae	30 g
Herba Dendrobii	15 g
Radix Rehmanniae	30 g
Radix Astragali seu Hedysari	30 g
Rhizoma Polygonati	15 g
Poria	9 g

Rhizoma Atractylodis Macrocephalae	9 g
Radix Angelicae Sinensis	9 g
Radix Salviae Miltiorrhizae	15 g

(For making a decoction)

(5) Treatment for the Type of Noxious Heat Invading the Heart

Symptoms and Signs: This type is found among patients with heart diseases. The main symptoms include severe palpitation, dyspnea, choking sensation in the chest, spontaneous perspiration, insomnia, restlessness, pale complexion, clammy limbs, pale tongue with thin white coating, and thready, weak pulse, or slow pulse with irregular intervals.

Therapeutic Method: Supplement *Qi*, nourish the heart and tranquilize the spirit.

Recipe——modified *Yangxin Tang* (Formula 104).

Radix Pseudostellariae	15 g
Radix Glehniae	15 g
Radix Adenophorae	15 g
Radix Astragali seu Hedysari	30 g
Radix Angelicae Sinensis	9 g
Radix Rehmanniae	15 g
Radix Salviae Miltiorrhizae	15 g
Poria cum Ligno Hospite	9 g
Semen Ziziphi Spinosae (parched)	15 g
Semen Biotae	15 g
Fructus Schisandrae	9 g
Radix Polygalae	9 g
Concha Margaritifera Usta	30 g
Radix Glycyrrhizae	6 g

(6) Treatment for the Type Deficiency of Both the Spleen and Kidneys

Symptoms and Signs: This type is found mostly at the anaphase of renal lesions. The common symptoms are as follows: pale complexion, aversion to cold, clammy limbs, edema, acratia, listlessness, lassitude in the loin, abdominal distension, loss of appetite, scanty urine, loose stool and putty face, shoulders, and back. In some severe cases, there are even symptoms like hydrothorax ascites, cardio palms, shortness of breath, pale enlarged tongue with teethmarks, and deep thready pulse.

Therapeutic Method: Warm *Yang* for diuresis.

Recipe——modified *Jinkui Shenqi Wan* (Formula 105) plus *Erxian Tang* (Formula 96) and *Shenfu Tang* (Formula 106).

Radix Aconiti praeparata	9 g
Herba Epimedii	15 g
Rhizoma Curculiginis	10 g
Radix Morindae Officinalis	9 g
Semen Cuscutae	15 g
Radix Astragali seu Hedysari	15 g
Radix Codonopsis Pilosulae	15 g
Rhizoma Atractylodis Macrocephalae	9 g
Rhizoma Dioscoreae	15 g
Poria	9 g
Ramulus Cinnamomi	9 g
Polyporus Umbellatus	12 g
Rhizoma Alismatis	12 g

(for making a decoction)

2. External Treatment

(1) Apply *Shengj i Yuhong Gao* (Formula 128) onto the af-

fected part, twice or three times daily.

(2) Rub a mixture of *Mituoseng San* (Formula 107), Powder of Lithargyrum, and vinegar onto the affected part, twice or three times a day.

3. Additional Therapeutic Method

During the stage of acute attack or in severe cases, TCM treatment is often combined with western medical treatment for better results.

Nursing and Prevention

1. Avoid sun-burn.

2. Increase nourishment properly. Cases with edema should take non-salt or low salt diet.

3. Refrain from overwork, pay attention to warm-keeping, and, during the stage of acute attack, bed rest.

4. Refrain from excessive child-birth and too much sex.

10.2 Dermatasclerosis

Dermatasclerosis is a kind of desmosis, characterized by skin tumefaction, sclerema and, finally, atrophy. It is clinically divided into two types: the localized and the generalized. Its symptoms, belonging to the arthralgia-syndrome, are similar to those of 'pi bi' (numbness in the skin) as described in some TCM classics. It has a protracted course, and may attack people of all age-groups, with female patients outnumbering the male.

Etiology and Pathogenesis

This disease is caused by the following interrelating factors: insufficiency of the kidney-*Yang* and blood, the failure of superficial-*Qi* to protect the body against diseases, loose striae of skin and muscles, the invasion of pathogenic factors of wind, cold, and dampness (which accumulate in the channels, the skin, and the blood vessels causing the disharmony between *Ying* and *Wei*), the stagnation of *Qi* and blood, or the invasion of exogenous pathogenic factors into the *Zang—Fu* organs, causing the disharmony between the solid and hollow organs, and the stagnation of *Qi* and blood.

Clinical Manifestations

1. Localized Dermatasclerosis

The lesion involves only the skin except for some occasional invasion of the muscles beneath the skin, with no internal organs involved, and the prognosis is favourable. The common skin lesion usually takes three forms: macular, linear and spotty.

(1) Macular Dermatasclerosis: This type is the most common. It may occur on any part of the skin, the amount of the lesion varying with different cases, and the shape being non—symmetrical. At the beginning, the skin lesion is in the form of mild desmatous hard maculae, in the colour of pink, with clear edges. Gradually, the lesion expands into round, oval or irregular shapes; the colour of the central part fades away bit by bit, turning into yellowish white and slightly concave, surrounded by a thin narrow margin which is in the colour of violet red; the skin of the affected part is shiny as if it has been waxed. Besides, the muscles beneath it may also be hardened. As the course progresses, there ensue dermatrophia, loss of skin elasticity, telangiectasis, pigmentation mingled with depigmentation, mild desquamation and baldness. Normally, there are no subjective local symptoms, or sensation of tension and discomfort. The course is a protracted one, and may get a natural cure in a few years.

(2) Spotty Dermatasclerosis: This type is comparatively rare.

In most cases it attacks the neck and chest. It is in the form of numerous white or ivorycoloured hardened spots the size of soybeans, which are in clusters, round—shaped and a little concave, surrounded by light purplish aula. The affected skin will incur atrophy as the course progresses. This disease may exist together with localized dermatasclerosis.

(3) Linear Scleroderma and Morpha Linearis: The skin lesion of this type is similar to that of macular dermatasclerosis, but it is arranged in the shape of bands. Mostly, it attacks the face, head, torso, limbs, etc; the lesion is often arranged unilaterally. The lesion on the forehead may extend backward across the scalp and, with the progress of the course, it grows white, concave, atrophic, accompanied by trichomadesis, and the lesion takes on the appearance of chipping—marks. The lesion on the torso is often in the form of a half—ring round the torso. The lesion on a limb is often arranged along the long axis, but occasionally, it may also appear in ring—shaped arrangement.

2. Systemic Scleroderma

Apart from the invasion of the skin, the pathologic process of this disease often involves some internal organs and the prognosis is relatively unfavourable.

(1) Early—stage Symptoms: The onset is far from distinct. The patient may gradually feel listless and fatigued, grow thinner, have loss of appetite and suffer from arthralgia. Arteriospasm on the end of limbs (Raynaud's phenomenon) is often the premonitory symptom of this disease.

(2) Skin lesion: Starting from the free end of limbs or from the face, the lesion gradually spreads out all over the body, often arranged symmetrically. In severe cases, the lesion occurs

systemically even at the beginning. The pathological process consists of three stages: edema, sclerosis and atrophy. During the stage of edema, the skin shows non-concave edema, the cleavage lines disappear, the skin surface is smooth, yellowish, or yellowish-white. During the stage of sclerosis, the edematous part gradually becomes taut and hardened, the surface being smooth and showing a wax-like luster, accompanied by pigmentation, which may possibly be mingled with depigmentation, along with trichomadesis and retardation of perception. During the stage of atrophy, the skin becomes thinner due to atrophy, and the skin accessory organs will shrink and disappear. Other symptoms include trichomadesis, dyshidrosis and the darkening of the pigmentation. The skin lesion becomes hard as leather, and adheres fast to the bones.

(3) During the metaphase and anaphase, manifestations of different kinds appear, varying according to the different parts of the body it attacks: When the face is invaded, it becomes mask-like, accompanied by ochriasis and apathy. There is some difficulty in the movement of mouth and eye-lids. The lips become thinner, the mouth smaller with radial fissures, the teeth exposed, the nose slender and sharp-tipped as if it were whittled. The ears become thinner, too. There are also some other special facial features as well. When it invades the chest, the skin of the affected part is hardened as if it were covered with armour; and there is hypopnea. When it invades the limbs, there is ankylosis, and the movement of the joints is hampered. If the end of a limb is invaded, the finger tips become slender, and the fingers grow hard and stiff and look like the hooked claws of a hawk. Some patients may have ulceration on the tips of the fingers or toes,

which is usually persistent.

(4) Effect on the Internal Organs: The digestive tract is affected, the movement of the tongue is hindered, the esophagus becomes hardened and narrowed, and these are accompanied by dysphagia, nausea, vomiting, abdominal distension, diarrhea or constipation. When the heart is affected, the cardiac musles may become fibred, and there may also be such effects as arrhythmia, cardiectasis and even heart failure. If the lungs are affected, it may result in pulmonary fibrosis, reduction of vital capacity of the lungs, difficulty in breathing and secondary infections. If the kidneys are affected, it may lead to hypertension, proteinuria, and urinaemia.

(5) The course is a protracted one. In those systemic and progressive cases, death often results from cardionephric functional failure, dystrophy, or bronchopneumonia, etc.

(6) Laboratory Examination Discoveries: anemia; blood sedimentation quickened; serum protein increased among some cases; rheumatoid factor positive; antinuclear antibody positive; lupus erythematosus cells found among 7% of the cases; proteinuria, hematuria and cast found among cases with the kidneys affected; and spotty or patchy shadows (shown by X-ray examination) due to extensive calcium salt sediment in the subcutaneous soft tissues and muscles.

Type and Treatment

1. Internal Treatment

(1) Treatment for the Type Blood and *Qi* Stagnation

Symptoms and Signs: This type is found among cases of dermatasclerosis without general symptoms. The main symptoms include skin sclerosis and atrophy, pigmentation or depigmentation. It may be accompanied by acroarteriospasm. The tongue is dark coloured or shows some ecchymosis, the pulse is likely to be uneven.

Therapeutic Method: Promote blood circulation to remove blood stasis

Recipe——*Xiefu Zhuyu Tang* (Formula 108), modified.

Radix Rehmanniae	30 g
Semen Persicae	9 g
Flos Carthami	9 g
Radix Angelicae Sinensis	15 g
Radix Paeoniae Rubra	15 g
Radix Salviae Miltiorrhizae	15 g
Rhizoma Ligustici Chuanxiong	15 g
Rhizoma Sparganii	9 g
Radix Cyathulae	9 g
Caulis Spatholobi	30 g

(2) Treatment for the Type Insufficiency of Both the Spleen and the Kidneys

Symptoms and Signs: This type is found mostly among cases of systemic scleroderma. Among the main symptoms are derma-sclerosis, cacochroia, acrocyanosis, coldness of the body and extremities, lumbago, acratia, baldness, spontaneous perspiration, sexual impotence, spermatorrhea, loss of appetite, abdominal distension, enlarged tongue with teeth marks, and deep thready or slow pulse.

Therapeutic Method: Enhance the spleen and Kidneys, warm up *Yang* and regulate the channels.

Recipe——modified *YangHe Tang* (Formula 109).

Herba Ephedrae	6 g

Rhizoma Rehmanniae Praeparatae	15 g
Colla Cornus Cervi	9 g
Radix Aconiti Praeparata	9 g
Cortex Cinnamomi	9 g
Rhizoma Zingiberis	9 g
Semen Sinapis Albae	9 g
Radix Astragali seu Hedysari	15 g
Radix Clematidis	12 g
Poria	9 g
Caulis Spatholobi	15 g
Radix Glycyrrhizae	6 g

Modifications: For cases of *Qi* deficiency, add Radix Codonopsis Pilosulae 15 g and Rhizoma Polygonati 15 g; for cases of blood deficiency, add Radix Angelicae Sinensis 15 g, Radix Polygoni Multiflori 15 g and Colla Corii Asini 9 g; for those with loose stool, add Semen Plantaginis 15 g (wrapped in a cloth bag to be boiled).

Proprietaries: The following drugs may be used singly or by mixing them together. For cases of insufficiency of both the spleen and kidneys, administer *Jinkui Shenqi Wan* (Formula 105), to be taken twice a day, one or two pills each time; for cases of deficiency of both *Qi* and blood, administer *Shiquan Dabu Wan* (Formula 62), to be taken twice a day, one or two boluses each time; for cases with articular dyskinesia, administer *Xiao Huo luo Wan* (Formula 110), to be taken twice a day, one or two boluses each time, or *Shenj in Pian* (Formula 111), to be taken three times a day, three pills each time; for cases of *Qi* stagnation and blood stasis, administer *Huoxue Quyu Pian* (Formula 101) to be taken three times a day, 5～10 pills each time.

2. External Treatment

(1) Make a proper amount of decoction with the following drugs: Herba Lycopodii 30 g, Caulis Impatientis 30 g, Folium Artemisiae Argyi 15 g, Resina Boswelliae Carterii 6 g and Resina Commiphorae Myrrhae 6 g. Steam and bathe the affected part with this hot decoction twice a day, thirty minutes each time.

(2) Make a mixture of *Huiyang Yulong Gao* (Formula 93) and honey and apply this to the affected part. Then heat the area over a fire for twenty minutes each time, once a day.

10.3 Dermatomyositis

Dermatomyositis is a non-infective, diffuse and inflammatory pathological change in the skin and muscles, belonging to the scope of connective tissue diseases, with the following as its main symptoms: skin swelling, myalgia, acratia, tumefaction, and atrophy. This disease may also involve internal organs and become a generalized disease. So far, there is no exact equivalent term found in TCM classics, but according to its clinical manifestations, it is similar to *jibi* (stagnation-syndrome of *Qi* in the skin and muscles). As recorded in Plain Questions: "The disease, exiting in the skin and muscles and causing them to ache, is termed *jibi*, which results from cold-dampness." This disease is found mostly among females or those above middle age (the proportion of female cases to male cases is 2:1); children who contract this disease are usually below the age of ten years. The pathological process is a chronic one.

Etiology and Pathogenesis

This disease is due to a weak constitution and the failure of the superficial-*Qi* to protect the body against diseases, which allows the invasion of wind—heat or wind—cold—dampness into the skin and muscles. In acute cases, the wind—heat pathogenic factor may, apart from causing stagnation of *Qi* in the skin and muscles, invade *Zang—Fu* organs due to excessive noxious heat; in chronic cases, the disease is mostly due to the stagnation of wind—cold—dampness in the skin and muscles, which may obstruct the channels, cause disharmony between *Ying* and *Wei*, and hamper the circulation of *Qi* and blood. There are also cases due to excessive noxious heat caused by long stagnation of wind—cold—dampness. Whether it be acute or chronic, this disease will deplete and exhaust *Qi* and blood, and cause insuficiency of both *Qi* and blood if the pathological process is protracted.

Clinical Manifestations

Clinically, this disease is classified into two types——acute and chronic. The main symptoms of the acute type are as follows: At first there is general discomfort for a short period (usually a couple of days), later swelling and pain of the limbs occur abruptly, often accompanied by fever, dizziness, acratia, symmetrical pain in the muscles of the limbs, which will be aggravated when the patient exercises or carries something heavy; and there is tenderness as well. Generally speaking, the chronic type is latent. Most of the cases have upper respiratory tract infection at first; but there are also cases caused by exposure to the scotching sun or by catching cold. It is manifested by erythema on the face at the beginning, and later by lassitude, acratia, swelling, myalgia and arteriospasm on the limb—end as well.

1. Symptoms on the Skin

Edematous patches, which are reddish violet, usually appearing first on the face, especially on the eye—lids, known as reddish voliet eye—lids or reddish violet face, are characteristic of this disease. But, edema is a parenchymatous symptom, it does not sink under pressure and may expand to the neck, chest, shoulders, limbs, etc, and may merge into one another. Later, as the disease progresses, the lesion gradually dries up, followed by chaff—like desquamation, or mild skin atrophy and pigmentation, together with spotty depigmentation and telangiectasis. Therefore, it has the manifestions of heterochromous syndrome. It may also have pathological changes similar to those of dermatasclerosis, because there exist non—pitting edema, pachyderma, sclerosis, etc. Hair, especially that on the head, may shed and become sparse, thinner, and dull. Mucosal pathologic changes are also commonly found, such as swelling, erosion, and ulcer, etc.

2. Muscular Symptoms

Muscular symptoms are among the main symptoms of this disease. The affected muscles are usually multiple and symmetrical, but may occasionally be localized. They may occur with skin lesion either simultaneously or otherwise. The two kinds of symptoms may differ in intensity. The muscles near the upper end of limbs are the most vulnerable, other vulnerable parts include scapular regions, the neck, face, throat, etc. There exist the following main muscular symptoms: severe asthenia, tension, spontaneous pain and tenderness which are likely to be intensified by movements. The patient often feels difficulty in sitting down, getting up, climbing up stairs, and walking. A severe case may have to be confined to bed, and may even have difficulty in turning the body. Clinical manifestations vary with muscles of different parts. For instance, when muscles of the neck are affected, the neck will be difficult to keep erect; when muscles of the throat and esophagus are affected, dysphagia will result; when expiratory muscles are affected, it will cause abnormal phonation and dyspneic respiration; when the heart is affected, it is usually manifested by myocarditis and heart failure. In the early stage of the disease, muscles of the affected part show swelling, and decline in muscular power, whereas in the anaphase, atrophy, sclerosis, hindrance to activity, or even flaccidity, may ensue.

3. General Symptoms

Irregular fever, lassitude, asthenia, polyhidrosis, pthologic leanness, anemia, lymphadenectasis, hepatosplenomegaly, arteriospasm on the extremities, and symptoms similar to those of rheumatoid arthritis. About 20% of the patients have malignant tumour as a complicating disease. Reportedly, the rate of dermatomyositis—patients who contract cancer as a complicating disease is as high as 52.2%.

4. Laboratory Examination

The following discoveries are made in lab examination: leukocytosis; blood sedimentation quickened: noticeable increase in the urinal creatine (according to a 24-hour determination); decrease in the output of creatinine; increase in the number of globulins in serum enzyme, especially in creatine phosphokinase, aldolase, lactic dehydrogenase, glutamic oxaloacetic transaminase and glutamic-pyruvic transaminase; pathologic change of myositis shown by myogenic electromyogram and by examining living muscular tissue.

Type and Treatment

1. Internal Treatment

(1) Treatment for the Type Excessive Noxious Heat

Symptoms and Signs: This type is found during the acute active stage. The onset is abrupt, with vivid erythema, diffusion, high fever, hyperhidrosis, dizziness, thirst, bitter taste in the mouth, dry throat, myalgia, asthenia, reddened tongue with yellow thick coating, full and rapid pulse, etc.

Therapeutic Method: Clear away heat and toxic material from the blood, and nourish *Yin*.

Recipe——modified *Qingwen Baidu Ying* (Formula 73).

Radix Rehmanniae	30 g
Cortex Moutan Radicis	9 g
Radix Paeoniae Rubra	15 g
Radix Scutellariae	9 g
Rhizoma Coptidis	6 g
Fructus Capejasmine	9 g
Fructus Forsythiae	9 g
Radix Isatidis	30 g
Gypsum Fibrosum	30 g
Rhizoma Anemarrhenae	9 g
Radix Scrophulariae	15 g
Fructus Arctii	9 g
Radix Glycyrrhizae	6 g

Modifications: For cases with persistent high fever, add Cornu Antelopis 0.3—0.6 g (in powder form, to be added into the boiling decoction of other ingredients); for cases with obvious swelling, add Semen Plantaginis 12 g, to be put in a package for boiling and Rhizoma Alismatis 15 g; for cases with arthralgia and myalgia, add Radix Gentianae Macrophyllae 9 g and Radix Clematidis 9 g.

(2) Treatment for the Stagnated Damp—heat Type

Main Symptoms and Signs: Medium-degree fever or low fever, lassitude, acratia, loss of appetite, abdominal distension, constipation, yellow urine, flush swelling and pain on the skin, yellow and sticky tongue coating, soft and rapid pulse. These are found mostly during acute, subacute and active stages.

Therapeutic Method: Clear away heat and toxic material, promote diuresis to alleviate edema.

Recipe——modified *Yinchen Hao Tang* (Formula 112) plus *Bij ie Chenshi Tang* (Formula 53).

Herba Artemisiae Capillaris	15 g
Capejasmine	9 g
Radix et Rhizoma Rhei	6 g
(to be added later)	
Cortex Phellodendri	9 g
Rhizoma Dioscoreae Septemlobae	9 g
Poria	12 g
Semen Coicis	30 g
Semen Plantaginis	9 g
(contained in a small cloth bag for boiling)	
Rhizoma Alismatis	15 g
Talcum	15 g
Medulla Tetrapanacis	6 g
Cortex Moutan Radicis	9 g
Radix Glycyrrhizae	6 g

Modifications: For cases with loss of appetite, add Fructus Crataegi 15 g and Fructus Aurantii 9 g; for cases with persistent low fever, add Radix Stellariae 9 g and Cortex Lycii Radicis 12 g.

(3) Treatment for the Type Deficiency of *Qi* and Blood

Symptoms and Signs: Dark red skin lesion, pigmentation,

xerosis cutis, desquamation, atrophoderma, derma-sclerosis, lassitude, acratia, lassitude in loin and knees, aversion to cold, spontaneous perspiration and night sweat, sore-throat, xerostomia, abdominal distension, loss of appetite, pale or reddened tongue with thin fur or even without fur, tooth-prints on the edge of the tongue, deep and weak pulse. These symptoms are found mostly during the stationary phase.

Therapeutic Method: Strengthen *Qi* and nourish the blood, promote blood circulation and regulate channels.

Recipe——modified *Shiquan Dabu Wan* (Formula 62).

Radix Astragali seu Hedysari	15 g
Radix Codonopsis Pilosulae	12 g
Rhizoma Atractylodis Macrocephalae	9 g
Poria	12 g
Radix Angelicae Sinensis	15 g
Radix Rehmanniae Praeparata	15 g
Radix Paeoniae Rubra	12 g
Radix Paeoniae Alba	12 g
Caulis Spatholobi	15 g
Radix Salviae Miltiorrhizae	15 g
Radix Clematidis	9 g
Radix Glycyrrhizae	6 g

Modifications: For cases with sore-throat, xerostomia and reddened tongue without fur, add Radix Rehmanniae 15 g, Radix Ophiopogonis 12 g and Herba Dendrobii 12 g; for cases with aversion to cold, cold limbs, arthralgia myalgia and acroarteriosposm, add Ramulus Cinnamomi 9 g, Herba Asari 3 g and Rhizoma Ligustici Chuanxiong 9 g; for cases with spontaneous perspiration and night sweat, add Fructus Tritici Levis 30 g and Fructus Schisandrae 9 g.

Proprietaries: During the Stationary phase, the following proprietaries may be administered: *Renshen jianpi Wan* (Formula 113) or *Shiquan Danbu Wan* (Formula 62) or *Jinkui Shenqi Wan* (Formula 105)——these are to be taken twice a day, one or two boluses each time,; or *Shenjin Pian* (Formula 111) which is taken three times daily, six boluses each time, but in the case of babies the amount should be reduced.

2. External Treatment

Therapies like massage, physiotherapy and acupuncture may be employed as supplement for preventing or reducing muscular atrophy.

3. Other Treatment

Some relevant western medical treatment may be employed depending on the condition of the case during the acute stage.

Nursing and Prevention

1. During the acute stage, the patient should rest in bed with a quiet environment. When the condition becomes alleviated, some activities and movement are necessary.

2. Avoid scorching sunshine and bitter cold.

3. The diet for the patient should be nourishing, digestible and proteinrich.

4. Avoid pregnancy lest the condition should be worsened or relapse.

11 Disease of Cutaneous Appendages

11.1 Acne Vulgaris

This is a disease of the hair follicle sebaceous glands commonly found among young people during their adolessence, mostly on the face, breast and back. In TCM works they are termed *Cuo* (acne) or *Fen Ci* (comedo), etc.

Etiology and Pathogenesis

This disease is caused by heat in the blood and the lung Channel, which affects the face, or by heat accumulated in the spleen and stomach due to uncontrolled diet and too much intake of heavy food, plus noxious wind that has invaded and stagnated in the body.

Clinical Manifestaions

1. Mostly it attacks the adolescents with the male patients outnumbering the female.

2. The skin rash tends to appear on the face, shoulders, breast and back, where sebaceous glands are plentiful.

3. At first, comedo appears, which is, in fact, papular eruptions the size of a needle—end. Those in greyish—white or skin—colour are referred to as white—headed comedo while those with black top are called black—headed comedo. When they are pressed with fingers, cream—white or yellowish—white lipid droplets can be squeezed out. With secondary infection, comedo may turn into red papular eruption the size of a millet grain or a

phaseolus angularis. The top of some of the red papular eruptions may develop small pus-pockets, and some may develop various kinds of lesion such as nodes, abscess, cystis and scar, often accompanied by excessive seborrhea.

4. In most cases, there are no subjective symptoms, but in severe cases, there is an itching sensation of various degrees.

5. The clinical course is slow. The skin rash appears in one place after another. When the stage of adolescence comes to an end, most cases will have a natural cure or become alleviated.

Type and Treatment

Mild cases need no treatment, or, if necessary, only some external treatment. But some severe cases may require internal treatment.

1. Internal Treatment

(1) Treatment for the Type Damp-heat in the Lungs and Stomach

Symptoms and Signs: The face is flush and greasy. The skin rash is mainly in the form of red papular eruption and pus-pockets. It is often accompanied, to varying degrees, by itching and pain. Other possible symptoms include ozostomia, an inclination towards cold drinks, constipation, reddened tongue with yellow or yellow greasy tongue coat, taut and slippery pulse or slippery and rapid pulse.

Therapeutic Method: Remove damp-heat from lungs and stomach; clear away heat and toxic material from the blood.

Recipe——modified *Pipa Qingfei Yin* (Formula 114).

Folium Eriobotryae	9 g
Cortex Mori Radicis	9 g
Radix Scutellariae	9 g

Cortex Phellodendri	9 g
Rhizoma Coptidis	6 g
Fructus Capejasmine	9 g
Radix Rehmanniae	15 g
Cortex Moutan Radicis	9 g
Radix Paeoniae Rubra	15 g
Gypsum Fibrosum	15 g
Herba Artemisiae Capillaris	15 g
Radix Glycyrrhizae	6 g

Modifications: For cases with obvious pus-pockets and with intense toxic-heat, add Flos Lonicerae 30 g, Herba Taraxaci 30 g, Herba Violae 15 g; for cases with constipation, add Radix et Rhizoma Rhei 6 g (to be added after other drugs have been boiled for some time); for cases with obvious seborrhea, add Semen Coicis 30 g, Rhizoma Atractylodis Macrocephalae 12 g and Herba Plantaginis 30 g.

(2) Treatment for the Type Phlegm Stagnancy

Symptoms and Signs: Repeated relapse and persistent course of disease. The skin rash mainly takes the form of node, cystis and scar.

Therapeutic Method: Promote blood circulation by removing blood stasis; remove thick stagnant phlegm to soften lumps.

Recipe——modifed *Haizao Yuhu Tang* (Formula 115).

Radix Angelicae Sinensis	12 g
Rhizoma Ligustici Chuanxiong	12 g
Radix Paeoniae Rubra	15 g
Radix Salviae Miltiorrhizae	15 g
Pericarpium Citri Reticulatae Viride	9 g

Pericarpium Citri Reticulatae	9 g
Rhizoma Pinelliae	9 g
Zhejiang Bulbus Fritillariae	9 g
Thallus Laminariae seu Eckloniae	15 g
Sargassum	15 g
Spica Prunellae	15 g
Fructus Forsythiae	12 g

[margin note: *Thunbergi?*]

Proprietaries: *Fanfen Tongshen Wan* (Formula 54) or *Longdang Xiegan Wan* (Formula 8) for cases of the type damp—heat in lungs and stomach (to be taken 6 g at a time, twice a day); *Sanjie Pian* (Formula 116) for cases of phlegm stagnancy (10 tablets at a time, three times daily).

2. External Treatment

Make a paste by mixing an appropriate amount of *Diandao San* (Formula 19) with decoction of tea and apply the paste to the affected part before going to bed, but wash it clean the next morning.

Nursing and Prevention

1. Wash the face frequently with warm water and soap.
2. Do not press or squeez the affected part.
3. Take less amount of greasy, sweet food, refrain from drinking wine or eating irritating food with a pungent taste; eat more vegetables, fruit and try to keep the digestive canal free from disturbance.

11.2 Brandy Nose

Brandy nose, called distiller—grain nose in TCM, is a chronic skin disease on the nose, the name so gained because is the nose purplish red like distiller's grains. The skin lesion is characterized by skin flush, papular eruptions, pus pockets and telangiectasis. It has been suggested recently that the disease be called trichocryptosis dermatitis because trichocryptosis has been discovered in the skin lesion of brandy nose.

Etiology and Pathogenesis

This disease is due to either blood—heat in the lung channel, too much alcoholic drinking causing pathogenic heat to affect the face, or too much intake of heavy or pungent—tasting food causing accumulated heat in the stomach and intestines to move upward. These factors, plus the intrusion of pathogenic windcold, cause blood stasis, which in turn results in brandy nose.

Clinical Manifestations

1. Most victims of this disease are middle—aged.

2. The skin eruptions are found in the center of the face, mainly on the nose—tip and nose—flanks, but sometimes may also be found on the cheeks and forehead. In some rare cases, it is confined only to the cheeks and forehead while the nose proper remains intact.

3. Three stages may be classified as follows, according to the course of the skin eruption, but there is no obvious distinction between them:

(1) The Stage of Erythema: At first, there appear temporary and paroxysmal erythema in diffusion. It tends to become notable when exposed to cold wind or when the patient has taken irritating food or experienced emotional strain. The erythema may last a long period, accompanied by mild telangiectasis in the shape of twigs. Some will develop into papular eruption and another stage begins.

(2) The Stage of Papular Eruption: A great many comedo-like small papular eruptions are spread over the basis of the erythema, some eruptions may turn into pus-pockets, especially those on the nose-tip. The skin colour changes gradually from bright red to purplish brown. During this stage, there is notable telangiectasis in the shape of a spider web, hence this stage is also called the stage of telangiectasis. It may last several years, and, in some rare cases, even develop into the stage of minophyma.

(3) The Stage of Rhinophyma: Rhinophyma is found among a few patients during the anaphase. It is formed by harmartoplasia in the nose and nodular hypertrophy develope from papular eruption, the surface being rough and uneven.

In most cases, it is accompanied by seborrhea which causes the face to be greasy as if oil has been rubbed on it.

4. The course is a protracted one, usually without notable subjective symptoms but possibly with some mild itching.

Type and Treatment

1. Internal Treatment

(1) Treatment for the Type Damp-heat in the Lungs and Stomach

Symptoms and Signs: During the erythema stage and papular eruption stage, the skin rash mainly takes the form of erythema, papular eruption and telangiectasis, possibly accompanied by itching, inclination for cold drinks, oliguria, dark urine, constipation, reddened tongue with thin yellow fur, slippery and rapid pulse, etc.

Therapeutic Method: Remove heat from the blood, clear away dampness and promote blood circulation.

Recipe——modified *Pipa Qinfei Yin* (Formula 114).

Folium Eriobotryae	9 g
Flos Sophorae	9 g
Cortex Mori Radicis	9 g
Gypsum Fibrosum	30 g
Radix Scutellariae	9 g
Rhizoma Coptidis	6 g
Capejasmine Fruit	9 g
Cortex Moutan Radicis	9 g
Radix Rehmanniae	15 g
Radix Paeoniae Rubra	15 g
Rhizoma Imperatae	30 g
Flos Carthami	9 g

Modifications: For patients with notable pus-pockets, add Herba Taraxaci 30 g and Flos Chrysanthemi Indici 15 g; for those with constipation, add Radix et Rhizoma Rhei 6 g (to be added after other drugs have been boiled for some time).

(2) Treatment for the Type Blood-stasis

Symptoms and Signs: The nose shows dark red or reddish purple, the skin is thickened and sometimes rhinophyma results, the tongue is dark red or with ecchymosis, and the pulse is taut or uneven.

Therapeutic Method: Promote blood circulation to remove blood-stasis.

Recipe——modified *Tongqiao Huoxue Tang* (Formula 100).

Radix Angelicae Sinensis	15 g
Radix Paeoniae Rubra	15 g
Semen Persicae	9 g
Flos Carthami	9 g

Rhizoma Ligustici Chuanxiong	9 g
Faeces Trogopterorum	9 g
Pollen Typhae	9 g
Cortex Mori Radicis	9 g
Pericarpium Citri Reticulatae	9 g
Radix Angelicae Dahuricae	9 g
Bulbus Allii Fistulosi	9 g
Rhizoma Zingiberis Recens	6 g

Proprietaries: For cases with serious blood stasis, administer *Dahuang Zhechong Wan* (Formula 117), to be taken one pill at a time morning and evening.

2. External Treatment

(1) Sulphur Ointment (5–10% sulphur by weight) for external application, twice or three times daily; or *Diandao San* (Formula 19) to be mixed with water into a thin paste for application before sleep, but it is to be removed by washing the following morning.

(2) Make a mixture of Semen Hydnocapi, Hydrargyrum and Semen Juglandis (each weighing 6 g) by first grinding the Semen Hydnocapi and Semen Juglandis into a soft mass, then mixing the mass with Hydnocapi, and beating the mixture until the Hydnocapi can no longer be seen; wrap the mixture in gauze and then rub it over the affected part until there is a sensation of warmth. This application is done 4 or 5 times daily.

Nursing and Preventions

1. Take no heavy or irritating foods such as wine and pepper. Also, take care to avoid constipation.

2. Prevent the face from being irritated by hot or cold factors.

3. Refrain from being hot—tempered and maintain a stable mood.

11.3 Seborrhea and Seborrheic Dermatitis

Seborrhea is a common skin disease characterized by hypersteatosis while seborrheic dermatitis is a chronic dermatitis developed from seborrhea. Secondary eczematoid pathogenic change is termed seborrheic eczema. In some TCM works, *Baixie Feng* and *Mianyou Feng* are terms used respectively of cases with skin lesion on the head and those with lesion on the face. They are found mostly among the young and middle—aged though they may also be found among the new—born.

Etiology and Pathogenensis

In the case of dry skin lesion, the disease is caused by the accumulation and stagnation of pathogenic factors of wind dryness and heat which impair blood, resulting in malnutrition of the skin; in the case of moist skin lesion, it is caused by too much intake of heavy, pungent—tasting food or wine, which gives rise to the accumulation of damp—heat in the intestines and stomach. This, plus the invasion of pathogenic wind, results in the stagnancy of *Qi* in the skin and muscles.

Clinical Manifestations

1. Seborrhea

(1) Seborrhea among the Young and the Middle—aged: It occurs mainly on those parts of the body with plenty of sebaceous glands, like the scalp, the face, etc. Clinically, it is classified into seborrhea oleosa and seborrhea sicca. In the case of seborrhea oleosa, there are the following manifestations: hypersteatosis, greasy shining hair, scalp, and face (especially the nose), visible

expansion of follicular orifice, yellowish white lipid emboli that can easily be squeezed out; in the case of seborrhea sicca, the manifestations are as follows: the whole scalp is covered with tiny greyish white scales, which shed easily (as with combing or scratching), but are soon produced again. In time, the hair usually grows thinner, softer, and sheds, which is termed seborrheic baldness.

(2) Seborrhea among the New-born: It is found mostly among those infants who have had excellent nourishment yet too much intake of fat. On their scalp, a thick yellow crust can be found. There is flush on the cheeks, which are covered with greasy scales.

2. Seborrheic dermatitis

(1) It is liable to occur on those parts of the body with plenty of sebaceous glands, such as the scalp, face, external ears, fossa axillaris, breast and back, often starting from the head and then spreading downward and, in severe cases, all over the body.

(2) The skin rash is in the form of yellowish red or pink papulae of varying sizes and uneven edges. Clinically, it is classified into scale type and scab type. In the case of the scale type, the skin rash takes the form of patches covered with greasy scales, while in the case of scab type, a thick yellow scab is formed from the greasy scales mixed with exudation. The latter type is found mostly among infants.

(3) The manifestations vary with different affected parts of the body: On the head, the lesion mainly takes the form of red papulae with an uneven edge, greasy scales and scab; besides, erosion and exudation may result from scratching. On the face, the most frequently affected parts are wings of the nose, nasolabial

and superciliary arch, with the lesion in the form of light erythema covered with greasy scales; On the ears, the lesion is in the form of erosion, yellow scab or rhagas; On the torso, the most frequently affected part is the skin between the breast and scapula, the lesion being in the form of reddish yellow or pink patches in a round or oval shape and covered with greasy scales. While a few patches may appear separately, most patches are mingled with each other, or tend to have a healed center, hence forming shapes of a ring or multi—ring, like the eruption of pityriasis rosea; on rugose areas such as the groin inguen, axilliary fossa, fissure between buttocks, scrotum and the area under a female's breast, the lesion is usually in the form of reddish yellow scaly patches, often with eczemotid erosion.

(4) The course is a protracted one, often accompanied by various degrees of itching. After a long time, the patient's skin becomes thick and moist, taking on the pathologic change of chronic dermatitis.

Type and Treatment

1. Internal Treatment

(1) Treatment for the Damp—heat Type

Symptoms and Signs: The skin rash shows flushed, and is covered with greasy scales or erosion, exduation and scab. There is a sensation of itching, possibly accompanied by a choking sensation in the chest, bitter taste and a loss of appetite. The tongue shows reddened, with a greasy yellow coating, and the pulse is rapid and slippery.

Therapeutic Method: Clear away heat and remove dampness, remove pathogenic wind to stop itching.

Recipe: modified *Longdan Xiegan Tang* (Formula 8).

Radix Gentianae	9 g
Radix Scutellariae	9 g
Cortex Phellodendri	9 g
Fructus Capejasmine	9 g
Radix Sophorae Flavescentis	9 g
Cortex Dictamni Radicis	15 g
Fructus Kochiae	15 g
Radix Bupleuri	9 g
Cortex Magnoliae Officinalis	9 g
Semen Plantaginis	9 g
Herba Artemisiae Capillaris	15 g
Rhizoma Alismatis	12 g
Caulis Aristalachiae Manshuriensis	6 g

(2) Treatment for the Wind—dryness Type

Symptoms and Signs: Dry scales, mild inflammation, or rough, dry and thick skin, considerable itching, or possibly trichoxerosis and trichomadesis; reddened tongue with scanty fur, and taut pulse.

Therapeutic Method: Nourish the blood to expel wind and moisten dryness.

Recipe: modified *Danggui Yinzi* (Formula 4).

Radix Angelicae Sinensis	15 g
Radix Rehmanniae	30 g
Radix Polygoni Multiflori	30 g
Rhizoma Ligustici Chuanxiong	9 g
Radix Paeoniae Rubra	9 g
Radix Paeoniae Alba	9 g
Cortex Moutan Radicis	9 g
Radix Scrophulariae	15 g

Radix Ophiopogonis	15 g
Fructus Tribuli	15 g
Radix Ledebouriellae	9 g
Cacumen Biotae	9 g

2. External Treatment

(1) Make a decoction by boiling the *Zhaoshi Xiyao* (Formula 59), with which to wash the affected part; or dissolve the *Xiaofan xiyao* (Formula 16) in hot water and then wash the affected part with it once or twice a day, 20 to 30 minutes each time.

(2) For cases with erosion and exudation, make a decoction by boiling the *Zhaoshi Xiyao* (Formula 59) and then cool it down for wet dressing; during the interval of wet dressing, mix *Huangbai San* (Formula 17), with sesame and then apply the paste-like mixture onto the affected part.

(3) For cases with erythema in the main but without erosion or exudation, use for external application sulphur ointment (5 to 10% sulphur by weight) or *Diandaosan* lotion which is a mixture of *Sulfur* 7.5 g, Radix et Rhizoma Rhei 7.5 g and lime water (100 ml); the application is done twice or three times a day.

11.4 Alopecia Areata

Alopecia Areata is a disease of cutaneous appendages, characterized by abrupt patch-like trichomadesis on the head with no inflammation or subjective symptoms on the affected part. It is termed *Youfeng* in TCM works.

Etiology and Pathogenesis

This disease is often caused by deficiency of blood, which fails to cooperate with *Qi* in nourishing the skin. The striae of skin and muscles in turn become loose, and the opening of the sweat glands is loose, hence, pathogenic wind intrudes from outside, causing blood—dryness and malnutrition of the hair. Besides, the mood of depression, stagnation of the liver—Qi, and overwork may impair the heart—Qi and cause stagnation of Qi and blood—stasis so that Qi and blood cannot nourish the hair, hence the occurence of the disease; deficiency of the liver—Qi and kidney—Qi may also cause this disease, because the liver stores the blood whose state can be manifested by the hair while the kidneys produce bone marrow which is also responsible for the growth of hair.

Clinical Manifestations

1. This disease may attack people of any age group although most of the patients are the young and middle—aged.

2. It often results from overwork, insufficiency of sleep or from mental irritation.

3. The onset is abrupt; it is often by chance that the patch—like trichomadesis is discovered either by the patient himself or by other people. The trichomadesis area is shaped round, oval, or irregular, the size ranging from a finger—nail to a coin or even bigger, and the number varying between one and several. The surface is smooth, slightly shining and with a clear edge. The alopecia—areata—affected spot may stay unchanged for a long time, but may also expand gradually.

4. A severe case may have the whole head involved so that most of the hair or even all the hair on the head may be lost, which is called complete alopecia. If it is hair all over the body, including eye—brow, eyelash, beard, axillary hair, pubisure and fine hair, it is termed general trichomadesis.

5. The affected part usually shows no subjective symptoms.

6. The course is a protracted one. It may gradually have a natural cure but may have relapses.

Type and Treatment

1. Internal Treatment

(1) Treatment for the Blood-deficiency and Wind-dryness Type

Symptoms and Signs: Apart from trichomadesis, there also exist dizziness, light-headedness, restlessness, insomnia, too much dreaming, pale tongue-fur and thready pulse.

Therapeutic Method: Nourish the blood to expel wind

Recipe——Modified *Shenying Yangzheng Dan* (Formula 12).

Radix Angelicae Sinensis	15 g
Radix Paeoniae Alba	12 g
Radix Rehmanniae Praeparatae	15 g
Radix Polygoni Multiflori	30 g
Rhizoma Ligustici Chuanxiong	9 g
Flos Carthami	9 g
Fructus Ligustri Lucidi	12 g
Semen Cuscutae	12 g
Rhizoma seu Radix Notoptergii	9 g
Rhizoma Gastrodiae	6 g

Modification: For cases with insomnia and too much dreaming, add Semen Ziziphi Spinosae 15 g, Poria cum Ligno Hospite 9 g and Radix Polygalae 9 g; for those already having contracted the disease for a long time, or with such symptoms as general trichomadesis or complete alopecia, lassitude in loin and knees, tinnitus, blurring of vission, seminal emission with night sweat, pale tongue with scanty fur, and weak thready pulse, add Fructus Lycii 15 g, Fructus Mori 15 g and Herba Ecliptae 15 g.

Proprietaries: *Yangxue Shengfa Pian* (Formula 118), to be taken 10 tablets each time, 3 times daily; or *Qibao Meiran Dan* (Formula 119), to be taken one bolus each time, 3 times a day.

(2) Treatment for the Type *Qi*-Stagnation and Blood-stasis

Symptoms and Signs: Persistent alopecia defying treatment, dim blackish complexion, and possibly, headache, chest pain, and hypochondria pain; dark-red tongue or tongue with petechia, uneven or taut thready pulse. The affected part may have a record of external injury with hematoma.

Therapeutic Method: Activate blood flow to remove blood stasis.

Recipe: modified *Tongqiao Huoxue Tang* (Formula 100).

Radix Angelicae Sinensis	9 g
Radix Paeoniae Rubra	9 g
Rhizoma Ligustici Chuanxiong	9 g
Semen Persicae	9 g
Flos Carthami	9 g
Rhizoma Sparganii	9 g
Rhizoma Zedoariae	9 g
Radix Bupleuri	9 g
Radix Curcumae	9 g
Rhizoma Curcumae Longae	9 g
Rhizoma Zingiberis Recens	6 g
Bulbus Allii Fistulosi	9 g

Proprietaries: Huoxue Quyu Pian (Formula 101), 5 to 10 pills each time, 3 times daily.

2. External Treatment

1) *Bugu Zhiding* (Tincture of Fructus Psoraleae) for external application, 3 times a day.

2) Rub the affected part rapidly with the cross-section of a ginger-root.

3) Beat appropriately the affected part with plum-blossom hammer, twice a day.

11.5 Tragomaschalia

Tragomaschalia is a skin disease characterized by fox-like smell of the sweat in the arm pits, known popularly as fox-smell, in TCM-works, it is also termed axilla smell or body smell, based on its characteristics. For instance, *the Encyclopedia of Surgery* (compiled in the Qing Dynasty) states in the chapter *Axilla Smell*: "Axilla smell, commonly known as fox-smell, is inherited from birth. There are pores in the armpits from which foul smell comes. Almost no drugs can cure it completely."

Etiology and Pathogenesis

This disease is inherited from birth in most cases, though the accumulation of damp-heat may also cause foul smell to flow out from the pores. Modern medicine holds that the foul smell of tragomaschalia results from the decomposition of large sweat gland secretion by germs.

Clinical Manifestations

1. This disease is mostly found among the young people, especially among young females. There may be persons with the same disease among his or her relatives.

2. In most cases, it is found in the armpit, but in severe cases, it may also be found on the areola mammae, navel, external genitalia, anus and groins, where there are large sweat glands.

3. The armpits have some strip-like pores which produce sweat profusely with some foul smell. Since the sweat is yellow, it

soils one's underwear easily, especially in summer when sweating is frequent. A mild case may almost have no foul smell at all when there's no sweating. This disease starts in adolescence and gradually abates or disappears during senility.

Type and Treatment

Usually it requires no internal treatment; but if there are quite a few diseased parts, and if the sweat is sticky greasy, yellow, with strong foul smell or accompanied by abdominal distension, loss of appetite, loose stool, scanty dark urine, yellow greasy tongue-coating, slippery and rapid pulse, it is due to the accumulation of damp-heat inside, causing foul smell to be expelled. In this case, internal treatment as a supplement is also advisable.

Therapeutic Method: Clear away heat and remove dampness by means of aromatics.

Recipe——modified *Ganlu Xiaodu Yin* (Formula 120).

Herba Agastachis	9 g
Herba Menthae	9 g
Semen Amomi Cardamomi	9 g
Rhizoma Acori Graminei	12 g
Radix Scutellariae	9 g
Fructus Forsythiae	9 g
Rhizoma Smilacis Glabrae	15 g
Herba Artemisiae Capillaris	15 g
Rhizoma Atractylodis	9 g
Talcum	1.5g
Caulis Aristolochiae Manshuriensis	6 g
Rhizoma Alismatis	9 g

(To be boiled into a decoction before taking it.)

2. External Treatment

(1) Rubbing the diseased part with *Mituo Sengsan* (Formula 107) or with Powder of Alumen Exsiccatum, several times a day.

(2) Grinding into a powder—mixture the three drugs: Alumen Exsiccatum 30 g, powder of Mactra quadrangularis Deshayes 15 g and Camphora 15 g, to be rubbed over the diseased part twice a day, morning and evening.

Nursing and Prevention

1. Keep the diseased part clean and dry, take frequent baths, change clothes regularly, wash the diseased part frequently with scented soap and warm water.

2. Watch one's diet and avoid food with a pungent taste, it is advisable to give up the habit of smoking and alcoholic drinking.

12 Pigmentary Dermatoses

12.1 Vitiligo

Vitiligo is a kind of dematosis characterized by the appearance of white patches which give no subjective symptoms but on which the hair may turn white. In TCM-works, it is known as Baidian or Baibo Feng. For instance, the *General Treatise on the Causes and Symptoms of Diseases* records in the chapter *Symptoms of Baidian*:"The skin of the affected part is white, different from that of flesh, with no itching or pain. This is due to the invasion of the skin by pathogenic wind causing the disharmony between Qi and blood."

Etiology and Pathogenesis

This disease is caused by depressed emotions and results in the stagnation of liver—Qi and the disturbance of visceral functions, or by disharmony between the Qi and blood due to deficiency of kideny—Yin and the invasion of pathogenic wind into the skin. This results in the disharmony between Qi and blood or the stagnation of Qi and blood, which fails to nourish the skin.

Clinical Manifestations

1. It may attack people of any age, though in most cases it attacks young adults.

2. It may occur on any part of the body, but mostly it attacks such local areas as the face, neck, and dorsum of the hand, etc. The patches may be arranged in a symmetrical manner or just unilaterally; sometimes, they are distributed segmentally or in a

band-shaped manner.

3. The skin lesion takes the form of round, oval or irregular white patches with clear boundaries and in different sizes. The pigment around the patch is usually quite dark, the surface of the patch feels smooth, the hair within it may turn white or remain normal. The number of patches varies with different cases from single to a multitude, and they may also become merged into a large area.

4. Usually there are no subjective symptoms, though a few cases may give a sensation of itching during the course. When the affected part has been exposed to the sun for some time, it will turn red and give a sensation of burning heat and itching.

5. The development of the skin rash may sometimes be very quick, but there are also times when the condition stays unchanged for a long time and the course is a protracted one. A few patients, especially in the case of children, may have a natural cure.

Type and Treatment

1. Internal Treatment

Therapeutic Method: Expel pathogenic wind, nourish the blood, promote blood circulation and strengthen the kidney.

Recipe——modified *Baibo Pian* (Formula 121).

Radix Ledebouriellae	9 g
Fructus Tribuli	30 g
Herba Spirodelae	15 g
Rhizoma Ligustici Chuanxiong	9 g
Radix Paeoniae Rubra	9 g
Flos Carthami	9 g
Radix Angelicae Sinensis	9 g

Caulis Spatholobi	15 g
Fructus Psoraleae	9 g
Husk of Glycine Max	15 g
Pericarpium Citri Reticulatae	9 g

(To be boiled in water into a decoction)

Proprietaries: *Baibo Pian* (Formula 121) or *Xixian Wan* (Formula 122), to be taken one or two pills at a time, twice a day; *Fufang Jili Pian* (Formula 123), to be taken ten pills at a time, three times a day.

2. External Treatment

(1) Make a mixture of *Mituoseng San* (Formula 107) and a proper amount of vinegar to be applied to the affected part, three times a day.

(2) Apply *Buguzhi Ding* (Tincture of 25% Fructus Psoraleae by weight) to the affected part, three times a day.

12.2 Chloasma

Chloasma is a skin disease characterized by facial pigment hyperplasia, commonly known as butterfly spot. In some TCM—works it is named facial dust or dark patch.

Etiology and Pathogenesis

Anxiety and depression cause stagnation of liver—Qi and, consequently, blood stasis on the face; or it is due to improper diet causing damp—heat in the spleen and stomach which in turn affects the face; or due to deficiency of kidney—Yin causing flaring—up of fire of the deficiency type to stagnate in the skin, and hence the disease.

Clinical Manifestations

1. Mostly, it attacks married women, though a few men and

virgin girls may also be the victims. Some cases may have a secondary disease resulting from hepatic diseases, tuberculosis, or other chronic diseases.

2. The skin lesion is usually found on the face, neck, nose or around the mouth, often in symmetrical patterns.

3. The skin lesion shows yellowish brown or dark brown, with the boundary being either clear or indistinct. The patches vary in size; sometimes they merge into each other, forming a larger patch, the surface of the patches is smooth. Too much exposure to sun—light may aggravate the case. This is why the colour of the patch is darkened in spring and summer.

4. The course of the disease is a protracted one, with no subjective local symptoms; a few may have a natural cure.

Type and Treatment

1. Internal Treatment

(1) Treatment for the Type of Liver—*Qi* Stagnation and Blood Stasis

Symptoms and Signs: This disease is mostly found among climacteric women, or women who suffer from hepatic diseases or diseases of the reproductive system. Apart from symmetrical brown patches on the face, other symptoms include irritability, melancholy, fullness in the chest and hypochondrium, menstrual disorder, thin and pale tongue coating, possible patches of blood stasis on the tongue, and taut pulse.

Therapeutic Method: Soothe the liver and regulate the circulation of *Qi*, promote blood circulation by removing blood stasis.

Recipe——modified *Xiaoyao San* (Formula 124).

Radix Bupleuri	12 g
Radix Angelicae Sinensis	12 g

Radix Paeoniae Rubra	9 g
Radix Paeoniae Alba	9 g
Rhizoma Atractylodis Macrocephalae	9 g
Poria	9 g
Pericarpium Citri Reticulatae Viride	9 g
Pericarpium Citri Reticulatae	9 g
Rhizoma Cyperi	9 g
Radix Salviae Miltiorrhizae	15 g
Flos Carthami	9 g
Herba Menthae	6 g

(To be boiled into a decoction)

Proprietary: *Xiaoyao Wan* (Formula 124) 6 g a time, twice a day.

(2) Treatment for the Type Damp-heat in the Sleen and Stomach

Symptoms and Signs: The patch is Yellowish brown and distinct. Other symptoms include loss of appetite, abdominal distension, thirst, ozostomia, loose stool, scanty dark urine, yellow greasy tongue coating and slippery rapid pulse.

Therapeutic Method: Clear away heat and eliminate dampness.

Recipe——modified *Qingj i Shenshi Tang* (Formula 125).

Rhizoma Atractylodis	9 g
Rhizoma Atractylodis Macrocephalae	9 g
Cortex Magnoliae Officinalis	9 g
Pericarpium Citri Reticulatae	9 g
Radix Bupleuri	9 g
Caulis Akebiae	6 g
Rhizoma Alismatis	9 g

Radix Angelicae Dahuricae	9 g
Rhizoma Cimicifugae	9 g
Capejasmine Fruit	9 g
Rhizoma Coptidis	6 g
Radix Scutellariae	9 g

(To be boiled into a decoction)

Modification: For cases with constipation add Radix et Rhizoma Rhei 6 g, (to be added after other drugs have been boiled for some time).

Proprietary: *Sanhuang Wan* (Formula 126), to be taken 4.5 g at a time, twice a day.

(3) Treatment for Fire Flaring-up of the Deficiency Type

Symptoms and Signs: The patch is yellow and vague. Possibly, the patient also suffers from tuberculosis or other chronic diseases. Other symptoms may include low fever, night sweat, dysphoria with feverish sensation in chest, palms and soles, lassitude in loin and legs, insomnia, excessive dreaming, reddened tongue with yellow coating, and thready and rapid pulse.

Therapeutic Method: Nourish *Yin* to reduce pathogenic fire

Recipe——Modified *Zhibai Dihuang Tang* (Formula 70).

Radix Rehmanniae	15 g
Radix Rehmanniae Praeparata	15 g
Radix Scrophulariae	15 g
Cortex Moutan Radicis	9 g
Cortex Lycii Radicis	9 g
Radix Paeoniae Rubra	15 g
Rhizoma Dioscoreae	15 g
Fructus Corni	12 g
Rhizoma Alismatis	9 g

    Poria   9 g
    Cortex Phellodendri   9 g
    Rhizoma Anemarrhenae   9 g

Proprietaries: *Liuwei Dihuang Wan* (Formula 79) or *Zhi Bai Dihuang Wan*, to be taken one or two pills at a time, twice a day.

2. Exteranl Treatment

(1) Grind into powder the following drugs: Rhizoma Typhonii, Radix Angelicae Dahuricae and Talcum (250 g of each), and apply the powder onto the affected part after washing the face, twice a day, morning and evening.

(2) Pick some green tender persimon leaves and dry them by sunning before grinding them into powder. Mix 30 g of the powder with 30 g of vaseline into an ointment and apply it onto the affected part before going to bed at night but wash it clean the following morning.

12.3 Freckle

It is commonly known as sparrow spot, owing to the fact that the face is dotted with spots the size of a sesame seed, and coloured like a sparrow's egg. It is also known as summer spot. The face, neck and dorsum manus are the places it is most likely to attack. The usual colour of the spot is yellowish brown or dark brown. This disease has a genetic predisposition.

Etiology and Pathogensis

Freckles are due to an inherent defect, the failure of kidney—*Yin* to nourish the face, the accumulation of fire, or the combination of pathogenic wind and fire, resulting from the stagnation of fire in channels and vessels and the invasion of wind pathogen.

Clinical Manifestations

1. Freckles are found among people of both sexes, with females being the majority. They usually start from childhood, increase in number during adolesence and stop further development when the affected person has grown into an adult.

2. The face, neck, and dorsum manus are the places where freckles are most likely to be found, though they may also be found on the chest and the anterior portion of the limbs, usually existing in symmetry.

3. The size of freckles ranges from a millet grain to a sesame seed coloured brown or dark brown, with distinct boundary. They are non-prominent, dispersed either densely or sparsely, and never mingled together. In summer, the number grows and the colour darkens after exposure to the sun, whereas in winter, the number diminishes and the colour pales.

4. There are no subjective symptoms.

Type and Treatment

1. Internal Treatment

Therapeutic Method: Nourish *Yin* to reduce pathogenic fire.

Recipe——Modified *Zhi Bai Dihuang Tang* (Formula 70).

Radix Rehmanniae	150 g
Radix Rehmanniae Praeparata	150g
Fructus Corni	60 g
Cortex Moutan Radicis	50 g
Rhizoma Alismatis	50 g
Poria	60 g
Rhizoma Dioscoreae	90 g
Radix Scrophulariae	90 g
Radix Ampelopsis	60 g

Rhizoma Typhonii　　　　　　　　　　40 g

(To be mixed with honey into boluses, each weighing 10 g, taken twice a day, morning and evening)

Proprietariess: *Liuwei Dihuang Wan* (Formula 79) or *Zhi Bai Dihuang Wan* (Formula 70), to be taken twice a day, one or two pills at a time.

2. External Treatment

(1) Grind into fine powder 30 g of Semen Pharbitidis, make a paste by mixing a little amount of the powder with egg white, and apply the paste to the affected part before going to bed, but wash it clean with warm water the following morning and this should be continued for five to seven weeks.

(2) Make a paste by mixing *Shizhen Zhengrong San* (Formula 127) and water, apply the paste to the affected part before going to bed and wash it clean the following morning.

Nursing and Prevention

Avoid strong sunlight in spring and summer, wear hats with a broad rim in out-door activities.

附

Formula Index

方 剂 索 引

Angong Ninhuang Wan 安宫牛黄丸(36) 49,101,148,336
(Bezoar Bolus for Resurrection). 364,387
    Source: Treatise on Differentiation and Treatment of Epidemic Febrile Diseases 《温病条辨》
Composition:

Calculus Bovis	牛黄	(*Niuhuang*)
Radix Curcumae	郁金	(*YuJin*)
Cornu Rhinocerotis	犀角	(*XiJiao*)
Rhizoma Coptidis	黄连	(*Huanglian*)
Cinnabaris	朱砂	(*Zhusha*)
Fructus Capejasmine	栀子	(*Zhizi*)
Realgar	雄黄	(*Xionghuang*)
Radix Scutellariae	黄芩	(*Huangqin*)
Margarita	珍珠	(*Zhenzhu*)
Borneolum	冰片	(*Bingpian*)
gold foil	金箔	(*Jinbo*)
Moschus	麝香	(*Shexiang*)

    Administration: Take one pill each time, once to three times daily.
    Actions: Clearing away heat and toxic material; inducing re-

suscitation and tranquilization.

Uses: Erysipelas, allergic drug rash, lupus erythematosus, etc. which are caused by invasion of heat into the blood. marked by coma, delirium and rest lessness.

用法：每服1丸，日1～3次。
功用：清热解毒，宣窍安神。
主治：丹毒、药疹、红斑性狼疮等热入营血出现神昏谵语、烦躁不宁者。

Baibo Pian　白驳片(121)　　　　　　　187,188,407
(*Baibo* Bolus)

Source: a practical proved recipe (经验方)
Composition:

Radix Arnebiae seu Lithospermi 紫草　(*Zicao*)
Lignum Dalbergiae Odoriferae 降香　(*Jiangxiang*)
Paris Polyphylla Smith 草河车(*Caoheche*)
Radix Stephaniae Cepharanthae 白药子(*Baiyaozi*)
Rhizoma Typhonii 白附子(*Baifuzi*)
Rhizoma Atractylodis 苍术　(*Cangzhu*)
Os Sepiella seu Sepiae 海螵蛸(*Haipiaoxiao*)
Radix Polygoni Multiflori 生首乌(*Shengshouwu*)
Radix Gentianae 龙胆草(*Longdancao*)
Flos Carthami 红花　(*Honghua*)
Semen Persicae 桃仁　(*Taoren*)
Fructus Tribuli 刺蒺藜(*Chijili*)
Radix Glycyrrhizae 甘草　(*Gancao*)

Manufacture: Grind the drugs together into fine powder to make boluses, each bolus weighing 0.5g.

Administration: 10 tablets each time, twice daily.

Actions: Clearing away heat; expelling wind and activating blood flow.

Uses: Vitiligo.

制法:共为细末,制成片, 每片重 0.5 克。

用法:每服 10 片, 每日 2 次。

功用:清热散风活血。

主治:白癜风。

Baixianpi Yin 白鲜皮饮(80)   112,117,130,370
(Decoction of Cortex Dictamni Radicis)   372,379

Source: a prescription of the Affiliated Hospital of Shandong TCM College (山东中医学院附属医院方)

Composition:

Cortex Dictamni Radicis 15 g	白藓皮 (*Baixianpi*)
Radix Rehmanniae 15 g	生地 (*Shengdi*)
Radix Paeoniae Rubra 15 g	赤芍 (*Chishao*)
Radix Salviae Miltiorrhizae 15 g	丹参 (*Danshen*)
Radix Scutellariae 15 g	黄芩 (*Huangqin*)
Periostracum Cicade 9 g	蝉蜕 (*Chantui*)
Radix Angelicae Sinensis 12 g	当归 (*Danggui*)
Rhizoma Atractylodis 9 g	苍术 (*Cangzhu*)
Herba Schizonepetae 9 g	荆芥 (*Jinjie*)
Radix Ledebouriellae 9 g	防风 (*Fangfeng*)
Flos Lonicerae 15 g	金银花 (*Jinyinhua*)
Radix Arnebiae seu Lithospermi 9 g	紫草 (*Zicao*)

Actions: Nourishing the blood, promoting blood circulation, dispelling wind and arresting itching.

Uses: Urticaria, neurodermatitis, pityriasis rosea, seborrheic dermatitis, etc.

功用:养血活血，祛风止痒。

主治:荨麻疹、神经性皮炎、玫瑰糠疹、脂溢性皮炎等疾病。

Bishu Gao 必舒膏(39)   65,345
(Bishu Ointment)

Source: a prescription of Shanghai Ninth Pharmaceutical Factory （上海第九制药厂方）

Composition:

Camphor	樟脑	(Zhangnao)
Herba Menthae 5 g	薄荷脑	(Bohenao)
Ilex Pedunculosa oil 5 ml	冬青油	(Dongqingyou)
Ointment base 85 g	软膏基质	(Ruangao Jizhi)

Manufacture: Mix the above drugs thoroughly.

Administration: External application.

Actions: Destroy parasites, subdue swelling, relieve itching.

Uses: Insect dermatitis, papular urticaria, neurodermatitis. pruritus, and so on.

制法:上药混和搅匀备用。

用法:外涂患处。

功用:杀虫，消肿，止痒。

主治:虫咬皮炎、丘疹性荨麻疹、神经性皮炎、瘙痒症等。

Bixie Shenshi Tang 萆薢渗湿汤(53)   52,76,122,164
(Decoction of Rhizoma Dioscoreae   338,352,375,394
Septemlobae)

Source: Clinical Experience in External Medicine 《疡科心

得集》

Composition:

Rhizoma Dioscoreae Septemlobae 9 g	萆薢 (*Bijie*)
Semen Coicis 15 g	苡仁 (*Yiren*)
Cortex Phellodendri 12 g	黄柏 (*Huangbai*)
Poria 12 g	茯苓 (*Fuling*)
Cortex Moutan Radicis 12 g	丹皮 (*Danpi*)
Rhizoma Alismatis 9 g	泽泻 (*Zexie*)
Talcum 9 g	滑石 (*Huashi*)
Tetrapanacis 6 g	通草 (*Tongcao*)

Actions: Clearing away heat and promoting diuresis.

Uses: Erysipelas on the lower limbs, eczema, allergic drug rash and secondary pyogenic infection from HongKong foot.

功用:清利湿热。

主治:用于下肢丹毒、湿疹、药疹及足癣继发化脓性感染等。

Chaihu Shugan Tang 柴胡疏肝汤(33)　　34,146,329,386
(Radix Bupleuri Decoction for Dispersing the Depressed Liver)

Source: Complete Works by Zhang Jingyue 《景岳全书》

Composition:

Radix Bupleuri 9 g	柴胡 (*Chaihu*)
Fructus Aurantii 9 g	枳壳 (*Jike*)
Radix paeoniae Alba 15 g	白芍 (*Baishao*)
Rhizoma Cyperi 9 g	香附 (*Xiangfu*)
Rhizoma Ligustici Chuanxiong 9 g	川芎 (*Chuanxiong*)
Pericarpium Citri Reticulatae Viride 9 g	青皮 (*Qingpi*)
Radix Glycyrrhizae 6 g	甘草 (*Gancao*)

Actions: Soothing the liver; regulating the circulation of Qi as well as the function of the liver and stomach.

Indications: chronic lupus erythematosus discoides, sequelae of herpes zoster, leukoplakia, etc.

功用:疏肝理气，调和肝脾。

主治:慢性盘状红斑狼疮、带状疱疹后遗痛、粘膜白斑等。

Dahuang Zhechong Wan 大黄䗪虫丸(117)   174,399
(Bolus of Radix et Rhizoma Rhei and Eupolyphagaseu Steleophaga)

Source: Synopsis of Prescriptions of Golden Chamber 《金匮要略》

Composition:

Radix et Rhizoma Rhei	大黄(*Dahuang*)
Eupolyphagaseu Steleophaga	䗪虫(*Zhechong*)
Radix Paeoniae Alba	芍药(*Shaoyao*)
dried gum of Rhus Verniciflua Stokes	干漆(*Ganqi*)
Radix Rehmanniae	生地(*Shengdi*)
Radix Scutellariae	黄芩(*Huangqin*)
Semen Persicae	桃仁(*Taoren*)
Semen Armeniacae Amarum	杏仁(*Xingren*)
Tabanus	虻虫(*Manchong*)
Hirudo	水蛭(*Shuizhi*)
Holotrichia Diomphalia	蛴螬(*Qicao*)
Radix Glycyrrhizae	甘草(*Gancao*)

Manufacture: Grind the drugs into fine powder and make boluses by mixing the powder with honey, each bolus weighing 3 g.

Administration: 1 pill each time, three times daily.

Actions: Promoting blood circulation and removing blood stasis; subduing swelling and softening hard masses.

Uses: Keloid, prurigo nodularis, dermatasclerosis, acne, rosacea, and so on.

制法:上药共末,炼蜜为丸,每丸重3克。

用法:每次1丸,日服3次。

功用:活血破瘀,消肿软坚。

主治:瘢痕疙瘩、结节性痒疹、硬皮病、痤疮、酒渣鼻等。

Danggui Sini Tang 当归四逆汤(43) 68,123,127,346
(Chinese Angelica Decoction for Restoring *Yang*) 375,377

Source: Treatise on Febrile Diseases 《伤寒论》

Composition:

Radix Angelicae Sinensis 12 g	当归	(*Danggui*)
Radix Paeoniae Alba 15 g	白芍	(*Baishao*)
Ramulus Cinnamoni 9 g	桂枝	(*Guizhi*)
Herba Asari 3 g	细辛	(*Xixin*)
Tetrapanacis 6 g	通草	(*Tongcao*)
Fructus Ziziphi Jujubae 3 dates	大枣	(*Dazao*)
Prepared Radix Glycyrrhizae 6 g	炙甘草	(*Zhigancao*)

Actions: Expelling pathogenic cold from channels; promoting blood circulation to remove obstruction in the channels.

Uses: Chilblain, cold erythema multiforme, cold urticaria and so on.

功用:温经散寒,活血通脉。

主治:冻疮、寒冷性多形红斑、冷性荨麻疹等。

Danggui Yinzi 当归饮子(4) 21,77,83,90,101,113,118
(Decoction of Radix Ledebouriellae 178,352,355,358,364
and Other Ingredients) 370,373,402

Source: Orthodox Manual of External Diseases 《外科正宗》

Composition:

Radix Ledebouriellae 15 g	当归	(*Danggui*)
Rhizoma Ligustici Chuanxiong 12 g	川芎	(*Chuanxiong*)
Radix Paeoniae Alba 15 g	白芍	(*Baishao*)
Radix Rehmanniae 15 g	生地	(*Shengdi*)
Radix Ledebouriellae 9 g	防风	(*Fangfeng*)
Herba Schizonepetae 9 g	荆芥	(*Jingjie*)
Fructus Tribuli 12 g	白蒺藜	(*Baijili*)
Radix Polygoni Multiflori 15 g	何首乌	(*Heshouwu*)
Radix Astragali seu Hedysari 15 g	黄芪	(*Huangqi*)
Radix Glycyrrhizae 6 g	甘草	(*Gancao*)

Actions: Enriching the blood and moistening dryness; dispelling wind and arresting itching.

Uses: Eczema, urticaria, cutaneous pruritus, neurodermatitis, seborrheic dermatitis, etc., due to deficiency of blood and wind-dryness.

功用:养血润燥,祛风止痒。

主治:血虚风燥型的湿疹、荨麻疹、皮肤瘙痒症、神经性皮炎、脂溢性皮炎等。

Dan Zhi Xiaoyao San 丹栀消遥散(84) 118,372
(Ease Powder of Moutan Bark and Cape Jasmine Fruit)

Source: Essentials of Internal Medicine 《内科摘要》

Composition:
Radix Angelicae Sinensis 12 g　　　当归(*Danggui*)
Poria 9 g　　　茯苓(*Fuling*)
Radix Paeoniae Alba 15 g　　　白芍(*Baishao*)
Rhizoma Atractylodis Macrocephalae 9 g　白术(*Baizhu*)
Radix Bupleuri 9 g　　　柴胡(*Chaihu*)
Cortex Moutan Radicis 9 g　　　丹皮(*Danpi*)
Rhizoma Capejasmine 9 g　　　栀子(*Zhizi*)
roasted ginger 3 chips　　　煨姜(*Weijiang*)
Herba Menthae 6 g　　　薄荷(*Bohe*)
Radix Glycyrrhizae 6 g　　　甘草(*Gancao*)

Manufacture: Grind the drugs into fine powder and make pellets by mixing the powder with water.

Administration: 6 g each time, three times daily.

Uses: Chloasma, neurdermatitis, acne, lupus erythematosus, etc.

制法:共为细末，水泛为丸。
用法:每服6克，日服3次。
主治:黄褐斑、神经性皮炎、痤疮、红斑性狼疮等。

Daqing Gao 大青膏(30)　　　27,49,128 325
(Ointment of Folium Isatdis)　　　336,377

Source: a prescription of the Hospital Affiliated Shandong TCM College (山东中医学院附属医院方)

Composition:
Folium Isatidis 60 g　　　大青叶　(*Daqingye*)
Resina Olibani 30 g　　　乳香　(*Ruxiang*)
Myrrha 30 g　　　没药　(*Moyao*)

Radix et Rhizoma Rhei 30 g　　大黄　　(*Dahuang*)
Alumen 30 g　　　　　　　　明矾　　(*Mingfan*)
Pb304 30 g　　　　　　　　　漳丹　　(*Zhangdan*)
Rhizoma Coptidis 30 g　　　　黄连　　(*Huanglian*)
Chalcanthitum 30 g　　　　　 胆矾　　(*Danfan*)
Verdigris 30 g　　　　　　　　铜绿　　(*Tonglu*)
Folium Hibisci 30 g　　　　　 芙蓉叶　(*Furongye*)
Calla Chinensis 30 g　　　　　五倍子　(*Wubeizi*)

Actions: Clearing aways heat and toxic material; eliminating dampness and blood stasis; subduing swelling and pain.

Manufacture: Grind the above ingredients into fine powder and make an ointment by mixing the powder with vaseline.

Directions: Spread the ointment on sterilized gauze to be applied on the diseased part, once every other day.

Indications: Various kinds of acute, purulent, infectious diseases with local swelling and pain, such as furuncle, carbuncle, phlegmon, erysipelas, etc.

功用:清热解毒，燥湿祛瘀，消肿止痛。
制法:共研细末，加50～70%凡士林调膏。
用法:摊于消毒纱布上，外敷患处，隔日一次。
主治:一切急性化脓性感染疾患，局部红肿热痛者。如:疖、痈、蜂窝织炎丹毒等。

Diandao San　颠倒散(19)　　　　25,170,397,399
(Diandao Powder)

Source: The Golden Mirror of Medicine 《医宗金鉴》
Composition:
Rhizoma Rhei　　　　　　　大黄　　(*Dahuang*)

Sulphur 硫磺 (*Liuhuang*)
(both in the same amount)

Manufacture: Grind the medicinal herbs into fine powder for use.

Adiministration: Mix the powder with a cool tea decoction and apply it to the diseased part.

Uses: Acne, Brandy nose, etc.

制法:上药共研细末备用。

用法:用凉茶水调粉末外敷。

主治:痤疮、酒渣鼻等。

Dongchuang Gao 冻疮膏(45)   68,346
(Ointment for Chilblain)

Source: a practical proved prescription (经验方)

Compositon:

Calamine 15 g	炉甘石 (*Luganshi*)
Elephos maximus 12 g	象皮 (*Xiangpi*)
Os Draconis Fossilia Ossis Mastodi 12 g	龙骨 (*Longgu*)
Camphor 9 g	樟脑 (*Zhangnao*)
Cortex Cinnamoni 24 g	肉桂 (*Rougui*)
Paruffing 12 g	石蜡 (*Shila*)
vaseline 120 g	凡士林 (*Fanshiling*)

Manufacture: Grind the first five of the drugs into fine powder and then mix the powder thorougly with paraffin and vaseline.

Administration: External application

Actions: Expelling pathogenic cold from the channels, promoting tissue regeneration and wound healing.

Uses: Chilblain.

制法:以上前五味药共研细末,兑入石蜡,凡士林调匀成膏。

用法:外敷患处。

功用:温经散寒,生肌敛疮。

主治:冻疮。

Duhuo Jisheng Tang 独活寄生汤(74)　　106,138,366,382
(Decoction of Radix Angelicae Pubescentis and Ramulus Loranthi)

Source: Prescriptions Worth a Thousand Gold for Emergencies《千金方》

Composition:

Radix Angelicae Pubescentis 9 g	独活	(*Duhuo*)
Ramulus Loranthi 9 g	桑寄生	(*Sangjisheng*)
Cortex Eucommiae 9 g	杜仲	(*Duzhong*)
Radix Achyranthis Bidentatae 9 g	牛膝	(*Niuxi*)
Herba Asari 3 g	细辛	(*Xixin*)
Radix Gentianae Macrophyllae 9 g	秦艽	(*Qingjiu*)
Cortex Cinnamomi 6 g	肉桂心	(*Rouguixin*)
Poria 9 g	茯苓	(*Fuling*)
Radix Ledebouriellae 9 g	防风	(*Fangfeng*)
Rhizoma Ligustici Chuangxiong 9 g	川芎	(*Chuanxiong*)
Radix Codonopsis Pilosulae 9 g	党参	(*Dangshen*)
Radix Rehmanniae 12 g	干地黄	(*Gandihuang*)
Radix Glycyrrhizae 6 g	甘草	(*Gancao*)
Radix Angelicae Sinensis 12 g	当归	(*Danggui*)
Radix Paeoniae Alba 12 g	白芍	(*Baishao*)

Actions: Nourishing the blood and regulating the channels.
Uses: Psoriasis, dermatasclerosis, dendrolimiasis and so on.
功用:养血通络。
主治:银屑病、硬皮病、松毛虫病等。

Erhao Xiyao 二号洗药(90) 124,376
(No.2 Lotion)

Source: a prescription of the Hospital Affiliated to Shandong TCM College (山东中医学院附属医院方)

Composition:

Radix Aconiti 9 g	川乌	(*Chuanwu*)
Radix Aconiti Kusnezoffii 9 g	草乌	(*Caowu*)
Rhizoma Atractylodis 9 g	苍术	(*Cangzhu*)
Radix Angelicae Pubescentis 9 g	独活	(*Duhuo*)
Ramulus Cinnamomi 9 g	桂枝	(*Guizhi*)
Radix Ledebouriellae 9 g	防风	(*Fangfeng*)
Folium Artemisiae Argyi 9 g	艾叶	(*Aiye*)
Pericarpium Zanthoxyli 9 g	花椒	(*Huajiao*)
Artemisia anomala 9 g	刘寄奴	(*Liujinu*)
Flos Carthami 9 g	红花	(*Honghua*)
Speranskia Tuberculata 9 g	透骨草	(*Tougucao*)
Herba Lycopodii 9 g	伸筋草	(*Shenjincao*)

Manufacture: Grind the drugs into coarse granules.

Administration: Decoct the drugs and rinse the diseased part with the decoction.

Actions: Expelling pathogenic cold from the channels; promoting blood circulation; removing obstruction from the channels.

Uses: Erythema nodosum, dermatasclerosis, erysipelas anaphase, etc.

制法:共研粗末。
用法:煎汤熏洗患处。
功用:温经散寒,活血通络。
主治:结节性红斑、硬皮病、丹毒后期等。

Erxian Tang 二仙汤(96)   137,151,382,388
(Decoction of Rhizoma Curculiginis and Herba Epimedii)

Source: a practical proved recipe(经验方)
Composition:

Rhizoma Curculiginis 9 g	仙茅	(*Xianmao*)
Herba Epimedii 9 g	仙灵脾	(*Xianlingpi*)
Radix Morindae Officinalis 9 g	巴戟天	(*Bajitian*)
Cortex Phellodendri 9 g	黄柏	(*Huangbai*)
Rhizoma Anemarrhema 9 g	知母	(*Zhimu*)
Radix Angelicae Sinensis 12 g	当归	(*Danggui*)

Actions: Warming Kidney−*Yang*, tonifying kidney−*Yin*, regulating and controlling the *Chong* and *Ren* channels.

Uses: Urticaria, dermatasclerosis and lupus erythematosus which are due to the disharmony of the *Chong* and *Ren* channels.

功用:温肾阳,益肾阴,调摄冲任。
主治:用于调任不调所致的荨麻疹,硬皮病、红斑性狼疮。

Ezhangfeng Cujingji 鹅掌风醋浸剂(25)   26,52,54,325
(*Ezhangfang* Acetum−infusion)   338,339

Source: a practical proved prescription (经验方)
Composition:

Semen Hydnocarpi 9 g　　　　大枫子仁(*Defengziren*)
Pericarpium Zanthoxyli 9 g　　花椒　　(*Huajiao*)
Flos Impatiens Balsamina 9 g　鲜凤仙花(*Xianfengxianhua*)
Gleditschia horrida 15 g　　　皂角　　(*Zhaojia*)
Cortex Pseudolaricis 15 g　　 土槿皮　(*Tujinpi*)
Cortex Lycii Radicis 6 g　　　 地骨皮　(*Digupi*)
Herba Agastachis 11 g　　　　藿香　　(*Huoxiang*)
Alumen 12 g　　　　　　　　　明矾　　(*Mingfan*)
Vinegar 100 g　　　　　　　　食醋　　(*Shicu*)

　　Manufacturing Procedure: Soak the drugs in water for a week before filtering them out.

　　Administration: Soak the diseased part in the infusion, twice or three times daily, 20 to 30 minutes each time.

　　Actions: Destroying parasites and relieving itching.

　　Uses: Hand-foot tinea.

制法:将诸药浸入醋泡1周,滤药渣备用。

用法:浸泡患处,每日2~3次,每次20~30分钟。

功用:杀虫止痒。

主治:手足癣。

Fangfeng Tongsheng San 防风通圣散(54)
(Miraculous Powder of Ledebouriella)

77,82,83,89,93,94
107,113,118,140,170
352,355,358,360
367,370,372,383,397

　　Source: Elaboration on Neijing-Internal Classic 《宣明论》

　　Composition:

Radix Platycodi 30 g　　　　　桔梗(*Jugeng*)
Radix Glycyrrhizae 60 g　　　 甘草(*Gancao*)
Gypsum Fibrosum 30 g　　　　石膏(*Shigao*)

Talcum 90 g	滑石(*Huashi*)
Radix et Rhizoma Rhei 15 g	大黄(*Dahuang*)
Natrii Sulfas 15 g	芒硝(*Mangxiao*)
Rhizoma Ligustici ChuanXiong 15 g	川芎(*Chuanxiong*)
Radix Ledebouriellae 15 g	防风(*Fangfeng*)
Rhizoma Atractylodis Macrocephalae 15 g	白术(*Baizhu*)
Radix Angelicae Dahuricae 15 g	白芷(*Baizhi*)
Herba Schizonepetae 15 g	荆芥(*Jingjie*)
Herba Menthae 15 g	薄荷(*Bohe*)
Fructus Forsythiae 15 g	连翘(*Lianqiao*)
Radix Angelicae Sinensis 15 g	当归(*Danggui*)
Herba Ephedrae 15 g	麻黄(*Mahuang*)
Radix Scutellariae 30 g	黄芩(*Huangqin*)
Capejasmine Fruit 15 g	栀子(*Zhizi*)

Actions: Relieving exterior syndrome, regulating the function of the viscera, dispelling Wind and removing heat.

Uses: Urticaria, folliculitis, seborrheic dermatitis, eczema, skin pruritus and so on.

Fangfeng Tongsheng Wan 防风通圣丸
(Miraculous Pill of Ledebouriella, a proprietary of the same ingredients)

Composition: The same as in *Fangfeng Tongsheng San*

Manufacture: Grind the drugs together into powder and make pills by mixing the powder with water.

Administration: Take 6 g each time, twice or three times a day.

功用:解表通里，疏风清热。

主治:荨麻疹、毛囊炎、脂溢性皮炎、湿疹、皮肤瘙痒症等。

〔附〕防风通圣丸
制法:组成同上,共研末和匀,水泛为丸。
用法:每次服6克,每日2～3次。

Feizi Fen 痱子粉(51)　　　　　　　　　　　72,348
(Powder for Sudamen)

Source: a practical proved prescription (经验方)

Composition:

Salicylic acid 10–20 g	水杨酸	(*Shuiyangsuan*)
dry alum 50 g	明矾	(*Mingfan*)
Borax 50 g	硼砂	(*Pengsha*)
Herba Menthae 10 g	薄荷脑	(*Bohenao*)
Zinc Oxide 1000 g	氧化锌	(*Yanghuaxing*)
Talcum Pulveratum 1000 g	滑石粉	(*Huashifen*)

Manufacture: Grind the drugs into fine powder.

Administration: Apply the powder to the diseased part.

Actions: Removing dampness, relieving itching and protecting astringency.

Uses: Sudamen eczema, etc.

制法:研细末即可。

用法:直接外扑患处。

功用:干燥止痒,保护收敛。

主治:用于痱子、湿疹等。

Fengyou Jing 风油精(40)　　　　　　　　65,94,345,361
(*Fengyoujing* Oil)

Source: A Mannual of Practical Chinese Patent Medicine by Song Lianzhu (宋连柱编《实用中成药手册》)

Composition:

Herba Menthae	薄荷	(*Bohe*)
eucalyptus oil	桉叶油	(*Anyeyou*)
essential oil	香精油	(*Xiangjingyou*)
salicylic acid	水杨酸	(*Shuiyangsuan*)
methyl ester	甲酯	(*Jiazhi*)
powder of Flos Syzygii Aromatici	丁香粉	(*Dingxiangfen*)
chlorophyl	叶绿素	(*Yelusu*)
chloroform	氯仿	(*Lufang*)
camphor	樟脑	(*Zhangnao*)

Administration: For external use, rub it onto the diseased part; for oral administration, take four to six drops each time.

Actions: Clearing away heat, alleviating pain, relieving itching and removing wind.

Uses: Insect dermatitis.

用法:外用涂擦患处。口服每次4～6滴。

功用:清热镇痛,止痒消风。

主治:虫咬皮炎。

Fufang Huanglian You 复方黄连油(21)   26,324
(Composite Ointment of Rhizoma Coptidis)

Source: a practical proved prescription (经验方)

Composition:

Rhizoma Coptidis 30 g	黄连	(*Huanglian*)
Oleum Sesami 150 g	麻油	(*Mayou*)
Borneolum Syntheficum 1 g	冰片	(*Bingpian*)

Manufacture: Grind the Rhizoma Coptidis and Borneolum into fine powder to be mixed with sesame oil.

Administration: Apply it to the diseased part, twice or three times daily.

Actions: Detoxicating; alleviating pain.

Uses: Scald, general ulcer and impetigo herpetiformis.

制法:将黄连、冰片研末入麻油中调匀备用。

用法:涂患处，每日 2～3 次。

功用:解毒止痛。

主治:烫伤，一般性溃疡及脓疱疮。

Fufang Jiji Pian 复方蒺藜片(123)   188,407
(Composite Fructus Tribuli Bolus)

Source: a prescription of the Affiliated Hospital of Shandong TCM College (山东中医学院附属医院方)

Composition:

Fructus Tribuli 15 g 刺蒺藜(*Chijili*)
Herba Spirodelae 12 g 浮萍　(*Fuping*)
Scorpio 9 g 金蝎　(*Jinxie*)
Flos Carthami 9 g 红花　(*Honghua*)
Radix Angelicae Sinensis 12 g 当归　(*Danggui*)
Herba Leonuri 12 g 益母草(*Yimucao*)
Prepared Radix Polygoni Multiflor 15 g 制何首乌(*Zhiheshouwu*)
Rhizoma Ligustici Chuanxiong 12 g 川芎　(*Chuanxiong*)
centipede one dried centipede 蜈蚣　(*Wugong*)

Manufacture: Grind the drugs into fine powder to make boluses with, each bolus weighing 0.3 g.

Administration: 10 tablets each time, three times daily; the dose for infants should be reduced.

Action: Nourishing the blood, activating blood circulation and dispelling wind.

Uses: Vitiligo.
制法:共为细末，制成片，每片重 0.3 克。
用法:每次 10 片，日 3 次，儿童酌减。
功用:养血活血疏风。
主治:白癜风。

Fufang Tujingpi Din 复方土槿皮酊(24)   26,51,55,325
(Compound Tincture of Cortex Pseudolaricis)   338,340,342

Source: a practical proved prescription (经验方)
Composition:

Cortex Pseudolaricis 8 g	土槿皮	(*Tujinpi*)
Radix Stemonae 6 g	百部	(*Baibu*)
Fructus Mume 6 g	乌梅	(*Wumei*)
Camphor 4 g	樟脑	(*Zhangnao*)
75%alcohol 100 ml	酒精	(*Jiujing*)

Manufacturing Procedure: Soak the drugs in water for a week before filtering them out.

Administration: External application, twice or three times daily.

Actions: Destroying parasites and relieving itching.

Uses: Hand-foot tinea, tinea corporis, etc.
制法:浸泡 1 周，过滤去渣备用。
用法:外涂患处，每日 2~3 次。
功用:杀虫止痒。
主治:手足癣、体癣等。

Furong Gao 芙蓉膏(92)   128,377
(Ointment of Folium Hibisci)

Source: Practical Traditional Chinese External Medicine by

Shang Dejun 《实用中医外科学》

Composition:

Folium Hibisci 250 g　　　　芙蓉叶　(*Furongye*)
Radix et Rhizoma Rhei 60 g 生大黄　(*Shengdahuang*)
Semen Phaseoli 60 g　　　　赤小豆　(*Chixiaodou*)

Manufacture: Grind the drugs into a fine powder and make an ointment by mixing the powder with vaseline.

Administration: Spread the ointment on anticeptic gauze to be applied on the diseased part; change the dressing every other day.

Actions: Clearing away heat and toxic material; subduing swelling and alleviate pain.

Uses: Various acute suppurative infections; local red-swelling; pain with a burning-heat sensation.

制法:共研成细末，用凡士林调和成膏。

用法:摊于消毒纱布上，外敷患处，隔日换一次。

功用:清热解毒，消肿止痛。

主治:一切急性化脓性感染疾病，局部红肿热痛者。

Ganlu Xiaodu Dan 甘露消毒丹(120)　　　　184,404
(Sweet Dew Detoxication Pill)

Source: Compendium on Epidemic Febrile Diseases 《温热经纬》

Composition:

Talcum 45 g　　　　　　　　　　　　飞滑石　(*Feihuashi*)
Herba Artemisia Capillaris 36 g　　　茵陈　　(*Yinchen*)
Rhizoma Aconi Graminei 18 g　　　　石菖蒲　(*Shichangpu*)
Caulis Aristolochiae Manshuriensis 15 g 木通　(*Mutong*)

· 215 ·

Bulbus Fritillariae Cirrhose 15 g 川贝母 (*Chuanbeimu*)
Herba Agastachis 12 g 藿香 (*Huoxiang*)
Herba Menthae 12 g 薄荷 (*Bohe*)
Semen Amomi Cardamomi 12 g 白寇仁 (*Baikouren*)
Fructus Forsythiae 12 g 连翘 (*Lianqiao*)
Rhizoma Belamcandae 12 g 射干 (*Shegang*)

Manufacture: Grind the drugs into fine powder for application, or make boluses by mixing the powder with massa Fermentata Medicinalis, each bolus being as big as a semen Phaseoli.

Administration: 9 g each time, three times daily, washed down with boiled water.

Actions: Promoting diuresis and removing dampness; clearing away heat and toxic material.

Uses: Tragomaschalia, etc.

制法:上药共研细末,或以神曲糊丸,如赤豆大。
用法:每服9克,日3次,白水送下。
功用:利湿化浊,清热解毒。
主治:腋臭等。

Goupi Gao 狗皮膏(38)   65,120,345,373
(Dog-skin Ointment)

Source: Essential Chinese Patent Medicine 《中国基本中成药》
Composition:

It is a common proprietary composed of eighty-two drugs, including Fructus Aurantii 枳壳 (*Zhike*) Radix Ledebouriellae 防风 (*Fangfeng*)

and so on.

Manufacture: Spread the ointment on a piece of dog-skin, or cloth or paper, each weighing 15 g or 30 g.

Administration: Soften the ointment by heating and then stick it on the diseased part.

Actions: Removing toxic material and softening hard masses; clearing away blood stasis and alleviating pain.

Uses: Insect dermatitis, such as caterpillar bite.

制法:将膏摊狗皮、布或纸背上、每张净重15克或30克.

用法:外用。加温软化、贴患处。

功用:解毒软坚,祛瘀止痛。

主治:用于虫咬皮炎,如松毛虫叮咬等。

Guipi Tang 归脾汤(63) 91,109,359,367,368
(Decoction for Invigorating the Spleen and Nourishing the Heart)

Source: The Complete Effective Prescriptions for Women 《妇人良方》

Composition:

Radix Astragali seu Hedysari 15 g	黄芪(*Huangqi*)
Radix Ginseng 9 g	人参(*Renshen*)
Rhizoma Atractylodis 15 g	白术(*Baizhu*)
Radix Angelicae Sinensis 12 g	当归(*Danggui*)
Poria cwn Ligno Hospite 12 g	茯神(*Fushen*)
Radix Polygalae 9 g	远志(*Yuanzhi*)
Radix Aucklandiae 9 g	木香(*Muxiang*)
Rhizoma Zingiberis Recens 3 chips	生姜(*Shengjiang*)
Fructus Ziziphi Jujubae 3 dates	大枣(*Dazao*)
Radix Glycyrrihizae 6 g	甘草(*Gancao*)

Arillus Longan 9 g 龙眼肉(*Longyanrou*)
Semen Ziziphi Spinosae 15 g 酸枣仁(*Suanzaoren*)

Actions: Reinforcing the spleen, nourishing the heart, invigorating *Qi* and enriching the blood.

Uses: lupus erythematosus due to insufficiency of the spleen and deficiency of blood; dermatasclerosis, dermatomyositis. allergic purpura, alopecia areata, etc.

Guipi Wan

(Pill for Invigorating the Spleen and Heart).

Manufacture: Grind the above drugs into fine powder and make pills by mixing the powder with water.

Administration: Take 6 g each time, three times daily.

功用:补脾养心，益气补血。

主治:用于脾虚血少之红斑性狼疮、硬皮病、皮肌炎、过敏性紫癜、斑秃等。

〔附〕归脾丸即上方诸药，共研细末和匀，炼蜜为丸。

用法:每次 6 克，每日 3 次。

Haizao Yuhu Tang 海藻玉壶汤(115)
(Decoction of Sargassum)

Source: The Golden Mirror of Medicine 《医宗金鉴》

Composition:

Sargassum 12 g 海藻(*Haizao*)
Thallus Eckloniae 12 g 昆布(*Kunbu*)
sea-tangle 12 g 海带(*Haidai*)
Rhizoma Pinelliae 9 g 半夏(*Banxia*)
Pericarpium Citri Reticulatae 9 g 陈皮(*Chenpi*)
Pericarpium Citri Reticulatae Viride 9 g 青皮(*Qingpi*)

Fructus Forsythiae 15 g　　　　连翘(*Lianqiao*)
Bulbus Fritillariae 12 g　　　　象贝(*Xiangbei*)
Radix Angelicae Sinensis 12 g　　当归(*Danggui*)
Rhizoma Ligustici Chuangxiong 9 g　川芎(*Chuanxiong*)
Radix Angelicae Pubescentis 9 g　独活(*Duhuo*)
Radix Glycyrrhizae 6 g　　　　甘草(*Gancao*)

　　Actions: Promoting blood circulation and regulating the flow of *Qi;* resolving phlegm and softening hard masses.
　　Uses: Erythema nodosum, acne, keloid, etc.
功用:活血理气，化痰软坚。
主治:结节性红斑、痤疮、瘢痕疙瘩等。

Hali You 蛤蜊油(47)　　　　　　　　　　　70,347
(*Hali* Ointment, a common proprietary)

　　Source: a practical proved prescription (经验方)
　　Administration:
　　　　External application
　　Actions: Moistening the skin.
　　Uses: Rhagade.
用法:外涂患处。
功用:润肤。
主治:皲裂疮。

Heidou Liuyou 黑豆馏油(22)　　　　　　　26,324
(Oil of Semen Sojae Nigrum)

　　Source: a practical proved prescription (经验方)
　　Composition:
　　　　Semen Sojae Nigrum　　黑豆　(*Heidou*)

· 219 ·

Manufacture: By means of distillation.

Adiministration: External application, twice or three times daily.

Actions: Moistening the skin and reliveing itching.

Uses: Chronic eczema, neurodermatitis, etc.

制法:用馏油法制得。

用法:外涂患处，日 2~3 次。

功用:润肤止痒。

主治:慢性湿疹、神经性皮炎等。

Heidou Liuyou Ruan Gao 黑豆馏油软膏(58)
(Ointment of Unguentum picis fabae nigrae)

Source: External Medicine compiled by Guangzhou TCM College(广州中医学院主编《外科学》)

Composition:

Unguentum picis fabae nigrae 5 g—20 g	黑豆馏油 (*Heidouliuyou*)
lanolin 10 g	羊毛脂 (*Yangmaozhi*)
vaseline 100 g	凡士林 (*Fanshiling*)

Administration: External application, twice or three times daily.

Actions: Softening hard masses and relieving itching.

Uses: Chronic eczema, psoriasis, etc.

用法:外涂患处，日 2~3 次。

功用:软坚止痒。

主治:慢性湿疹、银屑病等。

Houzheng Wan 喉症丸(66)
(Houzhen Pill)

Source: A Mannual of Practical Chinese Patent Medicine 《实用中成药手册》

Composition:

Radix Isatidis	板蓝根	(*Banlangen*)
Venenum Bufonis	蟾酥	(*Chansu*)
Radix Scrophulariae	元明粉	(*Yuanmingfen*)
Calculus Bovis	牛黄	(*Niuhuang*)
Borneolum	冰片	(*Bingpian*)
fuligo e herbis	百草霜	(*Baicaoshuang*)
Realgar	雄草	(*Xionghuang*)
Borax	生硼砂	(*Shengpengsha*)
Indigo Naturalis	青黛	(*Qingdai*)
bile	胆汁	(*Danzhi*)

Manufacture: Grind the drugs into fine powder, and make pellets by mixing the medical powder with water.

Administration: Grind the pellet into powder and make a paste of it for external application.

Actions: Clearing away heat and toxic material; alleviating pain.

Uses: Papular urticaria, insect dermatitis, etc.

制法:共研极细末，水泛为丸。
用法:将丸研末，调成糊状，外涂患处。
功用:清热解毒，止痛。
主治:丘疹性荨麻疹、虫咬皮炎等。

Huaban Tang 化斑汤(102)   147,387
(Decoction for Removing Maculae).

Composition:

Gypsum Fibrosum 30 g	生石膏	(*Sheng shigao*)
Rhizoma Anemarrhenae 9 g	知母	(*Zhimu*)
Oryza sativa 15 g	粳米	(*Gengmi*)
Scrophularia ningpoensis 9 g	元参	(*Yuanshen*)
Cornu Rhinocerotis 3 g (tiny pieces to be added to the boiling decoction of other ingredients)	犀角	(*Xijiao*)
Radix Glycyrrhizae 4.5 g	甘草	(*Gancao*)

Actions: Removing heat and toxic material from the blood.

Indications: Skin diseases with noxious heat syndrome, such as allergic purpura and systemic lupus erythematosus.

功用:清热，凉血，解毒

主治:过敏性紫癜，系统性红斑狼疮等热毒炽盛之证。

Huangbai San 黄柏散(17)   25,30,45,78,94,179,327
(Powder of Cortex Phellodendri)   334,352,361,402

Source: a prescription of the Hospital Affiliated to Shandong TCM College (山东中医学院附属医院方)

Composition:

Cortex Phellodendri 30 g	黄柏	(*Huangbai*)
Rhizoma Coptidis 3 g	黄连	(*Huanglian*)
Aloe 6 g	芦荟	(*Luhui*)
Rhizoma Atractylodis 9 g	苍术	(*Cangzhu*)

Talcum 9 g　　　　　　　　滑石　(*Huashi*)
Colophonium 12 g　　　　　松香　(*Songxiang*)
Borneolum Syntheticum 0.6 g　冰片　(*Bingpian*)

Manufacture: Grind the medicinal herbs into fine powder for use.

Administration: Sprinkle it on the diseased part or mix the powder with sesame oil into ointment to be applied on the diseased part.

Actions: Clearing away heat and eliminating dampness.

Uses: Eczema, eczematoid dermatitis, impetigo herpetiformis, erosion, exudation, etc.

制法:共研细末备用。
用法:撒布于患处或香油调成膏，外敷患处。
功用:清热燥湿。
主治:湿疹、湿疹样皮炎、脓疱疮等、皮肤糜烂、渗液者。

Huanglian Gao 黄连膏(28)　　　　　　　27,325
(Ointment of Rhizoma Coptidis)

Source: The Golden Mirror of Medicine《医宗金鉴》
Composition:

Rhizoma Coptidis 9 g　　　　黄连　(*Huanglian*)
Cortex Phellodendri 9 g　　　黄柏　(*Huangbai*)
Curcumae Longne 9 g　　　　羌黄　(*Qianghuang*)
Radix Angelicae Sinensis 15 g　当归　(*Danggui*)
Radix Rehmanniae 30 g　　　生地　(*Shengdi*)
Olcum Sesami 360ml　　　　　麻油　(*Mayou*)
Cera Flava 120 g　　　　　　　黄蜡　(*Huangla*)

Manufacture:Fry over a soft fire the above drugs except

Cera Flava until they become brown, then filter the drugs out, add in the Cera Flava and stir it until it becomes cool and thickened.

Administration: External application.

Actions: Clearing away heat, dryness and toxic material; alleviating pain.

Uses: Impetigo herpetiformis, vulva ulcer, etc.

制法：上药除黄蜡外，文火熬煎至药枯，去渣滤清，再加入黄蜡，搅拌至冷凝为止。

用法：外敷患处。

功用：清热润燥，解毒止痛。

主治：脓疱疮、外阴溃疡等。

Huanglian Jeidu Tang 黄连解毒汤(6)　　　21,44,48,53,65
(Antidotal Decoction of Coptis)　　100,334,336,338,345,364

Source: The Medical Secrets of an Official 《外台秘要》

Composition:

Rhizoma Coptidis 9 g	黄连	(*Huanglian*)
Radix Scutellariae 15 g	黄芩	(*Huangqin*)
Fructus Capejasmine 9 g	栀子	(*Zhizi*)
Cortex Phellodendri 9 g	黄柏	(*Huangbai*)

Actions: Clearing away heat, purging intense heat and toxic material.

Uses: Impetigo herpetiformis, folliculitis, boil and furunculosis, erysipelas, acne, Behect's Syndrome, etc.

功用：清热泻火解毒。

主治：脓疱疮、毛囊炎、疖与疖病、丹毒痤疮、白塞氏病等。

Huanglian You 黄连油(89)
(Ointment of Berberine)

Source: a practical proved prescription (经验方)
Composition:
Berberine tablet 1–2 g   黄连素 (*Huangliansu*)
sesame oil 100 ml   麻油   (*Mayou*)

Manufacture: Grind berberine tablets into fine powder and mix it thoroughly with sesame oil.

Administration: External application twice or three times daily.

Actions: Clearing away heat and toxic material, moisturizing the skin.

Uses: Lactigo; impetigo

制法:将黄连素片研细入麻油中调匀。
用法:外涂患处,每日2～3次。
功用:清热解毒润肤。
主治:婴儿湿疹、脓疱疮。

Hueiyang Yulong Gao 回阳玉龙膏(93)
(Yang-restoring Ointment)

Source: Orthodox Mannual of External Diseases 《外科正宗》

Composition:
Radix Aconiti Kusnezoffii 90 g   草乌 (*Caowu*)
Rhizoma Zingiberis 90 g   干姜 (*Ganjiang*)
Radix Paeoniae Rubrum 30 g   赤芍 (*Chishao*)
Radix Angelicae Dahuricae 30 g 白芷 (*Baizhi*)
Rhizoma Arisaematis 30 g   南星 (*Nanxing*)

Cortex Cinnamomi 15 g　　　　　肉桂　(*Rougui*)

Actions: Warming the channels, promoting blood flow, expelling cold and resolving phlegm.

Manufacture: Grind the drugs into fine powder.

Administration: Mix it with hot wine before applying it to the diseased part, once every other day.

Uses: Skin diseases with sore or ulcer, which show *Yin*-syndrome.

功用:温经活血，散寒化痰。
制法:上方共研细末备用。
用法:热酒调敷患处，隔日一次。
主治:疮疡阴证。

Huosiang Cujinji 藿香醋浸剂(26)   26,52,54,325
(Acetum-infusion of Herba Agastachis)   338,339

Source: a practical proved prescription (经验方)

Composition:

Herba Agastachis 30 g　　　藿香　(*Huoxiang*)
Rhizoma Polygonati 10 g　　黄精　(*Huangjing*)
Rhizoma Rhei 12 g　　　　　生大黄　(*Shengdahuang*)
Melanterite 12 g　　　　　　皂矾　(*Zhaofan*)
Vinegar 1000 g　　　　　　　食醋　(*Shicu*)

Manufacture: Soak the drugs in vinegar for 5 to 7 days to make a liquid.

Adiministration: Soak the diseased part in the infusion, twice or three times daily, 20 to 30 minutes each time.

Actions: Destroying parasites and relieving itching.

Uses: Hand-foot tinea.

制法:上药混合浸泡 5～7 天后备用。
用法:浸泡患处，每日 2～3 次，每次 20～30 分钟。
功用:杀虫止痒。
主治:手足癣。

Huoxue Quyu Pian 活血祛瘀片(101)   147,158,182
(Bolus for Promoting Blood Circulation   386,392,404
and Removing Blood Stasis)

Source: a prescription of the Affiliated Hospital of Shandong TCM College (山东中医学院附属医院方)

Composition:

Radix Angelicae Sinensis 30 g	当归	(*Danggui*)
Radix Paeoniae Rubra 30 g	赤芍	(*Chishao*)
Semen Persicae 24 g	桃仁	(*Taoren*)
Flos Carthami 24 g	红花	(*Honghua*)
Squama Manitis 24 g	穿山甲	(*Chuanshanjia*)
Artemisia anomala 45 g	刘寄奴	(*Liujinu*)
Gleditschia horrida 24 g	皂刺	(*Zaoci*)
Pyrolusite 60 g	制无	(*Zhiwu*)
Radix Ancklandiae 18 g	木香	(*Muxiang*)
Flos Caryophylli 15 g	丁香	(*Dinxiang*)
Radix et Rhizoma Rhei 15 g	生大黄	(*Shengdahuang*)
Eupolyphaga Sinensis Walker 24 g	土元	(*Tuyuan*)

Manufacture: Grind the drugs into fine powder and make boluses with the powder, each bolus weighing 0.3 g.

Administration: Ten boluses each time for an adult, three times daily; for a child, the dose should be smaller.

Actions: Promoting blood circulation by removing blood

stasis; removing obstruction from the channels to relieve swelling.

Uses: Dermatasclerosis, erythema nodosum, etc, due to blood stasis.

制法:共为细末，制片，每片0.3克。
用法:成人每服10片，日3次，小儿酌减。
功用:活血化瘀，通络消肿。
主治:硬皮病、结节性红斑等证属血瘀者。

Huoxue Zhitong San 活血止痛散(44) 68,70,73,128
(Powder for Promoting Blood Circulation   346,347,349,377
and Arresting Pain)

Source: a prescription of the Hospital of Shandong TCM College (山东中医学院附属医院方)

Composition:

Speranskia Tuberculata 30 g	透骨草(*Tougucao*)
Fructus Meliae Toosendan 15 g	川楝子(*Chuandongzi*)
tail-end of Radix Angelicae Sinensis 15 g	归尾 (*Guiwei*)
Cortex Erythrinae 15 g	海桐 (*Haitong*)
Rhizoma Curcumae Longae 15 g	姜黄 (*Jianghuang*)
Radix Clematidis 15 g	威灵仙(*Weilingxian*)
Radix Achyranthis Bidentatae 15 g	怀牛膝(*Huainiuxi*)
Rhizoma Seu Radix Notopterygii 15 g	羌活 (*Qianghuo*)
Radix Angelicae Dahuricae 15 g	白芷 (*Baizhi*)
Lignum Sappan 15 g	苏木 (*Sumu*)
Cortex Acanthopanacis Radicis 15 g	五加皮(*Wujiapi*)
Flos Carthami 15 g	红花 (*Honghua*)
Rhizoma Smilacis Glabrae 15 g	土茯苓(*Tufuling*)
Pericarpium Zanthoxyli 6 g	花椒 (*Huajiao*)

Resina Olibani 6 g　　　　　　　乳香　(*Ruxiang*)

Adiministration: Decoct the drugs and rinse the diseased part in the decoction while it is still hot. A dose of it may be used for one or two days. It is applied once or twice daily, 30 minutes each time.

Actions: Promoting blood circulation to stop pain; resolving masses and subduing swelling.

Uses: Chilblain, hand-foot rhagades, corn, dermatasclerosis, erythema nodosum, and so on.

用法:煎汤乘热熏洗患处，每剂可熏洗1~2天，每天1~2次，每次30分钟。

功用:活血止痛，散结消肿。

主治:冻疮、手足皲裂、鸡眼、硬皮病、结节性红斑等。

Jiaoqi Fen 脚气粉(37)　　　　　　　52,338
(*Jiaoqi* Powder)

Source: Practical Traditional Chinese External Medicine by Shang Dejun (尚德俊主编《实用中医外科学》)

Composition:

Cortex Phellodendri 15 g	黄柏　(*Huangbai*)
Alumen Exsiccatum 15 g	枯矾　(*Kufan*)
Talcum 15 g	滑石　(*Huashi*)
Camphor 15 g	樟脑　(*Zhangnao*)

Manufacture: Grind the drugs into fine powder for use.

Administration: Apply the powder on the diseased part, twice or three times daily.

Actions: Clearing away heat and eliminating dampness; destroying parasites and relieving itching.

Uses: Hand-foot tinea; skin erosion; etc.

制法:上药共研细末。

用法:撒布患处,每日2~3次。

功用:清热燥湿,杀虫止痒。

主治:用于手足癣、皮肤糜烂等。

Jiedu Xiyao 解毒洗药(13)   25,44,51,78,324
(Detoxicating Lotion)   334,338,352

Source: a prescription of the Hospital Affiliated to Shandong TCM College (山东中医学院附属医院方)

Composition:

Herba Taraxaci 30 g	蒲公英(*Pugongying*)
Radix Sophorae Flavescentis 12 g	苦参 (*Kushen*)
Cortex Phellodendri 12 g	黄柏 (*Huangbai*)
Fructus Forsythiae 12 g	连翘 (*Lianqiao*)
Semen Morindicae 12 g	木鳖子(*Mubiezi*)
Flos Lonicerae 9 g	金银花(*Jinyinhua*)
Radix Angelicae Dahuricae 9 g	白芷 (*Baizhi*)
Radix Paeoniae Rubra 9 g	赤芍 (*Chishao*)
Cortex Moutan Radicis 9 g	丹皮 (*Danpi*)
Radix Glycyrrhizae 9 g	生甘草(*Shenggancao*)

Administration: Decoct the medicinal herbs and rinse the diseased part in the decoction while it is still hot, once or twice daily, 30 minutes each time. In the case of wound, routine change of dressing is required after each rinsing.

Actions: Clearing away heat and toxic material; promoting blood circulation to reduce swelling; expelling curd and evacuating pus.

Indications: Before or after the ulceration of acute suppurative infections; post-traumatic infections; pyogenic dermatosis; etc.

用法:上药煎汤,乘热熏洗患处。每日1~2次,每次30分钟。有疮口者,可每次熏洗后,常规换药。

功用:清热解毒,活血消肿,祛腐排脓。

主治:急性化脓性感染疾病的初期和溃后,以及外伤感染,化脓性皮肤病等。

Jingfang Baidu San 荆防败毒散(2)　　　　20,322
(Antiphlogistic Powder of Schizonepeta and Ledebouriella)

Source: A Collection of Effective Prescriptions 《摄生众妙方》

Composition:

Radix Ledebouriellae 9 g	防风	(*Fangfeng*)
Radix Bupleuri 9 g	柴胡	(*Chaihu*)
Herba Schizonepetae 9 g	荆芥	(*Jingjie*)
Rhizoma Seu Radix Notoptergyii 9 g	羌活	(*Qianghuo*)
Radix Angelicae Pubescentis 9 g	独活	(*Duhuo*)
Fructus Aurantii 9 g	枳壳	(*Zhike*)
parched Radix Platycodi 9 g	炒桔梗	(*Chaojugeng*)
Poria 9 g	茯苓	(*Fuling*)
Rhizoma Ligustici Chuanxiong 9 g	川芎	(*Chuanxiong*)
Radix Glycyrrhizae 6 g	甘草	(*Gancao*)

Uses: Pruritic dermatosis showing wind-cold syndrome, such as urticaria, papular urticaria, erythema multiforme, etc.

主治:风寒型荨麻疹、丘疹性荨麻疹、多形性红斑等瘙痒性皮肤病。

Jinhuang San and Jinhuang Gao 金黄散(膏)(29)
(Jinhuang Powder and Jinhuang Qintment)

Source: Orthodox Manual of External Diseases 《外科正宗》

Composition:

Radix Trichosanthis 48 g	天花粉 (Tianhuafen)
Cortex Phellodendri 48 g	黄柏　(Huangbai)
Radix et Rhizoma Rhei 48 g	大黄　(Dahuang)
Curcumae Longae 48 g	姜黄　(Jianghuang)
Radix Angelicae Dahuricae 30 g	白芷　(Baizhi)
Cortex Magnoliae Officinals 18 g	厚朴　(Houpu)
Pericarpium Citri Reticulatae 18 g	桔皮　(Jupi)
Rhizoma Atractylodis 18 g	苍术　(Cangzhu)
Rhizoma Arisaematis 18 g	生南星 (Shengnanxing)
Radix Glycyrrhizae 18 g	甘草　(Gancao)

Manufacture: Grind the above drugs into fine powder and mix it with vaseline (50—70% by weight).

Administration: Apply the powder directly onto the diseased part, or mix it with tea decoction, vinegar and sesame oil before application, or prepare a ready made ointment as such for application.

Actions: Removing heat and toxic material; subduing swelling and pain.

Indications: Acute, purulent and infectious diseases with local swelling and pain.

制法：上药共研极细末备用。加50～70%的凡士林调膏即金黄膏。

用法：直接外扑患处，亦可用茶水、醋、麻油调后外用。或用膏外敷患处。

功用:清热解毒,消肿止痛。

主治:急性化脓性感染疾病局部红肿热痛者。

Jinkui Shenqi Wan 金匮肾气丸(105)
(*Jinkui* Bolus for Strengthening Kidney-*Qi*)

Source: Synopsis of Prescriptions of the Golden Chamber 《金匮要略》

Composition:

Radix Rehmanniae Praeparata 21 g	熟地	(*Shudi*)
Rhizoma Dioscoreae 15 g	山药	(*Shanyao*)
Fructus Corni 9 g	山萸肉	(*Shanyurou*)
Radix Alismatis 9 g	泽泻	(*Zhexie*)
Poria 9 g	茯苓	(*Fuling*)
Cortex Moutan Radicis 9 g	丹皮	(*Danpi*)
Cortex Cinnamomi 9 g	肉桂	(*Rougui*)
Radix Aconiti Praeparata 9 g	熟附子	(*Shufuzi*)

Manufacture: Grind the drugs into fine powder and make boluses by mixing the powder with honey.

Administration: 6 to 9 g each time, twice to three times daily.

Actions: Warming and recuperating the kidney-*Yang*.

Uses: Chloasma, dermatasclerosis, lupus erythematosus and seborrheic dermatitis showing the syndrome of deficiency of the kidney.

制法:上药为末,炼蜜为丸。

用法:每服6~9克,每日2~3次。

功用:温补肾阳。

主治:肾虚型黄褐斑、硬皮病、红斑性狼疮、脂溢性皮炎等。

Ji Yan Gao 鸡眼膏(52)   73,349
(Ointment for Corn)

    Source: a practical proved prescription (经验方)
    Composition:

Salicylic acid 5 g	水杨酸	(*Shuiyangsuan*)
Pb304 3 g	广丹	(*Guangdan*)
benzocaine 2 g	笨唑卡因	(*Benzuokayin*)
white sugar 2 g	白糖	(*Baitang*)

    Manufacture: Grind the drugs into fine powder and make an ointment by mixing it with 75% alcohol.

    Administration: Cover the healthy tissues surrounding the corn with adhesive plaster before applying the ointment to the affected area, and then, too, cover the area with adhesive plaster. Change the dressing every five days.

    Actions: Corrosion.

    Uses: Corn, etc.

制法:共研细末，以75%酒精调成膏。

用法:先将患处周围正常组织用橡皮膏保护好，再将药涂于患处，然后外盖橡皮膏，每五天换药一次。

功用:腐蚀。

主治:用于鸡眼等。

Kang Liuyou 糠馏油(23)   26,324
(Oil of Millet Chaff)

    Source: a practical proved prescription (经验方)
    Composition:

millet chaff　　小米糠皮　(*Xiaomikangpi*)

Manufacture: By means of distillation.

Administration: External application, twice or three times daily.

Actions: Moistening the skin and relieving itching.

Uses: Chronic eczema, neurodermatitis, etc.

制法:馏油法制得。

用法:外涂患处，每日 2～3 次。

功用:润肤止痒。

主治:慢性湿疹、神经性皮炎等。

Keyin Wan 克银丸(99)　　　　　　　　　　140,383
Anti-psoriasis Bolus

Source: Essential Chinese Patent Medicine 《中国基本中成药》

Composition:

　Rhizoma Smilacis Glabrae　　　土茯苓　(*Tufuling*)

　Cortex Dictamni Radicis, etc.　　白藓皮　(*Baixianpi*)

Manufacture: Grind the drugs into fine powder and make boluses by mixing the powder with honey, a big bolus weighing 10 g, a packet of small boluses weighing 20 g.

Administration: Two big boluses or one packet of little boluses each time, twice to three times daily.

Actions: Expelling wind and clearing away heat; removing toxic substances and relieving itching.

Uses: Psoriasis

制法:诸药研细末，炼蜜为丸，大丸重 10 克，小丸每袋 20 克。

用法:每次服大丸2丸或小丸1袋,每日2～3次。
功用:祛风清热,解毒止痒。
主治:银屑病。

Liangxue Qingan Tang 凉血清肝汤(32)　　32,328
(Decoction for Clearing Away Heat from the Blood and Liver)

Source: a prescription of the Hospital Affiliated to Shandong TCM College (山东中医学院附属学院方)

Composition:

Flos Lonicerae 15 g	金银花 (*Jinyinhua*)
Fructus Forsythiae 15 g	连翘　(*Lianqiao*)
Radix Paeoniae Rubra 15 g	赤芍　(*Chishao*)
Cortex Moutan Radicis 15 g	丹皮　(*Danpi*)
Radix Bupleuri 9 g	柴胡　(*Chaihu*)
Rhizoma Ligustici Chuanxiong 9 g	川芎　(*Chuanxiong*)
Capejasmine Fruit 9 g	栀子　(*Zhizi*)
Radix Gentianae 6 g	龙胆草 (*Longdancao*)
Radix Arnebiae seu Lithospermi 9 g	紫草　(*Zicao*)
Pericarpium Citri Reticulatae Viride 9 g	青皮　(*Qingpi*)
Radix Glycyrrhizae 6 g	甘草　(*Gancao*)
Radix Scutellariae 9 g	黄芩　(*Huangqin*)
Radix Rehmanniae 18 g	生地　(*Shengdi*)

Actions: removing heat from the blood.
Indication: herpes zoster, etc.
功用:凉血清热。
主治:带状疱疹等。

Liuwei Dihuang Wan 六味地黄丸(79)
(Bolus of Six Drugs Including Rehmannia).

108,147,192,367
386,408,410

Source: Key to Therapeutics of Children's Diseases 《小儿药证直诀》

Composition:
  Poria 9 g   茯苓   (*Fuling*)
  Rhizoma Dioscoreae 15 g   山药   (*Shangyao*)
  Fructus Corni 9 g   山萸肉 (*Shangyurou*)
  Radix Rehmanniae Praeparatae 21 g 熟地 (*Shudi*)
  Rhizoma Alismatis 9 g   泽泻   (*Zexie*)
  Cortex Moutan Radicis 9 g   丹皮   (*Danpi*)

Manufacture: Grind the drugs into fine powder and make boluses by mixing the powder with honey.

Administration: Take 9 g each time; twice or three times daily.

Actions: Nourishing *Yin* and the kidney; reducing pathogenic fire.

Uses: alopecia areata due to deficiency of *Yin*, allergic drug rash, chloasma, allergic purpura, lupus erythemtosus, etc.

Liuwei Dihuang Tang 六味地黄汤
(another proprietary of the same ingredients)

Manufacture: Decoct the above drugs.
制法:上药共研细末，炼蜜为丸。
用法:每服9克，日2～3次。
功用:滋阴补肾，降虚火。
主治:用于阴虚型斑秃、药疹、黄褐斑、过敏性紫癜、红斑性狼疮等。

〔附〕六味地黄汤
即上方水煎服。

Liu Yi San 六一散(49)   72,348
(Six to One Powder)

Source: Diagonosis and Treatment of Febrile Diseases 《伤寒标本》

Composition:
    Talcum 60 g   滑石   (*Huashi*)
    Radix Glycyrrhizae 10 g   甘草   (*Gancao*)

Manufacture: Grind the drugs into fine powder.

Administration: Take 9 g of it each time, or decoct it with other drugs.

Actions: Clearing away summer-heat and eliminating dampness.

Uses: Eczema, papular urticaria, sudamen, and so on.

制法:共为细末。
用法:每服9克,或入汤剂包煎。
功用:清暑利湿。
主治:湿疹、丘疹性荨麻疹、痱子等。

Longdan Xiegan Tang 龙胆泻肝汤(8)   22,30,33,77,81
(Decoction of Gentiana for Purging   83,99,100,114,115,139
the Liver-fire)   170,327,329,352,354,355,363,371,382,397,401

Source: The Golden Mirror of Medicine 《医宗金鉴》

Composition:
Radix Gen tianae 6 g   龙胆草 (*Longdancao*)
Fructus Capejasmine 9 g   栀子   (*Zhizi*)

Radix Scutellariae 12 g　　　　　黄芩　(*Huangqin*)
Radix Bupleuri 9 g　　　　　　　柴胡　(*Chaihu*)
Radix Rehmanniae 15 g　　　　　生地　(*Shengdi*)
Semen Plantaginis 9 g　　　　　　车前子(*Cheqianzi*)
Rhizoma Alismatis 9 g　　　　　　泽泻　(*Zexie*)
Caulis Aristolochiae Manshuriensis 6 g　木通　(*Mutong*)
Radix Angelicae Sinensis 9 g　　　当归　(*Danggui*)
Radix Glycyrrhizae 6 g　　　　　　甘草　(*Gancao*)

Actions: Removing damp-heat from the liver and the gallbladder.

Indications: Herpes zoster, culosis, eczema, etc.

It is especially effective in the case of damp-heat syndrome in the sternocostal area and pudendum.

Longdan Xiegan Wan

(Pill of Gentiana for Purging the Liver-fire, a Proprietary of the same ingredients as above).

Manufacture: Grind the drugs into fine powder, stir them thoroughly, and make into pills by mixing the powder with water.

Uses: Twice or three times daily, 6 g each time, accompanied by cool boiled-water. Actions and Uses are the same as has been listed above.

功用:清利肝胆湿热。

主治:带状疱疹、丹毒、湿疹等,尤适用于胸胁部及外阴部的湿热证。

〔附〕龙胆泻肝丸

即上方诸药,共研细末和匀,以水泛为丸。

用法:每次 6 克,每日 2～3 次,温开水送服。

Luganshi Xiji 炉甘石洗剂(87)   124,131,375,379
(Lotion of Calamina)

Source: External Medicine compiled by Guangzhou TCM College(广州中医学院主编《外科学》)

Composition:

Calamina 10 g	炉甘石	(*Luganshi*)
zinc oxide 5 g	氧化锌	(*Yanghuaxing*)
carbolic acid 1 ml	石炭酸	(*Shitansuan*)
glycerin 5 ml	甘油	(*Ganyou*)
water (or saturated lime water)100 ml	水	(*Shui*)

Administration: External application, twice or three times daily.

Actions: Antiinflammation and arrest itching.

Uses: nonexudative acute pruritic dermatosis, ex. eczema.

用法:外涂患处，每日 2～3 次。

功用:消炎止痒。

主治:用于无渗出的急性瘙痒性皮肤病如湿疹。

MaGui Geban Tang 麻桂各半汤(60)   88,357
(Decoction of Herba Ephedrae and Ramulus Cinnamami)

Source: Treatise on Febrile Diseases 《伤寒论》

Composition:

Ramulus Cinnamomi 9 g	桂枝	(*Guizhi*)
Radix Paeoniae Alba 12 g	芍药	(*Shaoyao*)
Rhizoma Zingiberis Recens 3 pieces	生姜	(*Shengjiang*)
fried Radix Glycyrrhizae 6 g	炙甘草	(*Zhigancao*)
Herba Ephedrae 6 g	麻黄	(*Mahuang*)
Fructus Ziziphi Jujubae 3 dates	大枣	(*Dazhao*)

Semen Armeniacae Amarum 9 g　　　杏仁　　(*Xingren*)

Actions: Regulating *Ying* and *Wei*, dispelling wind and arresting itching.

Uses: Urticaria, eczema, erythema multiforme, etc.

功用:调和营卫，祛风止痒。

主治:荨麻疹、湿疹、多形性红斑等。

Mituoseng Sang 密陀僧散(107)　　152,188,388,405,407
(Powder of Lithargyrum)

Source: Orthodox Mannual of External Diseases 《外科正宗》

Composition:

Sulphur 6 g	硫黄	(*Liuhuang*)
Realagr 6 g	雄黄	(*Xionghuang*)
Fructus Cnidii 6 g	蛇床子	(*Shechuangzi*)
Realgar 3 g	石黄	(*Shihuang*)
Lithargyrum 3 g	密陀僧	(*Mituoseng*)
Calomeas 1.5 g	轻粉	(*Qingfen*)

Manufacture: Grind the drugs together into fine powder.

Administration: Directly apply the powder to the diseased part or mix the medical powder with vinegar before application.

Action: Dispelling wind, destroying parasites and arresting itching.

Uses: Dermatomycosis microsporina, vitiligo tragomaschalia and so on.

制法:共为细末备用。

用法:直接外扑或醋调涂患处。

功用:祛风杀虫止痒。

主治:花斑癬、白癜风、腋臭等。

Nantong Sheyao Pian 南通蛇药片(42)   65,345
(a common proprietary for snake-poisoning)

Source: A mannual of Practical Chinese Patent Medicine 《实用中成药手册》

Adiministration: For the first time, take 5—20 pills, accompanied by an equal amount of liquor and warm water, then, every six hours, take 5—10 pills till the symptoms disappear.

Actions: Clear away heat and toxic material, subdue swelling and alleviate pain.

Uses: Snake-bite and other insect dermatitis with general symptoms

功用:清热解毒，消肿止痛。

主治:毒蛇咬伤等虫咬皮炎有全身症状者。

Pifu Ruan Gao 皮肤软膏(85)   55,120,141,340,373,383
(Ointment for Dermapathic USE)

Source: a prescription of the Affiliated Hospital of Shandong TCM College (山东中医学院附属医院方)

Composition:

    Salicylic acid 40 g   水杨酸   (*Shuiyangsuan*)
    benzoic acid 40 g   安息香酸(*Anxixiangsuan*)
    Sulphur Powder 40 g   硫磺粉   (*Liuhuangfen*)
    vaseline 500 g   凡士林   (*Fanshiling*)

Manufacture: Mix the above drugs thoroughly into an ointment.

Administration: Apply the ointment onto the diseased part,

once or twice daily.

Actions: Destroying parasites and arresting itching.

Uses: Hand-foot tinea, neurodermatitis, Psoriasis, and so on.

Huangsheng Pifu Ruan Gao
(another proprietary of the same ingredients)

Manufacture: Mix 3 g of Huangsheng Bolus with 30 g of each the above drugs.

Actions: The same as above, but with greater power of destroying parasites and arresting itching.

制法:将上药混合均匀,用凡士林调合成膏。

用法:外涂患处,日1~2次。

功用:杀虫止痒。

主治:手足癣、神经性皮炎、银屑病等。

〔附〕黄升皮肤软膏

即上药每30克药膏加入黄升丹3克即成。

功用:同上,唯杀虫、止痒作用更强。

Pipa Qing Fei Yin 枇杷清肺饮(114)　　168,172,397,399
(Decoction of Folium Eriobotryae for Removing Heat from the Lung)

Source: The Golden Mirror of Medicine 《医宗金鉴》

Composition:

Radix Ginseng 9 g	人参	(*Renshen*)
Folium Eriobotryae 12 g	枇杷叶	(*Pipaye*)
Rhizoma Coptidis 9 g	黄连	(*Huanglian*)
Cortex Phellodendri 9 g	黄柏	(*Huangbai*)
Cortex Mori Radicis 9 g	桑白皮	(*Sangbaipi*)

  Radix Glycyrrhizae 6 g   甘草 (*Gancao*)

Actions: Dispelling wind and clearing away lung-heat

Uses: Acne, rosacea, etc.

功用:疏风清肺。

主治:痤疮、酒渣鼻等。

Puji Xiaodu Yin 普济消毒饮(34)   47,335
(General Antiphlogistic Decoction)

Source: A Ten-volume Medical Book by Li Dong-huan 《东垣十书》

Composition:

Radix Scutellariae 15 g	黄芩	(*Huangqin*)
Rhizoma Coptidis 9 g	黄连	(*Huanglian*)
Radix Glycyrrhizae 6 g	生甘草	(*Shenggancao*)
Radix Scrophulariae 12 g	玄参	(*Xuanshen*)
Fructus Forsythiae 15 g	连翘	(*Lianqiao*)
Radix Isatidis 15 g	板蓝根	(*Banlangen*)
Lasiosphaera seu Calvatia 9 g	马勃	(*Mabo*)
Fructus Arctii 9 g	牛蒡子	(*Niubangzi*)
Herba Menthae 9 g	薄荷	(*Bohe*)
Bombyx Batryticatus 9 g	僵蚕	(*Jiangcan*)
Rhizoma Cimicifugae 6 g	升麻	(*Shengma*)
Radix Bupleuri 9 g	柴胡	(*Chaihu*)
Radix Platycodi 9 g	桔梗	(*Jugeng*)
Pericarpium Citri Reticulatae 9 g	陈皮	(*Chenpi*)

Actions: Removing heat and toxic material; expelling wind to subdue swelling.

Indications: skin and diseases showing yang syndrome; facial erysipelas, acute cervical lymphadenitis, etc.

功用:清热解毒，疏风消肿。

主治:疮疡阳证及颜面丹毒，急性颈部淋巴结炎。

Qibao Meiran Dan 七宝美髯丹(119)　　　　182,403
(Bolus of Seven Drugs for Nourishing Hair)

Source: A Collection of Prescriptions by Shao Yingjie 《邵应节方》

Composition:

Radix Polygoni Multiflori	首乌	(*Shouwu*)
Radix Achyranthis Bidentatae	牛膝	(*Niuxi*)
Radix Angelicae Sinensis	当归	(*Danggui*)
Fructus Psoraleae	补骨脂	(*Buguzhi*)
Poria	茯苓	(*Fuling*)
Semen Cuscutae	菟丝子	(*Tusizi*)
Fructus Lycil	枸杞子	(*Gouqizi*)

Manufacture: Grind the drugs into fine powder and make boluses by mixing the powder with honey.

Administration: 9 g each time, twice to 3 times daily.

Actions: Enriching the blood; strengthening the body; nourishing hair.

Uses: Hoary hair, alopecia areata, seborrheic dermatitis, etc.

制法:共研细末，炼蜜为丸。

用法:每服9克，日服2~3次。

功用:补血强身，乌须生发。

主治:白发、斑秃、脂溢性脱发等。

Qingge San 青蛤散(18)   25,324
(Powder of Indigo Naturalis and Calcining Rana Temporarie)

Source: The Golden Mirror of Medicine 《医宗金鉴》
Composition:

calcined Gypsum Fibrosum 30 g	煅石膏	(*Duanshigao*)
calcined Rana Temporaria 30 g	煅蛤粉	(*Duangefen*)
Indigo Naturalis 9 g	青黛	(*Qingdai*)
Cortex Phellodendri 1.5 g	黄柏	(*Huangbai*)
Calomeas 1.5 g	轻粉	(*Qingfen*)

Manufacture: Grind the medicinal herbs into fine powder for use.

Adiministration: In the case of exudation, sprinkle the powder on the diseased part, but in the case of pachyderma with xerosis cutis, mix the powder with sesame oil into an ointment for external application.

Action: Clearing away heat and eliminating dampness.

Uses: Eczema, especially infantile eczema.

制法:共研细末备用。
用法:局部渗液者，用药粉撒布患处，如皮肤肥厚干裂者，可以用麻油调和外搽患处。
功用:清热燥湿。
主治:湿疹，尤对婴儿湿疹有良好疗效。

Qingji Shenshi Tang 清肌渗湿汤(125)   190,408
(Decoction for Easing the Skin and Excreting Dampness)

Source: The Golden Mirror of Medicine 《医宗金鉴》
Composition:

Rhizoma Atractylodis 9 g　　　　　苍术(Cangzhu)
Cortex Magnoliae Officinalis 9 g　　厚朴(Houpu)
Pericarpium Citri Reticulatae 9 g　　陈皮(Chenpi)
Radix Glycyrrhizae 6 g　　　　　　甘草(Gancao)
Radix Bupleuri 9 g　　　　　　　　柴胡(Chaihu)
Caulis Aristolochiae Manshuriensis 6 g　木通(Mutong)
Rhizoma Alismatis 9 g　　　　　　　泽泻(Zhexie)
Radix Angelicae Dahuricae 9 g　　　白芷(Baizhi)
Rhizoma Cimicifugae 6 g　　　　　　升麻(Shenma)
Rhizoma Atractylodis 9 g　　　　　　白术(Baizhu)
Fructus Capejasmine 9 g　　　　　　栀子(Zhizi)
Rhizoma Coptidis 9 g　　　　　　　黄连(Huanglian)

Action: Easion the skin and excreting dampness; strengthening the spleen and stomach.

Uses: Erythema multiforme, etc.

功用:清肌渗湿，健脾和胃。

主治:多形性红斑等。

Qing Pi Chushi Yin 清脾除湿饮(77)　　　　107,367
(Decoction for Clearing away Heat and Dampness from the Spleen)

Source: The Golden Mirror of Medicine 《医宗金鉴》

Composition:

Rhizoma Atractylodis 9 g　　　　　　　　苍术　(Cangzhu)
Rhizoma Atractylodis Macrocephalae 9 g　白术　(Baizhu)
Radix Paeoniae Rubra 9 g　　　　　　　　赤芍　(Chishao)
Cortex Phellodendri 9 g　　　　　　　　　黄柏　(Huangbai)
Fructus Capejasmine 9 g　　　　　　　　栀子　(Zhizi)

Herba Artemisiae Capillaris 9 g　　茵陈　(*Yinchen*)
Fructus Aurantii 9 g　　枳壳　(*Jike*)
Rhizoma Alismatis 9 g　　泽泻　(*Zhexie*)
Fructus Forsythiae 12 g　　连翘　(*Lianqiao*)
Radix Rehmanniae 12 g　　生地　(*Shengdi*)
Radix Ophiopogonis 9 g　　麦冬　(*Maidong*)
Radix Glycyrrhizae 6 g　　甘草　(*Gancao*)
Herba Lopatheri 9 g　　竹叶　(*Zhuye*)
Medulla Junci 3 g　　灯心草　(*Dengxingcao*)
Natrii Sulfas Exsiccatus 3 g　　玄明粉　(*Xuanmingfen*)

Actions: Clearing away heat and toxic material; strengthening the spleen and stomach.

Uses: Acute eczema, seborrheic dermatitis, herpetic dermatosis, and so on.

功用:清热解毒，健脾和胃。

主治:急性湿疹、脂溢性皮炎、疱疹性皮肤病等。

Qingshu Tang 清暑汤(48)　　　　　　　　　71,348
(Decoction for Clearing Away Summer-heat)

Source: Life-saving Mannual of Diagonosis and Treatment of External Diseases 《外科全生集》

Composition:

Fructus Forsythiae 21 g　　连翘　(*Lianqiao*)
Radix Trichosanthis 15 g　　花粉　(*Huafen*)
Radix Paeoniae Rubra 15 g　　赤芍　(*Chishao*)
Talcum 9 g　　滑石　(*Huashi*)
Semen Plantaginis 9 g　　车前子　(*Cheqianzi*)
Flos Lonicerae 21 g　　金银花　(*Jinyinhua*)

Rhizoma Alismatis 9 g　　　泽泻　(Zexie)
Herba Lophatheri 9 g　　　竹叶　(Zhuye)
Radix Glycyrrhizae 6 g　　　甘草　(Gancao)

Actions: Clearing away summer-heat, eliminating dampness and reducing fever.

Uses: Impetigo herpetiformis, sudamen, summer boil and so on.

功用:清暑、解热、化湿。

主治:脓疱疮、痱子、暑疖等。

Qingwen Baidu Yin 清温败毒饮(73)　　　105,163,366,394
(Antipyretic and Antitoxic Decoction)

Source: A View of Epidemic Febrile Diseases with Rashes 《疫疹一得》

Composition:

Gypsum Fibrosum　　　生石膏　(Shengshigao)
Radix Rehmanniae　　　生地黄　(Shengdihuang)
Cornu Rhinocerotis　　　犀角　(Xijiao)
Herba Lophatheri　　　鲜竹叶　(Xiaozhuye)
Rhizoma Coptidis　　　黄连　(Huanglian)
Fructus Capejasmine　　　栀子　(Zhizi)
Radix Platycodi　　　桔梗　(Jugeng)
Radix Scutellariae　　　黄芩　(Huangqin)
Rhizoma Anemarrhenae　　　知母　(Zhimu)
Radix Scrophulariae　　　玄参　(Xuanshen)
Fructus Forsythiae　　　连翘　(Lianqiao)
Radix Glycyrrhizae　　　甘草　(Gancao)
Cortex Moutan Radicis　　　丹皮　(Danpi)

Actions: Removing pathogenic heat and toxic material from the blood.

Uses: Contact dermatitis, dermatitis medicamentosa, lupus erythematosus, and that which show syndrome of excessive noxious heat.

Qingwen Baidu Wan
(another proprietary, pill of the same ingredients)

Manufacture: Grind the drugs into fine powder and make pellets with it.

功用:清热凉血解毒。

主治:接触性皮炎、药物性皮炎、红斑性狼疮而热毒炽盛者。

〔附〕清瘟败毒丸
　　　即上药研末制丸。

Qingying Tang 清营汤(98) 140,383
(Decoction for Clearing Heat in the Ying System)

Source: Treatise on Differentiation and Treatment of Epidemic Febrile Diseases 《温病条辨》

Composition:

Cornu Rhinocerotis 6 g	犀角	(*Xijiao*)
Radix Rehmenniae 21 g	生地	(*Shengdi*)
Radix Scrophulariae 15 g	玄参	(*Xuanshen*)
Herba Lophatheri 9 g	竹叶心	(*Zhuyexing*)
Flos Lonicerae 30 g	金银花	(*Jinyinhua*)
Fructus Forsythiae 21 g	连翘	(*Lianqiao*)
Rhizoma Coptidis 9 g	黄连	(*Huanglian*)
Radix Salviae Miltiorrhize 15 g	丹参	(*Danshen*)

Radix Ophiopogonis 15 g 麦冬 (*Maidong*)

Actions: Clearing up the *Ying* system and removing toxic substances; replenishing the vital essence and removing heat.

Uses: Dermatitis medicamentosa, erysipelas, purpura, lupus erythematosus, chickenpox, etc.

功用:清营解毒，养阴泄热。

主治:药物性皮炎、丹毒、紫癜、红斑性狼疮、水痘等。

Qinjiu Wan 秦艽丸(55) 78,84,114,352,355,370,373
(Pill of Radix Gentianae Macrophyllae)

Source: The Golden Mirror of Medicine 《医宗金鉴》
Composition:

Radix Gentianae Macrophyllae 30 g 秦艽 (*Qinjiu*)
Radix Sophorae Flavenscentis 30 g 苦参 (*Kushen*)
Radix et Rhizoma Rhei 30 g 大黄 (*Dahuang*)
Radix Astragali seu Hedysari 60 g 黄芪 (*Huangqi*)
Radix Ledebouriellae 45 g 防风 (*Fangfeng*)
Radix Rhapontici seu Echinopsis 45 g 漏芦 (*Loulu*)
Rhizoma Coptidis 45 g 黄连 (*Huanglian*)
Zaocys 15 g 乌蛇肉(*Wusherou*)

Manufacture: Grind the drugs into fine powder, make pellets by mixing the medical powder with honey, each pellet weighing 9 g.

Administration: Take one pill each time, twice daily accompanied by warm boiled water.

Actions: Dispelling wind, arresting itching and regulating *Qi* and blood.

Uses: Lupus erythematosus discoides, neurodermatitis,

chronicity eczema, skin pruritus, lupus rulgaris, systemic lupus erythematosus, dermatasclerosis; and as assisting treatment for dermatomyositis during convalescence.

制法:共为细粉,炼蜜为丸,每丸重9克。
用法:每服1丸,日2次,温开水送服。
功用:散风止痒,调和气血。
主治:盘状红斑性狼疮、神经性皮炎、慢性湿疹、皮肤瘙痒症、寻常狼疮、以及系统红斑性狼疮、硬皮病、皮肌炎恢复期的辅助治疗

Qufeng Xiyao 祛风洗药(15)   25,51,84,115,119,
(Lotion for Dispelling Wind)   338,356,371,373

Source: a prescription of the Hospital Affiliated to Shandong TCM College (山东中医学院附属医院方)

Composition:

Radix Aconiti 15 g	生川乌 (*Shengchuanwu*)
Radix Aconiti Kusnezoffii 10 g	生草乌 (*Shengcaowu*)
Spina Gleditsiae 15 g	皂角 (*Zaojiao*)
Fructus Arctii 15 g	牛蒡子 (*Niubangzi*)
Herba Schizonepetae 15 g	荆芥 (*Jingjie*)
Radix Ledebouriellae 15 g	防风 (*Fangfeng*)
Herba Lycopi 15 g	泽兰叶 (*Zelanye*)
Radix Sophrae Flavenscentis 15 g	苦参 (*Kushen*)
Fructus Cnidii 15 g	蛇床子 (*Shechuangzi*)
Radix Paeoniae Rubra 15 g	赤芍 (*Chishao*)
Pericarpium Zanthoxyli 15 g	川椒 (*Chuanjiao*)
Cortex Dictamni Radicis 15 g	白藓皮 (*Baixianpi*)
Fructus Carpesii 15 g	鹤虱 (*Heshi*)

Semen Hydnocarpi 24 g 大枫子(*Dafengzi*)
Cortex Moutan Radicis 10 g 丹皮 (*Danpi*)

Administration: Decoct the drugs and rinse the diseased part in the decoction while it is still hot; Once or twice daily, 30 minuntes each time.

Actions: Dispelling pathogenic wind, eliminating dampness, destroying parasites and relieving itching.

Uses: Hand-foot tinea, tinea cruris, tinea corporis, cutaneous pruritus, neurodermatitis, chronic eczema, and so on.

用法：上药煎汤，乘热熏洗患处，每日1~2次，每次30分钟。
功用：祛风燥湿，杀虫止痒。
主治：手足癣、股癣、体癣等，以及皮肤瘙痒病、神经性皮炎、慢性湿疹等。

Renshen Jianpi Wan 人参健脾丸(113)　　109,166,368,395
(Bolus of Ginseng for Strengthening the Spleen).

Source: Complete Works of Zhang Jingyue 《景岳全书》
Composition:

Radix Ginseng 9 g	人参	(*Renshen*)
Fructus Amomi 9 g	砂仁	(*Sharen*)
Fructus Aurantii 9 g	枳壳	(*Zhike*)
Radix Glycyrrhizae 6 g	甘草	(*Gancao*)
Rhizoma Dioscoreae 12 g	山药	(*Shanyao*)
Rhizoma Atractylodis Macrocephalae 12 g	木香	(*MuXiang*)
Fructus Oryzae Germinatus 12 g	薏苡仁	(*Yiyiren*)
Semen Dolichoris Album 9 g	山楂	(*Shanzha*)
Semen Euryales 9 g	白术	(*Baizhu*)
Semen Nelumbinis 9 g	谷芽	(*Guya*)

Pericarpium Citri Reticulatae 9 g　　　白扁豆(*Baibiandou*)
Pericarpium Citri Reticulatae Viride 9 g　芡实　(*Qianshi*)
Radix Angelicae Sinensis 9 g　　　　　莲子肉(*Lianzirou*)
Massa Fermentata Medicinalis 9 g　　　陈皮　(*Chenpi*)
Fructus Crataegi 15 g　　　　　　　　青皮　(*Qingpi*)
Radix Aucklandiae 9 g　　　　　　　　当归　(*Danggui*)
Semem Coicis 15 g　　　　　　　　　六神曲(*Liushenqu*)

　　Manufacture: Grind the drugs into fine powder and make boluses by mixing the powder with honey, each bolus weighing 6 g.

　　Administration: One or two boluses each time, twice to 3 times daily.

　　Actions: Strengthening the spleen and stomach; preventing vomiting.

　　Uses: Protracted dermatoses or other serious diseases showing morbid condition of weakness of the spleen and stomach.

制法:共研细末，炼蜜为丸，每丸重6克
用法:每服1～2丸，日2～3次。
功用:健脾，和胃，止呕。
主治:皮肤病久病或重病，出现脾胃虚弱之证者。

Runfu Gao 润肤膏(27)　　　　　　　27,70,325,347
(Ointment for Moistening the Skin)

　　Source: a prescription of the Hospital Affiliated to Shandong TCM College (山东中医学院附属医院方)

　　Composition:
　　　Radix Angelicae Dahuricas 9 g　　　白芷　(*Baizhi*)
　　　Radix Angelicae Sinensis 9 g　　　　当归　(*Danggui*)

  Colophonium 6 g   松香 (*Shongxiang*)
  Oleum Sesami 30 g   麻油 (*Mayou*)
  Pig Fat 30 g   猪油 (*Zhuyou*)
  Cera Flava 30 g   蜂蜡 (*Fengla*)

  Manufacture: Fry the Radix Angelicae Dahuricae and Radix Angelicae Simensis in sesame oil and pig fat, then remove the drugs from the oil, put the Cera Flava in and stir it until the cera flava is dissolved, then, after moving it away from ppthe fire, put in the powder of Colophonium and stir it again.

  Adiministration: External application.

  Actions: Moisturizing the skin and promoting tissue regeneration.

  Uses: Rhagades of hand and foot.

  制法:麻油猪油炸白芷、当归，去渣，纳入蜂蜡搅至溶化，离火再入松香粉搅匀即成。

  用法:外涂患处，润肤生肌。

  主治:手足皲裂。

Runfu Wan 润肤丸(56)   78,84,119,352,355,373
(Pills for Nourishing the Skin)

  Source: a prescription of the Dermatology Section of Beijing TCM Hospital (北京中医医院皮肤科方)

  Composition:

 Semen Persicae 30 g   桃仁 (*Taoren*)
 Flos Carthami 30 g   红花 (*Honghua*)
 Radix Rehmanniae Praeparatae 30 g   熟地 (*Shudi*)
 Radix Angelicae Pubescentis 30 g   独活 (*Duhuo*)
 Radix Ledebouriellae 30 g   防风 (*Fangfeng*)

Radix Stephaniae Tetrandrae 30 g　　防己　(Fangji)
Rhizoma Ligustici Chuangxiong 45 g　川芎　(Chuanxiong)
Radix Angelicae Sinensis 45 g　　　 当归　(Danggui)
Cortex Moutan Radicis 45 g　　　　 丹皮　(Danpi)
Rhizoma seu Radix Notopterygii 60 g　羌活　(Qianghuo)
Radix Rehmanniae 60 g　　　　　　 生地　(Shengdi)
Cortex Dictamni Radicis 60 g　　　　白藓皮(Baixianpi)

Manufacture: Grind the drugs into fine powder, and make pellets by mixing the medical powder with water

Administration: Take 3 g to 6 g each time, twice daily accompanied by warm boiled water.

Actions: Promoting blood circulation and moisturizing the skin, dispelling wind and arresting itching.

Uses: Psoriasis, ichthyosiform, seborrheic eczema, eczema rhagadiforme, and other keratosis, hypertrophica dermatosis.

制法:共为细粉，水泛小丸。
用法:每服3～6克，日服2次，温开水送服。
功用:活血润肤，散风止痒。
主治:银屑病、鱼鳞病、脂溢性湿疹、皲裂性湿疹等。

Runji Gao 润肌膏(46)　　　　　　　　　　70,347
(Ointment for Nourishing the Skin and Muscles)

Source: Orthodox Mannual of External Diseases 《外科正宗》

Composition:
Oleum Sesami 120 ml　　　　　　　　麻油　(Mayou)
Radix Angelicae Sinensis 15 g　　　　 当归　(Danggui)
Radix Arnebiae seu Lithospermi 3 g　　紫草　(Zicao)

Cera Flava 15 g　　　　　　黄蜡　(*Huangla*)

Manufacture: Fry the Radix Angelicae Sinensis and Radix Arnebiae in the Oleum Sesami till they become brown, then filter them out, add the Cera Flava in the oil to be melted, and then pour it into a bowl to be cooled down for use.

Administration: External application, once or twice daily.

Actions: Moistening the skin, removing heat from the blood and relieving itching.

Uses: Rhagade, ptogtrudive metacarpophalangeal keratosis, etc.

制法:前三药同熬至药枯滤清，将油再熬入黄蜡化尽，倾入碗内，待冷而成。

用法:外涂患处，每天1~2次。

功用:润肤、凉血、止痒。

主治:皲裂疮、白屑风等证。

Sang Ju Yin 桑菊饮(71)
(Decoction of Mulberry Leaf and Chrysanthemum)

Source: Treatise on Differentiation and Treafment of Epidemic Febrile Diseases 《温病条辨》

Composition:

Folium Mori 9 g	桑叶	(*Sangye*)
Flos Chrysanthemi 9 g	菊花	(*Juhua*)
Semen Armeniacae Amarum 9 g	杏仁	(*Xingren*)
Fructus Forsythiae 15 g	连翘	(*Lianqiao*)
Herba Menthae 9 g	薄荷	(*Bohe*)
Radix Platycodi 9 g	桔梗	(*Jugeng*)
Rhizoma Phragmitis 15 g	芦根	(*Lugen*)

Radix Glycyrrhizae 6 g 甘草 (*Gancao*).

Actions: Dispelling wind and clearing away heat.

Uses: Urticaria, Pityriasis rosea, erythema multiforme, etc., showing wind-heat syndrome.

功用:疏风清热。

主治:风热型荨麻疹、玫瑰糠疹、多形红斑等。

San Huang Wan 三黄丸(126)   191,408
(Bolus of Three Ingredients)

Source: A Ten-volume Medical Book by Li Dong-huan 《东垣十书》

Composition:

  Rhizoma Coptidis 9 g   黄连 (*Huanglian*)
  Radix Scutellariae 15 g   黄芩 (*Huangqin*)
  Radix et Rhizoma Rhei 9 g   大黄 (*Dahuang*)

Manufacture: Grind the drugs into fine powder and make boluses by mixing the powder with honey or with rice-paste.

Administration: 6 g to 9 g each time, twice or 3 times daily.

Actions: Clearing away internal heat.

Uses: Dermatosis with oral ulcer, restlessness; loss of appetite; scanty dark urine, constipation.

制法:共研细末,炼蜜或米糊为丸。

用法:每服6~9克,日2~3次。

功用:清除内热。

主治:皮肤病伴口舌生疮,心烦纳呆,小便赤涩,大便秘结者。

San Jie Pian 散洁片 (116)
(Bolus for Resolving Hard Masses)

Source: a prescriptions of the Affiliated Hospital of Shandong TCM College (山东中医学院附属医院方)

Composition:

Radix Bupleuri	柴胡	(*Chaihu*)
Concha Ostreae	生牡蛎	(*Shengmuli*)
Radix Ranunculi Ternati	猫爪草	(*Maozhuacao*)
Radix Salviae Miltiorrhizae	丹参	(*Danshen*)
Radix Scrophulariae	玄参	(*Xunshen*)
Rhizoma Cyperi	香附	(*Xiangfu*)
Radix Paeoniae Alba	白芍	(*Baishao*)
Radix Curcumae	郁金	(*Yujin*)
Exocarpium Citri Reticulatae	桔红	(*Juhong*)
Bulbus Fritillariae	土贝母	(*Tubeimu*)
Flos Carthami	红花	(*Honghua*)
Rhizoma Pleionis	山慈菇	(*Shancigu*)
Rhizoma Ligustici Chuanxiong	川芎	(*Chuanxiong*)
Radix Angelicae Sinesis	当归	(*Danggui*)
Thallus Eckloniae	昆布	(*Kunbu*)
Spica Prunellae	夏枯草	(*Xiaokucao*)
Sargassum	海藻	(*Haizhao*)
Radix Scutellariae	黄芩	(*Huangqin*)
Radix Semiaquilegiae	天葵子	(*Tiankuizi*)

Manufacture: Obtain juice from Radix Bupleuri and Concha Ostreae, mix the juice with the powder of the other drugs to make boluses, each weighing 0.3 g.

Administration: 10 tablets each time, three times daily; the dose for infants should be reduced.

Actions: Relieving the depressed liver; resolving phlegm and softening hard masses.

Uses: Erythema nodosum, prurigo nodularis, tuberculoderm, keloid, etc.

制法：煎海藻、昆布取浓液，余药为细末，制片，每片0.3克。
用法：每次10片，每日3次，小儿酌减。
功用：舒肝理气，化痰散结。
主治：结节性红斑、结节性痒疹、皮肤结核、瘢痕疙瘩等。

Sanshi Shui 三石水(88)   124,375
(Sanshi Ointment)

Source: Collection of Clinical Experience of Zhu Yongkang 《朱仁康临床经验集》

Composition:

Calamina 90 g	炉甘石	(*Luganshi*)
Talcum 90 g	滑石	(*Huashi*)
Halloysitum Rubrum 90 g	赤石脂	(*Chishizhi*)
Borneolum 9 g	冰片	(*Binpian*)
glycerin 150 ml	甘油	(*Ganyou*)

Manufacture: Grind the above drugs except the glycer in into fine powder and then mix it with 10000 ml of distilled water and the glycerin.

Administration: External application, twice or three times daily.

Actions: Astringing dampness and arresting itching.

Uses: Nonexudative pruritic dermatosis, such as eczema, skin pruritus, etc.

制法:上药除甘油外研成细粉,加入蒸馏水10000毫升,再加甘油配成。
用法:外涂患处,每日2~3次。
功用:收湿止痒。
主治:湿疹、皮肤瘙痒症等瘙痒性皮肤病无渗液者。

Shen fu Tang 参附汤(106)　　　　　　　151,388
(Decoction of Ginseng and Prepared Aconite)

Source: The Complete Effective Prescriptions for Women 《妇人良方》

Composition:

Radix Ginseng 9 g	人参	(Renshen)
Radix Aconiti Praeparatae 15 g	熟附汤	(Shufutang)

Actions: Recuperating depleted *Yang* and rescuing the patient from collapse.

Uses: Allergic Drug rash, lupus erythematosus, etc, with cold clammy extremities and spontaneous cold perspiration.

功用:回阳救逆。
主治:药疹、红斑性狼疮等出现四肢厥冷、冷汗自出者。

Shengji Yuhong Gao 生肌玉红膏(128)　　　152,388
(Ointment for Replenishing the Skin and Flesh)

Source: Orthodox Mannual of External Diseases 《外科正宗》

Composition:

Radix Angelicae Sinensis 60 g	当归	(Danggui)
Radix Angelicae Dahuricae 15 g	白芷	(Baizhi)
honey 60 g	白蜡	(Baila)

Calomeas 12 g	轻粉	(*Qingfen*)
Resina Draconis 12 g	血竭	(*Xuejie*)
Radix Arnebiae seu Lithospermi 6 g	紫草	(*Zhicao*)
Radix Glycyrrhizae 36 g	甘草	(*Gancao*)
Oleum Sesami 500 g	麻油	(*Mayou*)

Manufacture: Soak in sesame oil for three days the following drugs; Radix Angelicae Sinensis and Radix Angelicae Dahuricae, then simmer it until they become brown before filtering them out. Afterwards, put in honey to be thoroughly melted. When the oil cools down slightly, put in the Resina Draconis and Calomeas, stir it to mix them thoroughly, and the ointment will be ready for use when the mixture has cooled down.

Administration: Spread the ointment evenly on a piece of gauze and apply it to the diseased part. Some pieces of the ointment gauze can be made beforehand for dressing change.

Actions: Removing slough and promoting tissue regeneration.

Uses: Chronic ulcer on the lower legs, Behcets syndrome, lupus erythematosus, etc.

制法：麻油浸当归、白芷、紫草、甘草3日，文火熬枯去渣，入白蜡化尽，待油温后，再入血竭、轻粉搅匀，冷后即成膏。

用法：将膏匀涂纱布上外敷患处。或制成玉红膏油纱布，以备换药用。

功用：祛腐生肌。

主治：小腿慢性溃疡、白塞氏综合征、红斑性狼疮等。

Shengmai San 生脉散(103) 149,387
(Pulse-activating Powder)

Source: Treatise on Internal and External Injuries 《内外伤辨惑论》

Composition:
Radix Ginseng 9 g	人参	(Renshen)
Radix Ophiopogonis 15 g	麦冬	(Maidong)
Fructus Schisandrae 9 g	五味子	(Wuweizi)

Actions: Supplementing *Qi* and promoting the production of body fluid.

Uses: Lupus erythematosus, dermatomysitis, dermatasclerosis and drug rash, due to deficiency of both *Qi* and *Yin*.

功用:益气生津。

主治:用于气阴不足之红斑性狼疮、皮肌炎、硬皮病、药疹等。

Shenjing Gao 伸筋膏(86) 120,373
(Shenjing Ointment)

Source: Practical Traditional Chinese External Medicine by Shang Dejun 《实用中医外科学》

Composition:

Thirty-two drugs including
Semen Strychni	马前子	(Maqianzi)
Lumbricus	地龙	(Dilong)

Manufacture: Fry the drugs in 2 kg of sesame oil until they become brown, then filter them out, heat the oil again, and when the temprature of the oil reaches the point where water, if added to it, would immediately turn into small spheres, put in 1 kg of Pb304.

Administration: Soften the ointment by soaking it in hot water and spread it on a piece of thick cloth before applying it to the diseased part.

Actions: Promoting blood circulation; removing blood stasis; relaxing muscles and tendons; alleviating pain.

Uses: Dermatomyositis, dermatasclerosis, lupus erythematosus, arthropsoriasis, neurodermatitis, etc.

制法:用麻油四斤将药炸枯，过滤去渣，再将油加热至滴水成珠时，下漳丹2斤即成。

用法:临用时将膏药用热水泡软，再均匀摊于厚布上，外贴患处。

功用:活血散瘀，舒筋止痛。

主治:皮肌炎、硬皮病、红斑性狼疮、关节型银屑病、神经性皮炎等。

Shenjingxing Piyan Yaoshui 神经性皮炎药水(83) (Medicine for Neurodermatitis)

Source: A Mannual of Practical Chinese Patent Medicine by Song Lianzhu 《实用中成药手册》

Composition:

Rumex Japonicus Houtt	羊蹄跟	(*Yangtigen*)
Rhizoma Pinelliae	生半夏	(*Shengbanxia*)
Rhizoma Arisaematis	生南星	(*Shengnanxing*)
Radix Aconiti	生川乌	(*Shengchuanwu*)
Radix Aconiti Kusnezoffii	生草乌	(*Shengcaowu*)
Rhododendron molle	闹洋花	(*Naoyanghua*)
Secretio bufonis	蟾酥	(*Chanshu*)
Fructus Piperis Longi	荜茇	(*Biba*)

Herba Asari　　　　　　　细辛　　(*Xixin*)
Cortex Pseudolaricis　　　土槿皮　(*Tujinpi*)

Manufacture: Soak the drugs in a proper amount of alcohol for a week before filtering them out, leaving the liquid for medical use.

Administration: Apply the medicine to the diseased part, twice or three times daily.

Actions: Dispelling wind, arresting itching and destroying parasites.

Uses: Neurodermatitis and all sorts of tinea.

制法:酒精适量，浸泡上药1周，过滤后备用。

用法:外涂患处，日2~3次。

功用:祛风止痒，杀虫。

主治:神经性皮炎及各种癣症。

Shen Jin Pian 伸筋片(111)　　　158,166,392,395
(*Shenjin* Pill)

Source: a prescription of the Affiliated Hospital of Shandong TCM College (山东中医学院附属医院方)

Composition:

Resina Olibani 9 g	乳香	(*Ruxiang*)
Myrrha 9 g	没药	(*Moyao*)
prepared Semen Strychni 1 g	制马前子	(*Zhimaqianzi*)
Herba Ephedrae 6 g	麻黄	(*Mahuang*)
Lumbricus 9 g	地龙	(*Dilong*)
Radix Ephedrae Charcoal 6 g	麻根炭	(*Magentan*)
Cortex Acanthopanacis Radicis 9 g	五加皮	(*Wujiapi*)
Resina Draconis 9 g	血竭	(*Xuejie*)

Radix Stephaniae Tetrandrae 9 g　　防己　　(*Fangji*)
Rhizoma Drynariae 9 g　　　　　　骨碎补　(*Gusuibu*)

Manufacture: Grind the drugs into fine powder and make pills with it, each pill weighing 0.3 g.

Administration: 6 tablets each time for adults, three times daily; the dose should be reduced for infants.

Actions: Promoting blood circulation and softening hard masses; promoting the flow of *Qi* by warming the channels; dispelling wind and relaxing muscles.

Uses: Psoriasis, dermatomyositis and erythema nodosum, etc. Which are accompanied by arthralgia and difficulty in bending and stretching the limbs.

制法:共为细末，制成0.3克片。
用法:成人每次服6片，日3次，小儿酌减。
功用:活血软坚，温经通络，散风舒筋。
主治:硬皮病、皮肌炎、结节性红斑等伴有关节酸痛、屈伸不利者。

Shenying Yangzhen Dan 神应养真丹(12)　　23,181,323,403
(Nourishing Bolus)

Source: Orthodox Manual of External Diseases 《外科正宗》

Composition:

Radix Angelicae Sinensis	当归	(*Danggui*)
Rhizoma Ligustici Chuangxiong	川芎	(*Chuanxiong*)
Radix Paeoniae Alba	白芍	(*Baishao*)
Radix Rehmanniae Praeparata	熟地	(*Shudi*)
Rhizoma Gastrodiae	天麻	(*Tianma*)

Rhizoma Seu Radix Notopterygii 羌活 (*Qianghuo*)
Semen Cuscutae 菟丝子 (*Tusizi*)
Fructus Chaenomelis 木瓜 (*Mugua*)

Actions: Enriching the blood, moistening dryness, expelling the wind and regulating blood flow.

Indications: Alopecia areata, seborrheic baldness, etc.

Manufacture: Grind the drugs into fine powder and make boluses by mixing the powder with water.

Administration: 9 g each time, three times daily.

功用:养血润燥，祛风活血。

主治:斑秃、脂溢性脱发等。

制法:上药共为细末，水泛为丸。

用法:每次9克，日3次。

Shihui Wan 十灰丸(72)　　　　　　　　105,366
(Pill made of Ashes of Ten Drugs)

Source: A miraculous Book of Ten Prescriptions 《十药神书》

Composition: (Ashes of the following drugs)

Herba seu Radix Cirsii Japonici 大蓟炭 (*Dajitan*)
Herba Cephalanoploris 小蓟炭 (*Xiaojitan*)
Cortex Moutan Radicis 牡丹皮炭 (*Mudanpitan*)
Cacumen Biotae 侧柏叶炭 (*Cebaiyetan*)
Radix et Rhizoma Rhei 大黄炭 (*Dahuangtan*)
Radix Rubiae 茜草炭 (*Xicaotan*)
Fructus Capejasmine 栀子炭 (*Zhizitan*)
Folium Nelumbinis 陈棕炭 (*Chenzhongtan*)
Palma 荷叶炭 (*Heyetan*)

Rhizoma Imperatae　　　　　白茅根炭(*Baimaogentan*)
(Same amount of each)

Manufacture: Grind the above ingredients into fine powder and make pellets by mixing the powder with the decoction of Rhizoma Bletillae.

Administration: 9 g each time, twice daily.

Actions: Removing pathogenic heat from blood; arresting bleeding.

Uses: Pigmented purpuric dermatosis

制法:共研细末，以白芨煎汤泛为丸。
用法:每次服9克，日服2次。
功用:清热凉血，涩血止血。
主治:色素性紫癜性皮肤病。

Shiquan Dabu Tang 十全大补汤(62)　　91,102,158,165,166
(Decoction of Ten Powerful Tonics)　　　359,360,392,395

Source: Medical Inventions 《医学发明》
Composition:

Radix Rehmanniae Preparata 15 g	熟地	(*Shudi*)
Radix Paeoniae Alba 15 g	白芍	(*Baishao*)
Radix Angelicae Sinensis 15 g	当归	(*Danggui*)
Rhizoma Ligustici Chuangxiong 12 g	川芎	(*Chuanxiong*)
Radix Codonopsis Pilosulae 15 g	党参	(*Dangshen*)
Rhizoma Atractylodis 15 g	白术	(*Baizhu*)
Poria 15 g	茯苓	(*Fuling*)
Radix Astragali seu Hedysari	黄芪	(*Huangqi*)
Cortex Cinnamomi 6 g	肉桂	(*Rougui*)
fried Radix Glycyrrihizae 6 g	炙甘草	(*Zhigancao*)

Actions: Invigorating *Qi* and blood

Uses: anaphase of pyogenic dermatosis; lupus erythematosus due to deficicency of both *Qi* and blood; dermatasclerosis, dermatomyositis, allergic drug rash, allergic purpura, etc.

Shiquan Dabu Wan
(Pill of Ten Powerful Tonics)

Manufacture: Grind the above drugs into fine powder, make pills by mixing the powder with honey.

Administration: Take 9 g each time, twice or three times daily.

功用:大补气血。

主治:用于化脓性皮肤病后期，及气血两亏的红斑性狼疮、硬皮病、皮肌炎、药疹、过敏性紫癜等。

〔附〕 十全大补丸

即上方诸药研末，炼蜜为丸。

用法:每次服9克，日2～3次。

Shizhen San 湿疹散(57)　　　　　78,94,119,352,361
(Powder for Eczema)

Source: a practical proved prescription (经验方)

Composition:

Rhizoma Coptidis 3 g	黄连	(*Huanglian*)
Cortex Phellodendri 9 g	黄柏	(*Huangbai*)
Indigo Naturalis 9 g	青黛	(*Qingdai*)
Borax 9 g	月石	(*Yueshi*)
Herba Menthae 3 g	薄荷	(*Bohe*)
Borneolum 3 g	冰片	(*Bingpian*)

Alumen Exsiccatum 12 g　　　枯矾　(Kufan)
Catechu 6 g　　　　　　　　　儿茶　(Ercha)

Manufacture: Grind the drugs into fine powder.

Administration: Spread the powder on the diseased part.

Actions: Clearing away heat and eliminating dampness.

Uses: Eczema, impetigo herpetiformis, and so on.

制法:共为细末备用。

用法:撒布于患处。

功用:清热燥湿。

主治:湿疹、脓疱疮等。

Shizhen Zhengrong San 时珍正容散(127)　　194,410
(Medical Powder for Facial Diseases)

Source: The Golden Mirror of Medicine 《医宗金鉴》

Composition:

Fructus Gleditsiae Abnormalis 30 g　猪牙皂角(Zhuyazhaojiao)
Herba Spirodelae 30 g　　　　　　　紫背浮萍(Zhibeifuping)
Fructus Pruni 30 g　　　　　　　　　白梅肉　(Baimeirou)
sweet cherry twigs 30 g　　　　　　　甜樱桃枝(Tianyintaozhi)
white substance of eagle-droppings 9 g　鹰粪白　(Yingfenbai)

Manufacture: Dry the first four drugs by baking them, mix them with the white substance of eagles droppings and then grind them together into fine powder.

Administration: Put a bit of the powder and some water in the middle of the palm to make a thick paste, then rub it on the face, and after some time wash the face with warm water.

Actions: tonifying the kidney, removing patches; letting out pathogenic wind; clearing away heat from the lung.

Uses: Freckle, chloasma, comedo, etc.
制法:前四味药焙干,兑鹰粪白,共研细末,备用。
用法:每日早晚用少许放在掌心,以水调浓,搓面部,良久以温水洗面。
功用:益肾消斑,疏风清肺。
主治:雀斑、黄褐斑、粉刺等。

Shuanghua Tuling Yin 双花土苓饮(94)   135,140,381,383
(Decoction of Flos Loncerae and Rhizoma Smilacis Glabrae)

Source: a prescription of the Affiliated Hospital of Shangdong TCM College (山东中医学院附属医院方)

Composition:

Flos Lonicerae 21 g	金银花(*Jinyinhua*)
Rhizoma Smilacis Glabrae 21 g	土茯苓(*Tufuling*)
Parched Flos Sophorae Immaturus 11 g	炒槐米(*Chaohuaimi*)
Radix Rehmanniae 15 g	生地 (*Shengdi*)
Radix Paeoniae Rubra 21 g	赤芍 (*Chishao*)
Radix Arnebiae seu Lithospermi 9 g	紫草 (*Zhicao*)
Radix Bupleuri 9 g	柴胡 (*Chaihu*)
Radix Scutellariae 15 g	黄芩 (*Huangqin*)
Periostracum Cicadae 12 g	蝉蜕 (*Changtui*)
Zaocys 9 g	乌梢蛇(*Wushaoshe*)
Radix Salviae Miltiorrhize 21 g	丹参 (*Danshen*)
Rhizoma Anemarrhenae 9 g	知母 (*Zhimu*)

Actions: Clearing away heat from the blood, dispelling wind and arresting itching.

Uses: Psoriasis, eczema, urticaria, and so on.

Xiao Yin Pian 消银片
(a proprietary of the same ingredients)

Manufacture: Grind the above drugs into fine powder, and make pills with it, each weighing 0.3 g.

Administration: Take 10 pills each time, twice or three time daily.

功用:清热凉血,祛风止痒。

主治:银屑病,湿疹、荨麻疹等。

〔附〕消银片
　　　即上方诸药共研细末，制片，每片 0.3 克，每次 10 片，每日 2～3 次。

Sichong Wan 四虫丸(82)   114,370
(Bolus of Four Insects)

Source: a prescription of the Affiliated Hospital of Shandong TCM College (山东中医学院附属医院方)

Composition (the same amount of each of the following):

Centipede	蜈蚣	(*Wugong*)
Scorpio	全蝎	(*Quanxie*)
Eupolyphagaseu Steleopage	土鳖虫	(*Tubiechong*)
Lumbricus	地龙	(*Dilong*)

Manufacture: Grind the drugs into fine powder, make boluses (the size of a Chinese parasol seed)by mixing the powder with water, and then dry them by leaving them in a shady place.

Administration: 3 g each time, twice or three times daily.

Actions: Removing blood stasis, clearing away obstruction from the channels, and relieving pain.

Uses: Chronic pruritic dermatosis.

制法:共为细末，水泛为丸，为梧子大,晾干备用。
用法:每服 3 克，日 2～3 次。
功用:通络祛瘀止痛。
主治:用于慢性瘙痒性皮肤病。

Simiao Wan 四妙丸(76)　　　　　　　　106,366
(Bolus of Four Drugs)

Source: A Mannual of Practical Chinese Patent Medicine by Song Lianzhu 《实用中成药手册》

Composition:

Rhizoma Atractylodis 9 g	苍术	(*Changzhu*)
Cortex Phellodendri 9 g	黄柏	(*Huangbai*)
Radix Achyranthis Bidentatae 9 g	牛膝	(*Niuxi*)
Semen Coicis 15 g	薏苡仁	(*Yiyiren*)

Manufacture: Grind the drugs into fine powder, make pellets by mixing the powder with water.

Administration: 6 g each time, three times daily.

Actions: Clearing away heat and eliminating dampness.

Uses: Chronic eczema, ulcer of calf and secondary infection from HongKong foot caused by downward flow of damp-heat.

制法:共为细末，水泛为丸。
用法:每次 6 克，日服 3 次。
功用:清热祛湿。
主治:湿热下注引起的慢性湿疹、小腿溃疡、足癣继发感染等。

Simiao Yangan Tang 四妙勇安汤(91)　　　　126,377
(Decoction of Four Wonderful Drugs for Quick Restoration of Health)

Source: New Compilation of Proved Recipes 《验方新编》

Composition:

Radix Scrophulariae 3 g	玄参	(*Xuansheng*)
Radix Angelicae Sinensis 21 g	当归	(*Danggui*)
Flos Lonicerae 30 g	金银花	(*Jinyinhua*)
Radix Glycyrrhizae 9 g	甘草	(*Gancao*)

Actions: Nourishing *Yin* and the blood; clearing away heat and toxic material.

Uses: erythema nodosum due to the accumulation of noxious heat; erythema multiform; allergic purpura; etc.

功用:滋阴养血，清热解毒。

主治:热毒蕴结所致之结节性红斑、多形红斑、过敏性紫癜等。

Siwu Tang 四物汤(97)   137,382
(Decoction of Four Ingredients)

Source: Prescription of Peaceful Benevolent Dispensary 《局方》

Composition:

Radix Angelicae Sinensis 15 g	当归	(*Danggui*)
Radix Rehmanniae 15 g	地黄	(*Dihuang*)
Radix Paoniae Alba 15 g	白芍	(*Baishao*)
Rhizoma Ligustici Chuanxiong 9 g	川芎	(*Chuanxiong*)

Actions: Enriching the blood.

Uses: urticaria, pruritus, alopecia areata, etc, which are due to deficiency of blood.

功用:补血养血。

主治:用于荨麻疹、皮肤瘙痒症、斑秃等。证属血虚者。

Siwu Xiaofeng San 四物消风散(3) 21,322
(Powder of Four Ingredients for Dispersing Pathogenic Wind)

Source: The Golden Mirror of Medicine 《医宗金鉴》
Composition:

Radix Rehmanniae 15 g	生地	(Shengdi)
Radix Angelicae Sinensis 12 g	当归	(Danggui)
Herba Schizonepetae 9 g	荆芥	(Jingjie)
Radix Ledebouriellae 9 g	防风	(Fangfeng)
Radix Paeoniae Rubra 12 g	赤芍	(Chishao)
Rhizoma Ligustici Chuangxiong 9 g	川芎	(Chuanxiong)
Cortex Dictamni Radicis 15 g	白藓皮	(Baixianpi)
Periostracum Cicadae 9 g	蝉蜕	(Chantui)
Herba Menthae 9 g	薄荷	(Bohe)
Radix Angelicae Pubescentis 9 g	独活	(Duhuo)
Radix Bupleuri 9 g	柴胡	(Chaihu)
Fructus Ziziphi Jujubae 3 dates	红枣	(Hongzao)

Actions: Nourishing the blood to expel wind.

Uses: Eczema, urticaria, neurodermatitis, etc., which are due to deficiency of blood and wind-dryness.

功用:养血祛风。

主治:血虚风燥之湿疹、荨麻疹、神经性皮炎等。

Taohong Erchen Tang 桃红二陈汤(11) 23,323
(Decoction of Semen Persicae and Other Ingredients)

Source: A Prescription of the Hospital Affiliated to Shandong TCM College (山东中医学院附属医院方)
Composition:

Semen Persicae 9 g 桃仁 (*Taoren*)
Flos Carthami 9 g 红花 (*Honghua*)
Pericarpium Citri Reticulatae 9 g 陈皮 (*Chenpi*)
Poria 9 g 茯苓 (*Fuling*)
Rhizoma Pinellia 9 g 半夏 (*Banxia*)
Radix Glycyrrhizae 6 g 甘草 (*Gancao*)

Actions: Removing blood stasis and softening hard masses.

Indications: Syndromes of phlegm stagnation and blood stasis such as tuberculoderm, verrucous vegetation, etc.

功用:祛瘀散结，化痰软坚。

主治:痰凝血瘀证，如皮肤结核、疣赘等。

Taohong Siwu Tang 桃红四物汤(10)　　22,137,323,382
(Decoction of Six Ingredients Including Semen Persicae and Flos Carthami)

Source: The Golden Mirror of Medicine 《医宗金鉴》

Composition:

Radix Angelicae Sinensis 15 g 当归 (*Danggui*)
Radix Paeoniae Rubra 15 g 赤芍 (*Chishao*)
Rhizoma Ligustici Chuangxiong 12 g 川芎 (*Chuanxiong*)
Radix Rehmanniae 15 g 生地 (*Shengdi*)
Semen Persicae 9 g 桃仁 (*Taoren*)
Flos Carthami 9 g 红花 (*Honghua*)

Actions: Promoting blood circulation by removing blood stasis, regulating and activating the channels and collaterals.

Indications: Purpura, erythema nodosum, urticaria, psoriasis, and so on.

功用:活血化瘀，通经活络。

主治:紫癜、结节性红斑、荨麻疹、银屑病等。

Tongqiao Huoxue Tang 通窍活血汤(100)   146,173,182
(Decoction for Activating Blood Circulation)   386,399,403

Source: Corrections on the Errors of Medical Works 《医林改错》

Composition:

Radix Paeoniae Rubra 15 g	赤芍	(*Chishao*)
Rhizoma Ligustici Chuangxiong 12 g	川芎	(*Chuanxiong*)
Semen Persicae 9 g	桃仁	(*Taoren*)
Flos Carthami 9 g	红花	(*Honghua*)
Moschus 0.5 g	麝香	(*Shexiang*)
Rhizoma Zingiberis Recens 3 chips	生姜	(*Shengjiang*)
Fructus Ziziphi Jujubae 5 dates	红枣	(*Hongzhao*)
Bulbus Allii Fistulosi (root) 10 cm	老葱	(*Laochong*)

Actions: Promoting blood circulation by removing blood stasis; Promoting the restoration of consciousness and regulating the channels.

Uses: Brandy nose, vitiligo, alopecia areata, and so on.

功用:活血化瘀,通窍。

主治:酒渣鼻、白癜风、斑秃等。

Wushen Tang 五神汤(9)   22,53,322,338
(Decoction of Five drugs)

Source: Essential Notes on External Medicine 《外科真诠》

Composition:

Flos Lonicerae 30 g	金银花	(*Jinyinhua*)
Herba Violae 30 g	紫地丁	(*Zididing*)

Semen Plantaginis 12 g　　　车前子　(*Cheqianzi*)
Poria 15 g　　　　　　　　　茯苓　　(*Fuling*)
Radix Achyranthis Bidentatae 9 g　牛膝　(*Niuxi*)

　　Actions: Clearing away heat and promoting diuresis.

　　Uses: Erysipelas, infection of Hongkong foot, eczema or ulcer of lower limbs, etc., due to accumulation of damp-heat.

　　功用:清热利湿。

　　主治:丹毒、足癣感染、下肢湿疹、下肢溃疡等由湿热凝结而成者。

Wuwei Xiaodu Yin 五味消毒饮(5)　　　44,63,65,71,139,334
(Antiphlogistic Decoction of Five Drugs)　　344,345,348,382

　　Source: The Golden Mirror of Medicine 《医宗金鉴》
　　Composition:
Flos Lonicerae 21 g　　　　　　金银花　(*Jinyinhua*)
Flos Chrysanthemi Indici 15 g　野菊花　(*Yejuhua*)
Herba Violae 15 g　　　　　　　紫地丁　(*Zididing*)
Radix Semiaquilegiae 9 g　　　 天葵子　(*Tiankuizi*)
Herba Taraxaci 21 g　　　　　　蒲公英　(*Pugongying*)

　　Actions: Clearing away heat and toxic material.

　　Uses: Pygenic dermatosis, such as impetigo herpetiformis, boil, etc.

　　功用:清热解毒。

　　主治:化脓性皮肤病,如脓疱疮、疖等。

Xianglian Wan 香连丸(78)　　　　　　　　107,367
(Bolus of Rhizoma Coptidis and Radix Aucklandiae)

　　Source: Prescriptions Collected by Yuebu 《岳部手集方》

Composition:
Rhizoma Coptidis 9 g　　　黄连　(*Huanglian*)
Radix Aucklandiae 9 g　　　木香　(*Muxiang*)

Manufacture: Grind the drugs into fine powder and make boluses by mixing the powder with water.

Administration: Take 6 g to 9 g each time, twice or three times daily.

Actions: Clearing away damp—heat in the stomach and intestine, promoting the circulation of *Qi* and alleviating pain.

Uses: dermapathic purpura, urticaria with gastrointestinal symptoms, etc.

制法:共为细末，醋糊为丸。
用法:每次 6～9 克，日 2～3 次。
功用:清胃肠湿热，行气止痛。
主治:用于肤性紫癜、有胃肠症状之荨麻疹等。

Xiaofan Xiyao 硝矾洗药(16)　　25,51,55,179,338
(Lotion of Mirabilitum and Alumen)　　340,402

Source: a prescription of the Hospital Affiliated to Shandong TCM College (山东中医学院附属医院方)

Composition:
Mirabilitum 12 g　　　朴硝　(*Puxiao*)
Borax 9 g　　　　　　月石　(*Yueshi*)
Alumen 9 g　　　　　 明矾　(*Mingfan*)

Adiministration: Dissolve it in boiling water and rinse the diseased parts while it is hot.

Actions: Antiinflammation; relieving itching; astringency, and removing verruca.

Uses: Hand-foot tinea and its like, seborrheic dermatitis, pompholyx, etc.

用法:用开水冲化后，趁热浸洗患处。

功用:消炎，止痒，收敛，除疣。

主治:手足癣等皮肤癣病，以及脂溢性皮炎、汗疱疹等。

Xiaofeng San 消风散(1)　　　20,82,87,98,321,355,357,363
(Powder for Dispersing Pathogenic Wind)

Source:Orthodox Manual of External Disease 《外科正宗》

Composition:

Herba Schizonepetae 9 g	荆芥	(Jingjie)
Radix Ledebouriellae 9 g	防风	(Fangfeng)
Fructus Arctii 9 g	牛蒡子	(Niubangzi)
Radix Rehmanniae 15 g	生地	(Shengdi)
Radix Sophorae Flavescentis 9 g	苦参	(Kushen)
Rhizoma Atractylodis 9 g	苍术	(Cangzhu)
Radix Angelicae Sinensis 9 g	当归	(Danggui)
Semen Sesamum inducum 9 g	大胡麻	(Dahuma)
Rhizoma Anemarrhema Asphodeloides 9 g	知母	(Zhimu)
Periostracum Cicadae 9 g	蝉蜕	(Chantui)
Gypsum Fibrosum 15 g	生石膏	(Shengshigao)
Caulis Aristolochiae Manshuriensis 9 g	木通	(Mutong)
Radix Glycyrrhizae 6 g	甘草	(Gancao)

Actions: Removing heat to expel wind; clearing away dampness to reduce swelling.

Uses: Eczema, urticaria, pityriasis, rosea, cutaneous pruritus, papular urticaria, etc.

功用:清热疏风，除湿消肿。

主治:湿疹、荨麻疹、玫瑰糠疹、皮肤瘙痒症、丘疹性荨麻疹等。

Xiao Huoluo Dan 小活络丹(110)   158,392
(Bolus for Activating Energy Flow in Channels and Collaterals)

Source: Prescription of Peaceful Benevolent Dispensary 《局方》

Composition:

Prepared Radix Aconiti	制川乌	(*Zhichuanwu*)
Lumbricus	地龙	(*Dilong*)
Prepared Rhizoma	制南星	(*Zhinanxing*)
Resina Olibani	乳香	(*Ruxiang*)
Myrrha	没药	(*Moyao*)

Manufacture: Grind the drugs into fine powder and make boluses by mixing the powder with honey, each bolus weighing 3 g.

Administration: 3 g each time, 2 to 3 times daily.

Actions: Dispelling wind and removing obstruction in the channels; removing dampness and alleviating pain.

Uses: Dermatomyositis and lupus erythematosus with arthralgia showing the syndrome of the accumulation of pathogenic cold.

制法:上药共为细末,炼蜜为丸,每丸重3克。

用法:每次3克,日2~3次。

功用:祛风通络,除湿止痛。

主治:阴寒型皮肌炎,红斑性狼疮伴有关节痛者。

Xiao Luo Tong 消络痛(75)   106,366
(Pills for Relieving Pain)

Source: A mannual of Practical Chinese Patent Medicine by Song Lianzhu 《实用中成药手册》

Administration:

3 tablets each time, three times daily.

Actions: Dispelling wind and dampness, and relieving pain.

Uses: Allergic Purpura accompanied by arthralgia; lupus erythematosus, etc.

用法：每次 3 片，日服 3 次。

功用：祛风湿，止痛。

主治：伴有关节痛的过敏性紫癜、红斑性狼疮等。

Xiaoyao San 逍遥散(124)   189,190,408
(Ease Powder)

Source: Prescription of Peaceful Benvolent Dispensary 《局方》

Composition:

Radix Bupleuri 9 g	柴胡(*Chaihu*)
Radix Angeliae Sinensis 12 g	当归(*Danggui*)
Radix Paeoniae Alba 15 g	白芍(*Baishao*)
Rhizoma Atractylodis Macrocephalae 12 g	白术(*Baizhu*)
Poria 9 g	茯苓(*Fuling*)
Radix Glycyrrhizae 6 g	甘草(*Gancao*)
Rhizoma Zingiberis Recens 3 chips	生姜(*Shengjiang*)
Herba Menthae 6 g	薄荷(*Bohe*)

Action: Relieving the depressed liver, nourishing the blood and strengthening the spleen.

Uses: Herpes zoster, erythema nodosum, neurodermatitis,

chloasma, alopecia areata, etc.

Xiaoyao Wan
(a proprietary of the same ingredients)

Manufacture: Grind the drugs into fine powder and make boluses by mixing the powder with water.

Administration: 6 g each time, 2 to 3 times daily.

功用:疏肝解郁，养血健脾。

主治:带状疱疹、结节性红斑、神经性皮炎、黄褐斑、斑秃等。

〔附〕逍遥丸

　　　即上方诸药研末，水泛为丸。

用法:每次 6 克，每日 2～3 次。

Xijiao Dihuang Tang 犀角地黄汤(7)   22,48,100,105,106
(Decoction of Rhinoceros Horn and   147,336,364
Rehmannia)   366,387

Source: Prescriptions Worth a Thousand Gold for Emergencies 《千金方》

Composition:

Cornu Rhinocerotis 9 g	犀角	(*Xijiao*)
Radix Rehmanniae 30 g	地黄	(*Dihuang*)
Radix Paeoniae Rubra 21 g	赤芍	(*Chishao*)
Cortex Rodicis 15 g	丹皮	(*Danpi*)

Actions: Clearing away heat and toxic material; removing heat from the blood and dissipating blood stasis.

Uses: Purpura, pigmented purpuric dermatosis, allergic drug rash, erythematous lupus, psoriasis, secondary hematosepsis from dermatosis, etc.

功用:清热解毒，凉血散瘀。

主治:紫癜、色素性紫癜性皮肤病、药疹、红斑性狼疮、银屑病、因皮肤病继发的败血症等。

Xijiao Huadu Wan 犀角化毒丸(65)　　　93,94,360
(Antiphlogistic Pill of Cornu Rhinocerotis)

Source: a prescription of Beijing Medicinal Company (北京市药材公司方)

Composition:

Cornu Rhinocerotis	犀角	(*Xijiao*)
Fructus Forsythiae	连翘	(*Lianqiao*)
Radix et Rhizoma Rhei	大黄	(*Dahuang*)
Cinnabaris	朱砂	(*Zhusha*)

Administration: One pill each time (each pill weighs 3 g), twice daily, accompanied by peppermint decoction or warm boiled water. The dose for infants under twelve months old should be less.

Actions: Clearing away heat and toxic material.

Uses: Infective diseases of infant skin, such as impetigo, herpetiformis lactigo and papular urticaria with infection.

用法:每服1丸(每丸重10克)，日2次薄荷汤或温开水送下，周岁以内小儿酌减。

功用:清热，化毒。

主治:小儿皮肤感染性疾患，如脓疱疮、婴儿湿疹、丘疹性荨麻疹伴有感染者。

Xiling Jiedu Wan 犀羚解毒丸(67)
(Antiphlogistic Bolus of Cornu Rhinocerotis and Cornu Saigae Tatariae)

Source: A Mannual of practical Chinese Patent Medicine 《实用中成药手册》

Composition:
Cornu Rhinocerotis	犀角	(*Xijiao*)
Cornu Saigae Taताricae	羚羊角	(*Lingyangjiao*)
Herba Menthae	薄荷	(*Bohe*)
Borneolum	冰片	(*Bingpian*)
Spica Schizonepetae	荆芥	(*Jingjie*)
Flos Lonicerae	金银花	(*Jingyinghua*)
Fructus Arctii	牛蒡子	(*Niubangzi*)
Radix Platycodi	桔梗	(*Jugen*)
Fructus Forsythiae	连翘	(*Lianqiao*)
Herba Lophatheri	淡竹叶	(*Danzhuye*)
Radix Glycyrrhizae	甘草	(*Gancao*)
Semen Sojae Fermentatum	淡豆豉	(*Dandougu*)

Adiministration: One pill each time, three times daily.

Actions: Clearing away heat and toxic material; dispelling wind and relieving exterior syndrome.

Uses: Allergic Purpura, erythema multiforme, lupus erythematosus, and so on.

用法:每次1丸，日3次。

功用:清热解毒，疏风解表。

主治:过敏性紫癜、多形性红斑、红斑性狼疮等。

Xinyi Qinfei Yin 辛荑清肺饮(31) 29,327
(Decoction of Flos Magnoliae for Eliminating Lung-heat)

Source: The Golden Mirror of Medicine 《医宗金鉴》
Composition:

Flos Magnoliae 9 g	辛夷	(*Xinyi*)
Calcined Gypsum Fibrosum 15 g	煅石膏	(*Duanshigao*)
Rhizoma Anemarrhenae 9 g	知母	(*Zhimu*)
Capejasmine Fruit 9 g	栀子	(*Zhizi*)
Radix Scutellariae 12 g	黄芩	(*Huangqin*)
Rhizoma Cimicifugae 6 g	升麻	(*Shengma*)
Folium Eriobotryae 9 g	枇杷叶	(*Pipaye*)
Bulbus Lilii 12 g	百合	(*Baihe*)
Radix Ophiopogonis 9 g	麦冬	(*Maidong*)
Radix Glycyrrhizae 6 g	生甘草	(*Shenggancao*)

Actions: Clearing away heat, Purging the pathogenic fire, and nourishing the lung.

Indications: Herpes simplex, acne, brandy nose, etc.

功用:清热，泻火，润肺。

主治:单纯疱疹、痤疮、酒渣鼻等。

Xixian Wan 豨莶丸(122) 188,407
(Bolus of Herba Siegesbeckiae)

Source: a practical proved recipe (经验方)
Composition:

Herba Siegesbeckia	豨莶草	(*Xixiancao*)

Manufacture: Grind the drugs into fine powder and make boluses by mixing the powder with honey, each bolus weighing 9 g.

Administration: 9 g each time, twice daily, washed down with warm boiled water.

Actions: Expelling wind and removing dampness.

Uses: psoriasis; lupus erythematosus accompanied by arthralagia; vitiligo; etc.

制法:研末，炼蜜为丸，每丸重9克。

用法:每服9克，日2次，温开水送服。

功用:驱风除湿。

主治:用于银屑病及红斑性狼疮伴发关节痛者，以及白癜风等。

Xuefu Zhuyu Tang 血府逐瘀汤(108)
(Decoction for Removing Blood Stasis in the Chest)

Source: Corrections on the Errors of Medical Works 《医林改错》

Composition:

Radix Angelicae Sinensis 15 g	当归	(Danggui)
Radix Rehmanniae 15 g	生地	(Shengdi)
Semen Persicae 9 g	桃仁	(Taoren)
Flos Carthami 9 g	红花	(Honghu)
Fructus Aurantii Immaturus 9 g	枳壳	(Zhike)
Radix Paeoniae Rubra 15 g	赤芍	(Chishao)
Radix Bupleuri 9 g	柴胡	(Chaih)
Radix Platycodi 9 g	桔梗	(Jugeng)
Rhizoma Ligustici Chuanxiong 12 g	川芎	(Chuanxiong)
Radix Achyranthis Bidentatae 9 g	牛膝	(Niuxi)
Radix Glycyrrhizae 6 g	甘草	(Gancao)

Actions: Promoting blood circulation to remove blood stasis;

clearing away obstruction in the channels to relieve pain.

Uses: Psoriasis, prurigo, erythema nodosum, etc. showing the syndrome of blood stasis.

功用:活血祛瘀，通络止痛。

主治:血瘀型银屑病、结节性痒疹、结节性红斑等。

Yanghe Tang 阳和汤(109) 157,391
(Yang-Activating Decoction)

Source: Life-saving Mannual of Diagnosis and Treatment of External Diseases 《外科全生集》

Composition:

Radix Rehmanniae Praeparatae 15 g	熟地	(*Shudi*)
Semen Sinapis Alba 9 g	白芥子	(*Baijiezi*)
baked Rhizoma Zingiberis Recens 6 g	炮姜炭	(*Paojiangtan*)
Herba Ephedrae 6 g	麻黄	(*Mahuang*)
Cortex Cinnamomi 6 g	肉桂	(*Rougui*)
Colla Cornus Cervi 6 g	鹿角胶	(*Lujiaojiao*)
Radix Glycyrrhizae 6 g	甘草	(*Gancao*)

Actions: Warming up *Yang*, dispelling cold and invigorating pulse-beat.

Uses: Psoriasis, cold urticaria, chilblain and angiopathy showing the syndrome of asthenia-cold.

功用:温阳散寒通脉。

主治:硬皮病、冷性荨麻疹、冻疮、虚寒性血管病等。

Yangxin Tang 养心汤(104) 150,388
(Decoction for Nourishing the Heart)

Source:Standards of Diagnosis and Treatment 《证治准绳》

Composition:
Radix Astragali seu Hedysari 15 g	黄芪 (*Huangqi*)
Poria 9 g	茯苓 (*Fuling*)
Poria cum Ligno Hospite 9 g	茯神 (*Fushen*)
Radix Angelicae Sinensis 12 g	当归 (*Danggui*)
Rhizoma Ligustici Chuanxiong 9 g	川芎 (*Chuanxiong*)
Bighead Atractylodes and Gastrodia 9 g	半夏曲 (*Banxiaqu*)
Semen Biotae 12 g	柏子仁 (*Baiziren*)
Semen Ziziphi Spinosae 15 g	酸枣仁 (*Suanzhaoren*)
Radix Polygalae 9 g	远志 (*Yuanzhi*)
Fructus Schisandrae 9 g	五味子 (*Wuweizi*)
Radix Ginseng 6 g	人参 (*Renshen*)
Cortex Cinnamomi 6 g	肉桂 (*Rougui*)
Radix Glycyrrhizae 6 g	甘草 (*Gancao*)

Actions: Nourishing the heart to calm the mind; invigorating *Qi* and enriching the blood.

Uses: Systemic lupus erythematosus showing the syndrome of noxious heat affecting the heart.

功用:养心安神,益气补血。

主治:系统性红斑狼疮之热毒扰心证。

Yangxue Anshen Wan 养血安神丸(81)   114,370
(Bolus for Nourishing the Blood and Tranquilizing).

Source: Essential Chinese Patent Medicine 《中国基本中成药》

Composition:
Herba Ecliptae	旱莲草 (*Hanliancao*)
Radix Rehmanniae Praeparatae	熟地 (*Shudi*)

Radix Rehmanniae	生地	(*Shengdi*)
Caulis Spatholobi	鸡血藤	(*Jixueteng*)
Herba Agrimoniae	仙鹤草	(*Xianhecao*)
Cortex Albiziae	合欢皮	(*Hehuanpi*)
Caulis Polygoni Multiflori	夜交藤	(*Yejiaoteng*)

Manufacture: Grind the drugs into fine powder and make boluses by mixing the powder with water.

Administration: Take 6 g each time, three times daily, with the stomach empty and accompanied by warm boiled water.

Actions: Enriching the blood and tranquilizing.

Uses: chronic, pruritic dermatosis.

制法:共研细末，水泛为丸。

用法:每服6克，日3次，空腹温开水送服。

功用:补阴血，交心神。

主治:用于慢性瘙痒性皮肤病。

Yangxue Runfu Yin 养血润肤饮(95)

(Decoction for Nourishing the blood and Moisturizing the Skin)

Source: Diagonosis and Treatment of External Diseases 《外科证治》

Composition:

Radix Rehmanniae 15 g	生地	(*Shengdi*)
Radix Angelicae Sinensis 15 g	当归	(*Danggui*)
Radix Paeoniae Rubra 15 g	赤芍	(*Chishao*)
Rhizoma Ligustici Chuanxiong 12 g	川芎	(*Chuanxiong*)
Radix Asparagi 9 g	天冬	(*Tiandong*)
Radix Ophiopogonis 9 g	麦冬	(*Maidong*)

Bombyx Batryticatus 9 g	僵蚕	(Jiangcan)
Radix Polygoni Multiflori 15 g	首乌	(Shouwu)
Cortex Moutan Radicis 12 g	丹皮	(Danpi)
Ramulus Mori 9 g	桑枝	(Sangzhi)

Actions: Enriching the blood, moistening dryness, nourishing *Yin* and relieving itching.

Uses: Pruritus of skin, chronic eczema, psoriasis, seborrheic dermatitis, acne dermatosis, etc.

功用:养血润燥，滋阴止痒。

主治:皮肤瘙痒症、慢性湿疹、银屑病、脂溢性皮炎、角化性皮肤病等。

Yangxue Shengfa Pian 养血生发片(118)　　181,402
(Bolus for Nourishing the Blood and Hair)

Source: a prescription of the Affiliated Hospital of Shandong TCM College (山东中医学院附属医院方)

Composition:

Radix Rehmanniae 15 g	生熟地	(Shengshudi)
Radix Polygoni Multifori 15 g	何首乌	(Heshouwu)
Semen Sojae Nigrum 30 g	黑豆	(Heidou)
Radix Paeoniae Alba 9 g	白芍	(Baishao)
Radix Angelicae Sinensis 15 g	当归	(Danggui)
Rhizoma Ligustici Chuanxiong 9 g	川芎	(Chuanxiong)
Radix Salviae Miltiorrhizae 15 g	丹参	(Danshen)
Flos Carthami 9 g	红花	(Honghua)
Semen Cuscutae 15 g	菟丝子	(Tusizi)
Fructus Ligustri Lucidi 12 g	女贞子	(Nüzhenzi)
Herba Ecliptae 12 g	旱莲草	(Hanliancao)

Rhizoma Gastrodiae 6 g　　　　　天麻　(*Tianma*)
Parched Semen Ziziphi Spinosae 15 g　炒枣仁　(*Chaozhaoren*)
Cacumen Biotae 9 g　　　　　　　侧柏叶　(*Cebaiye*)
Rhizoma seu Radix Notopterygii 6 g　羌活　(*Qianghuo*)
Fructus Chaenomelis 6 g　　　　　木瓜　(*Mugua*)
Radix Glycyrrhizae 6 g　　　　　　甘草　(*Gancao*)

Manufacture: Grind the drugs into fine powder to made boluses with, each bolus weighing 0.3 g.

Administration: 10 tablets each time, three times daily.

制法:上药共研细末制片，每片0.3克。

用法:每服10片，日3次。

Yinchenhao Tang 茵陈蒿汤(112)　　　　164,394
(Oriental Wormwood Decoction)

Source: Treatise on Febrile Diseases 《伤寒论》

Composition:

Herba Artemisiae Capillaris 9 g　　茵陈　(*Yinchen*)
Fructus Capejasmine 9 g　　　　　栀子　(*Zhizi*)
Radix et Rhizoma Rhei 9 g　　　　大黄　(*Dahuang*)

Actions: Clearing away heat and promoting diuresis.

Uses: Urticaria, dermatomyosite, acne, seborrheic dermatitis, etc, showing damp-heat syndrome.

功用:清热利湿。

主治:湿热型荨麻疹、皮肌炎、痤疮、脂溢性皮炎等。

Yupingfeng San 玉屏风散(61)　　　　90,91,358,359
(Jadescreen Powder)

Source: Effective Formulas Handed Down from Generations 《世医得效方》

Composition:

Radix Astragali seu Hedysaeri 15 g	黄芪(*Huangqi*)
Rhizoma Atractylodis Macrocephalae 15 g	白术(*Baizhu*)
Radix Ledebouriellae 9 g	防风(*Fangfeng*)

Actions: Invigorating *Qi*; strengthening the body surface resistance; hidroschesis.

Uses: Symptoms of urticara due to the failure of superficial—*Qi* to protect the body against diseases.

Yupingfeng Wan 玉屏风丸
(Yupingfeng Pill, a proprietary)

Manufacture: Grind the above drugs into fine powder, stir them thoroughly and make pills by mixing the powder with water.

Administration: Take 6 g each time, three times daily.

功用:补气，固表，止汗。

主治:荨麻疹之卫阳不固证。

〔附〕玉屏风丸

  即上方共研末和匀，水泛为丸。

用法:每次 6 克，每日 3 次。

Zaoshi Xiyao 燥湿洗药(59)
(Lotion for Clearing Away Dampness)

84,91,124,179,356, 359,375,402

Source: a prescription of the Hospital Affiliated to Shandong TCM College (山东中医学院附属医院方)

Composition:

Cortex Dictamni Radicis 30 g　　　白藓皮(*Baixianpi*)

Herba Portulacae 30 g 　　马齿苋(*Machijian*)
Radix Sophorae Flavenscentis 30 g 　苦参 (*Kushen*)
Cortex Phellodendri 15 g 　　黄柏 (*Huangbai*)
Rhizoma Atractylodis 15 g 　　苍术 (*Changzhu*)

Administration: Decoct the medicinal herbs and rinse the diseased part in the decoction.

Actions: Clearing away heat and eliminating dampness.

Uses: Eczema, contact dermatitis, hand-foot tinea, etc.

用法:煎汤熏洗患处。

功用:清热燥湿。

主治:湿疹、接触性皮炎、手足癣等。

Zengye Tang 增液汤(69)　　　　　　101,364
(Decoction for Increasing Fluid)

Source: Treatise on Differentiation and Treatment of Epidemic Febrile Diseases 《温病条辨》

Composition:

Radix Scrophulariae 15 g 　　玄参 (*Xuansheng*)
Radix Ophiopogonis 15 g 　　麦冬 (*Maidong*)
Radix Rehmanniae 15 g 　　生地 (*Shengdi*)

Actions: Increasing fluid for nourishing *Yin*.

Uses: Exfoliative dermatitis, syndrome of drug rash with *Yin* fluid impaired by noxious heat.

功用:增液养阴。

主治:剥脱性皮炎、药疹之热毒伤阴证。

Zhi Bai Dihuang Tang 知柏地黄汤(70)   102,108,148,191
(Decoction of Anemarrhena,   193,364,367,387,
Phellodendron and Rehmannia)   408,409,410

Source: The Golden Mirror of Medicine 《医宗金鉴》

Composition:

Poria	茯苓	(Fuling)
Rhizoma Dioscoreae	山药	(Shanyao)
Fructus Corni	山萸肉	(Shanyurou)
Radix Rehmanniae Praeparata	熟地	(Shudi)
Rhizoma Alismatis	泽泻	(Zexie)
Cortex Moutan Radicis	丹皮	(Danpi)
Rhizoma Anemarrhema	知母	(Zhimu)
Cortex Phellodendri	黄柏	(Huangbai)

Actions: Nourishing *Yin* to reduce pathogenic fire.

Uses: Lupus erythematosus due to deficiency of *Yin* and interior heat; dermatomyositis, allergic drug rash, allergic purpura, etc.

Zhi Bai Dihuang Wan 知柏地黄丸
(another proprietary of the same ingredients)

Manufacture: Grind the drugs into fine powder and make pellets by mixing the powder with honey.

Administration: 9 g each time, twice or three times daily.

功用:滋阴降火。

主治:阴虚内热之红斑性狼疮、皮肌炎、药疹、过敏性紫癜等。

〔附〕知柏地黄丸

即上药共研末，炼蜜为丸。

用法:每服9克, 日2～3次。

Zhibao Dan 至宝丹(68)   101,364
(Treasured Bolus)

Source: Prescription of Peaceful Benevolent Dispensary 《和剂局方》

Composition:

Cinnabaris	朱砂	(Zhusha)
Moschus	麝香	(Shexiang)
Cornu Rhinocertis	犀角	(Xijiao)
Borneolum	冰片	(Bingpian)
Calculus Bovis	牛黄	(Niuhuang)
Succinum	琥珀	(Hupo)
Realgar	雄黄	(Xionghuang)
Carapax Eretomochelydis	玳瑁	(Daimao)
gold foil	金箔	(Jinbo)
lead foil	铅箔	(Qianbo)
benzoin	安息香	(Anxixiang)

Manufacture: Grind the drugs into fine powder, stir it thoroughly, and make pellets by mixing the powder with honey (20-30% by weight).

Administration: One pill each time, twice daily.

Actions: Removing phlegm, inducing resuscitation and clearing away toxic material.

Uses: Severe drug rash due to excessive phlegm-heat affecting the pericardium; lupus erythematosus.

制法:上方研细末, 和匀, 加炼蜜20～30%为丸, 每丸重3克。

用法:每服1丸, 日2次。

功用:祛痰开窍，辟秽解毒。

主治:用于痰热亢盛扰及心包之重症药疹及红斑性狼疮等病。

Zhiyang Ding 止痒酊(41)   65,91,94,115,120,345,
(Tincture for Arresting Itching)   359,361,371,373

Source: a practical proved prescription (经验方)

Composition:

Fructus Cnidii 25 g	蛇床子	(*Shechuangzi*)
Radix Stemonae 25 g	百部	(*Baibu*)
75%alcohol 100 ml	酒精	(*Jiujing*)

Manufacture: Soak the above drugs in the alcohol for 24 hours to obtain a liquid for application.

Adiministration: External application, twice or three times daily.

Actions: Destroying parasites, expelling wind and relieving itching.

Uses: Pruritic dermatosis with no exudation, such as eczema, urticaria, allergic drug rash, papular urticaria, insect dermatitis, pruritus and so on.

制法:上药浸泡24小时，取汁备用。

用法:外涂患处，每日2～3次。

功用:杀虫祛风止痒。

主治:湿疹、荨麻疹、药疹、丘疹性荨麻疹、虫咬皮炎、瘙痒症等瘙痒性皮肤病无渗液者。

Zhi Yang Fen 止痒粉(64)   91,359
(Powder for Arresting Itching)

Source: Concise Traditional Chinese Dermatology 《简明中

医皮肤病学》

Composition:

Talcum 30 g	滑石	(*Huashi*)
Calcitun 9 g	寒水石	(*Hanshuishi*)
Borneolum 2.4 g	冰片	(*Bingpian*)

Manufacture: Grind the drugs into fine powder

Administration: Spread the powder on the diseased part.

Actions: Clearing away heat, relieving itching and removing dampness.

Uses: Sudamen, eczema, dermatitis and other pruritic dermatoses.

制法:上药共研为极细末。

用法:外扑。

功用:清凉，止痒，除湿。

主治:痱子、湿疹、皮炎以及其它瘙痒性皮肤病。

Zhiyang Pu Fen 止痒扑粉(50)   72,84,348,356
(Powder for Arresting Itching)

Source: a practical proved prescription(经验方)

Composition:

Semen Phaseoli Radiatus 50 g	绿豆	(*Lüdou*)
Zinc Oxide 5 g	氧化锌	(*Yanghuaxing*)
Talcum Pulveratum 44 g	滑石粉	(*Huashifen*)
Camphor 1 g	樟脑	(*Zhangnao*)

Manufacture: Grind the first three drugs into fine powder, add the camphor and grind again, mixing them thoroughly.

Administration: Apply the powder to the diseased part, 3 to 5 times daily.

Actions: Clearing away heat, arresting secretion, relieving itching.

Uses: Summer dermatitis, sudamen, allergic drug rash, neurodermatitis, pruritus, etc.

制法:将以上前三种药物研细后,再加入樟脑,研匀即可。
用法:干扑患处,每日3~5次。
功用:清热、收湿、止痒。
主治:夏季皮炎、痱子、湿疹、药疹、神经性皮炎、瘙痒症等。

Zhiyang Xiyao 止痒洗药(14)   25,51,78,84,91,115,119,324
(Lotion for Relieving Itching)   338,352,356,359,371,373

Source: a prescription of the Hospital Affiliated to Shandong TCM College (山东中医学院附属医院方)

Composition:

Fructus Cnidii 15 g	蛇床子	(Shechuangzi)
Fructus Kochiae 15 g	地肤子	(Difuzi)
Radix Sophorae Flavenscentis 15 g	苦参	(Kushen)
Cortex Phellodendri 15 g	黄柏	(Huangbai)
Fructus Carpesii 15 g	鹤虱	(Heshi)
Nidus Vespae 10 g	蜂房	(Fengfang)
Rhizoma Rhei 10 g	生大黄	(Shengdahuang)
Semen Armeniacae Amarum 10 g	生杏仁	(Shengxingren)
Alumen Exsiccatum 10 g	枯矾	(Kufan)
Cortex Dictamni Radicis 10 g	白藓皮	(Baixianpi)
Semen Hydnocarpi 10 g	大枫子	(Dafengzi)
Mirabilitum 10 g	朴硝	(Puxiao)
Periostracum Cicadae 10 g	蝉蜕	(Chantui)

Cortex Moutan Radicis 10 g　　　丹皮　　(*Danpi*)

Administration: Decoct the drugs and rinse the diseased part in the decoction while it is still hot, once or twice daily, 30 minutes each time.

Actions: Expelling wind, destroying parasites, clearing away heat, eliminating dampness and relieving itching.

Uses: Cutaneous pruritus, hand-foot tinea, neurodermatitis, psoriasis, eczema, and so on.

用法:上药煎汤，乘热熏洗患处。每日1～2次，每次30分钟。
功用:祛风杀虫，清热燥湿，止痒。
主治:皮肤瘙痒病、手足癣、神经性皮炎银屑病、湿疹等。

Zicao You 紫草油(20)　　　　　　　　　　　　25,324
(Ointment of Radix Arnebiae seu Lithospermi)

Source: a practical proved prescription (经验方)

Composition:

Radix Arnebiae Seu Lithospermi 50 g　　紫草　(*Zicao*)
Oleum Sesami 250 g　　　　　　　　　　麻油　(*Mayou*)

Manufacture: Grind the Radix Arnebiae Seu Lithospermi into fine powder and mix it with the sesame oil.

Administration: Apply it onto the diseased part, twice or three times daily.

Actions: Removing heat from the blood and eliminating blood stasis.

Uses: Scald, chronic ulcer.

制法:紫草研细粉，与麻油混合调匀。
用法:涂患处，每天2～3次。
功用:凉血化瘀。

主治:烫伤、慢性溃疡。

Zixue Dan 紫雪丹(35)   49,101,148,336,364,387
(Zixue Bolus)

Source: Prescription of Peaceful Benevolent Dispensary 《局方》

Composition:

Gypsum Fibrosum	生石膏 (Shengshigao)
Calcitum	寒水石 (Hanshuishi)
Talcum	滑石 (Huashi)
Radix Aristolochiae	青木香 (Qingmuxiang)
Lignum Aquilariae Resinatum	沉香 (Chenxiang)
Radix Scrophulariae	玄参 (Xuanshen)
Rhizoma Cimicifugae	升麻 (Shengma)
Flos Syzygii Aromatic	丁香 (Dingxiang)
Radix Glycyrrhizae	甘草 (Gancao)
Magnetitum	磁石 (Chishi)
Natrii Sulfas	芒硝 (Mangxiao)
Niter	火硝 (Huoxiao)
Cornu Rhinoceri	犀角 (Xijiao)
Cornu Antelopis	羚羊角 (Lingyangjiao)
Moschus	麝香 (Shexiang)
Cinnabaris	朱砂 (Zhusha)
Gold	黄金 (Huangjin)

Directions: Take 1.5 g each time, once or twice daily.

Actions: Clearing away heat and toxic material; relieving spasm and inducing resuscitation.

Indications: skin diseases due to pathogenic heat, accom-

panied by fever, restlessness, coma and fainting.
用法:每服1.5克，每日1～2次。
功用:清热解毒，镇痉开窍。
主治:皮肤病伴热邪内陷，高热烦躁，神昏惊厥等。

16
皮肤病学

序

《英汉实用中医药大全》即将问世，吾为之高兴。

歧黄之道，历经沧桑，永盛不衰。吾中华民族之强盛，由之。世界医学之丰富和发展，亦由之。然而，世界民族之差异，国别之不同，语言之障碍，使中医中药的传播和交流受到了严重束缚。当前，世界各国人民学习、研究、运用中医药的热潮方兴未艾。为使吾中华民族优秀文化遗产之一的歧黄之道走向世界，光大其业，为世界人民造福，徐象才君集省内外精英于一堂，主持编译了《英汉实用中医药大全》。是书之问世将使海内外同道欢呼雀跃。

世界医学发展之日，当是歧黄之道光大之时。

吾欣然序之。

中华人民共和国卫生部副部长
兼国家中医药管理局局长
世界针灸学会联合会主席
中国科学技术协会委员
中华全国中医学会副会长
中国针灸学会会长

胡熙明
1989年12月

序

中华民族有同疾病长期作斗争的光辉历程，故而有自己的传统医学——中国医药学。中国医药学有一套完整的从理论到实践的独特科学体系。几千年来，它不但被完好地保存下来，而且得到了发扬光大。它具有疗效显著、副作用小等优点，是人们防病治病，强身健体的有效工具。

任何一个国家在医学进步中所取得的成就，都是人类共同的财富，是没有国界的。医学成果的交流比任何其他科学成果的交流都应进行得更及时，更准确。我从事中医工作30多年来，一直盼望着有朝一日中国医药学能全面走向世界，为全人类解除病痛疾苦做出其应有的贡献。但由于用外语表达中医难度较大，中国医药学对外传播的速度一直不能令人满意。

山东中医学院的徐象才老师发起并主持了大型系列丛书《英汉实用中医药大全》的编译工作。这个工作是一项巨大工程，是一种大型科研活动，是一个大胆的尝试，是一件新事物。对徐象才老师及与其合作的全体编译者夜以继日地长期工作所付出的艰苦劳动，克服重重困难所表现出的坚韧不拔的毅力，以及因此而取得的重大成绩，我甚为敬佩。作为一个中医界的领导者，对他们的工作给予全力支持是我应尽的责任。

我相信《英汉实用中医药大全》无疑会在中国医学史和世界科学技术史上找到它应有的位置。

中华全国中医学会常务理事
山东省卫生厅副厅长

张奇文

1990年3月

出 版 前 言

　　中国医药学是我中华民族优秀文化遗产之一，建国以来由于党和国家对待中医药采取了正确的政策，使中医药理论宝库不断得到了发掘整理，取得了巨大的成绩。当前，世界各国人民对中国医药学的学习和研究热潮日益高涨，为促进这一热潮更加蓬勃的发展，为使中国医药学能更好地为全人类解除病痛服务，就必须促进中医中药在世界范围内的传播和交流，而要使这一传播和交流进行得更及时、更准确，就必须首先排除语言障碍。因此，编译一套英汉对照的中医药基本知识的书籍，供国内外学习、研究中医药时使用，已成为国内外医药学界和医药学教育界许多人士的迫切需要。

　　多年来，在卫生部门的号召下，在"中医英语表达研究"方面，已经作出了一些可喜的成绩。本书《英汉实用中医药大全》的编辑出版就是在调查上述研究工作的历史和现状的基础上，继续对中医药英语表达作较系统、较全面的研究，以适应中国医药学对外传播交流的需要。

　　这部"大全"的版本为英汉对照，共有21个分册，一个分册介绍论述中国医药学的一个分科。在编著上注意了中医药汉文稿的编写特色，在内容上注意了科学性、实用性、全面性和简明易读。汉文稿的执笔撰写者主要是有20年以上实践经验的教授、副教授、主任医师和副主任医师。各分册汉文稿撰写成后，均经各学科专家逐一审订。各分册英文主译、主审主要是国内既懂中医又懂英语的权威人士，还有许多中医院校的英语教师及医药卫生部门的专业翻译人员。英译稿脱稿后，经过了复审、终审，有些译稿还召开全国22所院校和单位人员参加的英译稿统稿定稿研讨会，对英译稿进行细致的研讨和推敲，对如何较全面、较系统、较准确地用英语表达中国医药学进行了探讨，从而推动整个译文达到较高水平，因此，这部"大全"可供中医院校高年级学生作为泛读教材使用。

这部"大全"的编纂得到了国家教育委员会、国家中医药管理局、山东省教育委员会、山东省卫生厅等各部门有关领导的支持。在国家教委高等教育司的指导下，成立了《英汉实用中医药大全》编译领导委员会。还得到了全国许多中医院校和中药生产厂家领导的支持。

希望这部"大全"的出版，对中医院校加强中医英语教学，对国内卫生界培养外向型中医药人才，以及在推动世界各国人民对中医药的学习和研究方面，都将产生良好的影响。

高等教育出版社

1990年3月

前　言

《英汉实用中医药大全》是一部以中医基本理论为基础，以中医临床为重点，较为全面系统、简明扼要、易读实用的中级英汉学术性著作。它的主要读者是：中医药院校高年级学生和中青年教师，中医院的中青年医生和中医药科研单位的科研人员，从事中医对外函授工作的人员和出国讲学或行医的中医人员，西学中人员，来华学习中医的外国留学生和各类进修人员。

由于中国医药学为我中华民族之独有，因此，英译便成了本《大全》编译工作的重点。为确保译文能准确表达中医的确切含义，我们邀集熟悉中医的英语人员、医学专业翻译人员、懂英语的中医药人员乃至医古文人员于一堂，共同翻译、共同对译文进行研讨推敲的集体翻译法，这样，就把众人之长融进了译文质量之中。然而，即使这样，也难确保译文都能尽如人意。汉文稿虽反映了中国医药学的精髓和概貌，但也难能十全十美。我衷心地盼望读者能提出批评和建议，以便《大全》再版时修改。

参加本《大全》编、译、审工作的人员达200余名，他们来自全国28个单位，其中有山东、北京、上海、天津、南京、浙江、安徽、河南、湖北、广西、贵阳、甘肃、成都、山西、长春等15所中医学院，还有中国中医研究院、山东省中医药研究所等中医药科研单位。

山东省教育委员会把本《大全》的编译列入了科研计划并拨发了科研经费，山东省卫生厅和一些中药生产厂家也给了很大支持，济南中药厂的资助为编译工作的开端提供了条件。

本《大全》的编译成功是全体编译审者集体劳动的结晶，是各有关单位主管领导支持的结果。在《大全》各分册即将陆续出版之际，我诚挚地感谢全体编译审者的真诚合作，感谢许多专家、教授、各级领导和生产厂家的热情支持。

愿本《大全》的出版能在培养通晓英语的中医人才和使中医早日全面走向世界方面起到我所期望的作用。

主编 徐象才

于山东中医学院

1990年3月

目 录

说明 ………………… 313

上篇 总 论

1 皮肤的中医生理……… 315
   1.1 皮肤与卫气学说 … 315
   1.2 皮肤与内脏的
       关系 ……………… 316
   1.3 皮肤与经络的
       关系 ……………… 317
2 皮肤病的中医病理 … 318
   2.1 风 ………………… 318
   2.2 湿 ………………… 319
   2.3 热 ………………… 319
   2.4 毒 ………………… 320
   2.5 燥 ………………… 320
   2.6 血瘀 ……………… 320
   2.7 肝肾不足 ………… 321
3 皮肤病的症状辨证 … 322
   3.1 自觉症状 ………… 322
   3.2 皮肤损害 ………… 323
4 皮肤病的中医治疗 … 325
   4.1 内治法 …………… 325
   4.2 外治法 …………… 327

下篇 各 论

1 病毒性皮肤病………… 330
   1.1 单纯疱疹 ………… 330
   1.2 带状疱疹 ………… 331
   1.3 疣 ………………… 333
2 细菌性皮肤病………… 337
   2.1 脓疱疮 …………… 337
   2.2 丹毒 ……………… 339
3 癣……………………… 341
   3.1 手足癣 …………… 341
   3.2 甲癣 ……………… 343
   3.3 体癣、股癣 ……… 343
   3.4 头癣 ……………… 344
   3.5 花斑癣 …………… 345
4 昆虫所致皮肤病……… 347
   4.1 疥疮 ……………… 347
   4.2 虫咬皮炎 ………… 348
5 物理性皮肤病………… 350
   5.1 冻疮 ……………… 350
   5.2 手足皲裂 ………… 351
   5.3 痱子 ……………… 352
   5.4 鸡眼 ……………… 353
6 变应性皮肤病………… 355
   6.1 接触性皮炎 ……… 355

6.2	湿疹	357
6.3	荨麻疹	360
6.4	丘疹性荨麻疹	363
6.5	药物性皮炎	365
6.6	过敏性紫癜	369

7 神经功能障碍性皮肤病 373
- 7.1 皮肤瘙痒症 373
- 7.2 神经性皮炎 375

8 红斑类皮肤病 378
- 8.1 多形性红斑 378
- 8.2 结节性红斑 380

9 红斑鳞屑性皮肤病 382
- 9.1 玫瑰糠疹 382
- 9.2 银屑病 383

10 结缔组织病 388
- 10.1 红斑性狼疮 388
- 10.2 硬皮病 393
- 10.3 皮肌炎 396

11 皮肤附属器疾病 400
- 11.1 寻常性痤疮 400
- 11.2 酒渣鼻 402
- 11.3 皮脂溢出症与脂溢性皮炎 404
- 11.4 斑秃 406
- 11.5 腋臭 408

12 色素性皮肤病 410
- 12.1 白癜风 410
- 12.2 黄褐斑 411
- 12.3 雀斑 413

英汉实用中医药大全（书目） 415

方剂索引（英汉对照） (195)

说　　明

《皮肤病学》是《英汉实用中医临床大全》的第十六分册。

中医文献内有关皮肤病的记载渊源已久，早在公元前14世纪的甲骨文中即有"疥"、"疕"类皮肤病的记述。隋《诸病源候论》中，对疣、癣、荨麻疹等几十种皮肤病已有了详细的描述。唐《千金要方》和《外台秘要》中，收载了很多利用雄黄、矾石、硫磺等中药治疗皮肤病的方法……。长期以来，历代医家创立了独特的诊疗皮肤病的方法，并积累了丰富的临床经验。因此，中医皮肤病学历史悠久，是中国医学宝库的重要组成部分。现代实践表明，许多现代医学方法疗效不佳或治疗无效的皮肤病，运用中医中药治疗可以收到满意效果。

因此中医皮肤病学日益受到国内外的重视。

本分册分上、下两篇。上篇总论共四章，简要介绍了皮肤的中医生理病理，皮肤病的症状辨证与中医治疗概要；下篇各论共十二章，介绍了近40种常见皮肤病。内容力求简明、扼要、实用、通俗。

在编译过程中，边天羽、雷希濂教授，以及美国学者Tracey L. Bailey教授，曾审阅本书；周行、杨阳、李笑蛮等同志也为本书做过有益的工作。谨表感谢。

编者

上篇 总 论

1 皮肤的中医生理

1.1 皮肤与卫气学说

2000多年前，中国医学就提出了脏腑、经、络、气、血、津液等生理学说。其中的气在中医学说中指的是构成人体和维持人体生命活动的最基本的物质之一，它对于人体具有十分重要的生理功能。气的含义涉及面较广泛，总的说来可归纳为两个方面：一是指体内流动着的富有营养的精微物质；二是泛指脏腑生理活动的能力。在人体各部分均分布有流动着的精微物质，由于分布的部位不同而有不同的名称，如聚于胸中的叫做宗气；发源于肾的叫做元气（或原气）；运行在血脉中的叫做营气；运行在脉外又宣发于肌肤腠理（指皮肤、肌肉、汗孔等）的叫做卫气。

在中医生理学中，与皮肤生理关系较密切的是卫气学说。《灵枢·本藏》说："卫气者，所以温分肉，充皮肤，肥腠理，司开阖者也。"又说："卫气和，则分肉解利，皮肤调柔，腠理致密矣"。概括而言，卫气的生理功能有三方面：一是护卫肌表，抗御外邪；二是温养内外（皮肤、毛发、肌肉、脏腑等）润泽皮肤；三是启闭汗孔，调节汗液分泌，维持体温相对恒定等。

卫气的强弱与皮肤的健康和对外邪的易感性有着密切的关系。卫气充盛，则皮肤柔润强固，肌肤丰满；腠理致密，外邪不得侵袭；卫气不足，则皮肤枯槁，毛发脱落，肌表不固，毛孔疏松，易出虚汗，外邪则易于乘虚而入，即所谓邪之所凑，其气必虚。因此说，卫气具有卫外而为固的重要生理功能。

1.2 皮肤与内脏的关系

人体是一个有机的整体，它的各种组织器官，虽然各有不同的功能，但却是互相联系、互相影响着的。换言之，一个器官的健康状况，能够影响到其他器官。皮肤（包括毛发、爪甲）是身体的重要组成部分，与其他器官密切关联。例如心主血脉，其华在面。心的功能正常与否，容易从面部色泽反应出来。正常时，面色红润有光泽；心气不足，循环不畅时，则面色㿠白或青紫。肝主筋，其华在爪（指、趾甲）。是指肝主管筋的活动，支配全身肌肉关节的运动。爪为筋之余，故爪和肝也有密切联系。肝血充足，筋强力壮，爪甲红润、坚韧；肝血不足，筋弱无力，爪甲枯槁、变色变形，容易脆裂。脾主运化，其华在唇。脾若能正常的运化水谷精微，滋养全身，则气血旺盛，四肢有力，肌肤健美，口唇红润；脾气虚弱，运化失常，则肌肤消瘦，四肢乏力，唇色淡白甚或萎黄无华。肺主气，外合皮毛。肺主气，即人身之气皆由肺所主。皮毛指一身之表，即皮肤、汗孔、毛发等组织。肺外合皮毛是指肺脏通过它的宣发作用，把水谷精微输布于皮毛，以滋养周身皮肤、毛发、肌肉等组织。其中卫气宣发到体表，可以发挥卫固体表，抗御外邪的作用。由于肺与皮肤紧密关联，故在病理上也常相互影响。如外邪入侵皮毛时，常同时侵犯肺脏，使皮肤和肺脏同时出现症状，如发热、怕冷、咳嗽等。如肺气虚弱，不能正常地宣发卫气，则可出现皮毛憔悴、枯槁，并使卫固体表，抵御外邪的功能下降，从而容易遭受外邪的侵袭。肾藏精，其华在发。发的生长与脱落、润泽与枯槁和肾的精气盛衰有关。肾脏精气充足，则毛发茂密乌黑而有光泽；肾脏精气不足，发失所养，则毛发易于枯脱或变白无光泽。

总之，皮肤与内脏关系十分密切。内脏功能的正常与否，常通过皮毛反映出来。反之，皮毛正常与否，也能反映内脏功能的盛衰。皮肤与内脏之间的这种密切关系部分是由经络连接和传导的。

1.3 皮肤与经络的关系

《素问·皮部论》中记载："凡十二经脉者，皮之部也。"说明皮肤是经络运行的重要部位。经络是人体组织结构的组成部分，它分布于全身各部，是经脉和络脉的总称。在生理上，经络具有运行营卫气血、沟通表里、抵御外邪、保卫机体的功能。

经络中的12经脉与脏腑直接相通，并分别循行在体表一定部位，与一定的内脏密切联系，各条经脉之间，通过经络相互沟通，从而使机体的各个组织器官联系成一个整体。由于经络内应脏腑，外联体表，因而病邪可通过经络在内脏与体表之间相互传变。如体表邪毒可由外传里，内攻脏腑，脏腑内在病变也可由里传表，从而在体表发生某些皮肤病。

依据皮肤病患病部位和经络在人体的循行分布，可以判断所属脏腑。这在皮肤病的辨证和按经用药上起着重要的指导作用。例如，鼻部属肺经，面颊部属胃经，因而酒渣鼻、面部痤疮常被推究为肺胃蕴热上蒸所致，此时可用清肺胃之热的方法治疗。耳部前后、胸胁部、阴部属肝胆经，因而耳部湿疹、胸胁部带状疱疹、阴囊湿疹可被推究为肝胆经湿热所致，此时可用清泻肝胆经湿热的方法治疗。

(杜锡贤)

2　皮肤病的中医病理

皮肤病的病种繁多，临床表现也多种多样，但究其病理变化，主要有风、湿、热、毒、燥、血瘀、肝肾不足等七种。这几种病理变化往往结合在一起发病，导致出现复杂的症状和皮肤损害。

2.1　风

1. 风的病理变化特点

(1) 发病急促，表现为突然发病，或病情进展迅速。如荨麻疹。

(2) 善行而数变，表现为皮损游走不定，或变化无常。如荨麻疹。

(3) 风性疏散，趋向外散上行。因此，由风所致的皮肤病，多发于人体头面和体表。如斑秃。

(4) 风善宿血分，风易犯血分，多与血热、血燥、血虚有密切关系。因此，不治血难以熄风，正如古人所说："治风先治血，血行风自灭"。

(5) 风为百病之长，风善于与他邪结合致病，故许多皮肤病具有风的病理特点。

2. 风的临床表现

皮肤损害多表现为风疹、丘疹、红斑。游走不定或泛发全身。常有突然发作，病情进展迅速，骤起骤消，瘙痒无度等特点。

2.2 湿

1. 湿的病理变化特点

(1) 湿性重浊，趋向下注和外渗。湿性下注表现在湿的病变多发于下肢或向下蔓延。湿性外渗表现在湿的病变易产生水疱、肿胀和渗液。

(2) 湿性粘滞留着难去，表现在湿的病变多迁延日久，反复发作，缠绵难愈。如湿疹。

(3) 湿常与风、热结合产生各种病理变化而致病。

2. 湿的临床表现

皮肤损害表现为皮肤肿胀、水疱、糜烂、渗出、皮脂分泌过多、脂性皮屑等。全身症状可有胸闷、纳呆、乏力等。局部常觉瘙痒。

2.3 热

1. 热的病理变化特点

(1) 热为阳邪，发病急促、暴烈。如丹毒、烫伤等。

(2) 热性上炎，常熏蒸头面部而致病。如酒渣鼻、青年痤疮等。

(3) 热易透达皮肤而致皮肤蕴热。如肝胆湿热透达皮肤可发生带状疱疹。

(4) 热势旺盛，易入营血，可引起全身发热。热盛灼肤，则红热灼痛，甚则肉腐成脓。

2. 热的临床表现

皮损色红、糜烂、脓疱、灼热、瘙痒、疼痛，可伴有身热口渴、便秘、溲赤等。

2.4 毒

毒，常见有药物毒、食物毒、虫毒、漆毒。

1. 毒的病理变化特点

(1) 禀性不耐者，毒邪易致病。

(2) 毒性暴烈，致病危重。或蕴结皮肤，出现多种皮损；或内攻脏腑，引起脏腑功能失调，甚则内脏损害；或毒陷营血，可引起高烧寒战等全身症状。如严重性药物性皮炎。

2. 毒的临床表现

皮肤损害可有红肿、紫斑、丘疹、风疹、水疱、糜烂、溃疡、表皮坏死与剥脱等多种形态。常发病突然，进展迅速，也可反复发作。局部灼热、瘙痒或疼痛。全身可有高热、疲倦不适等。

2.5 燥

1. 燥的病理变化特点

(1) 燥胜则干，易伤阴耗血，故常出现皮肤干燥、粗糙、鳞屑等皮损。

(2) 血虚可以化燥，血燥可以生风，风胜可以作痒。

(3) 燥的病理变化多出现在皮肤病的后期，多为慢性过程，病程较长。

2. 燥的临床表现

皮肤损害为皮肤干燥、粗糙、苔藓样变、皲裂、鳞屑、萎缩、毛发干枯脱落、指（趾）甲枯薄不荣等。自觉症状多为瘙痒。

2.6 血瘀

1. 血瘀的病理变化特点

(1) 瘀为实质性病变，或瘀积肌肤，或阻塞经脉，可瘀结成块，形成多种皮损和多种疾患。

(2) 血瘀的病理变化过程与气的关系非常密切，气行则血行，气滞则血瘀，血瘀也可导致气滞，故临床上治疗血瘀证常用行气活血法。

(3) 病变部位常固定不变，多为慢性病程。

2. 血瘀的临床表现

皮肤损害为瘀点、瘀斑、紫红或暗红斑、色素沉着斑、结节、肿块、毛细血管扩张、静脉曲张、肌肤甲错、肥厚变硬以及疣赘、瘢痕等。或伴有口唇青紫、舌有瘀斑、月经不调等。自觉症状可有疼痛、麻木、感觉迟钝等。

2.7 肝肾不足

1. 肝肾不足的病理变化特点
(1) 肝血虚不能养甲，则爪甲干枯。
(2) 肝血虚，血不养筋，筋气失荣则生疣目。
(3) 肝肾阴血虚，肤失濡养，可出现白斑。
(4) 肝肾精血不足，毛发失养，可致毛发干枯脱落或变白。
(5) 肾气虚，黑气上泛，则面生黧黑。

2. 肝肾不足的临床表现
(1) 色素性皮肤病，如黄褐斑、黑变病等
(2) 毛发爪甲病，如脱发、白发、甲营养不良症等。
(3) 结缔组织病，如系统性红斑狼疮、系统性硬皮病等。

自觉症状可有头晕目眩、耳鸣耳聋、腰膝酸软、阳萎早泄等。大多呈慢性病程。

3 皮肤病的症状辨证

皮肤病的症状分两部分。一是自觉症状,即病人对所患疾病的主观感觉。二是皮肤损害,即皮肤病的病理变化在皮肤或粘膜上的表现,是客观存在的病象,简称皮损或皮疹。

中医对皮肤病症状的认识,即中医对皮肤病的自觉症状和皮肤损害的辨证,是中医治疗皮肤病的理论基础。因此要对皮肤病进行辨证论治,重要的是认识皮肤病的症状和皮损,掌握中医对它的辨证。此外,还须了解病人的气血盛衰、脏腑虚实、禀性差异以及舌苔脉象的变化。

3.1 自觉症状

皮肤病的主要自觉症状是瘙痒,次为灼热、疼痛、麻木等。

1. 瘙痒

瘙痒主要由风、湿、热、燥、虫毒等五种病理变化作用于皮肤而引起,是皮肤病最普遍的症状。中医对瘙痒的辨证可分为:

(1) 风痒

风痒即以风的病理变化为主引起的瘙痒,多为遍身作痒或瘙痒无度,发病急,变化快,游走不定或泛发全身。如荨麻疹。

(2) 湿痒

湿痒即由湿的病理变化为主引起的瘙痒,多伴有皮肤肿胀、水疱、渗出、糜烂等皮损。如湿疹、足癣等。

(3) 热痒

热痒即由热的病理变化为主引起的瘙痒,多伴有皮肤焮红、灼热。如急性皮炎、湿疹类皮肤病。

(4) 燥痒

燥痒即因血虚化燥，血燥生风而引起的瘙痒，亦称血虚痒，多伴有皮肤干燥、粗糙、脱屑、苔藓样变。如神经性皮炎、慢性湿疹等。

(5) 虫痒

虫痒即因皮肤或粘膜感染虫毒而引起的瘙痒，表现为痒处固定，也可蔓延他处，常剧痒难忍，可有传染性。如疥疮、足癣等。

2. 疼痛

疼痛主要由气血瘀滞，经络阻塞不通而致。中医辨证分为：

(1) 热痛　痛处焮红灼热，遇冷痛轻。

(2) 寒痛　痛处皮色不变，得暖痛减。

(3) 气痛　痛无定处定时，喜缓怒甚。

(4) 血瘀痛　痛处固定，皮色红褐或紫青。

3. 麻木

麻木是皮肤经络阻隔，气血运行不畅而致局部气血虚弱，皮肤失养所致。多表现为肤色正常或略浅，或触觉、痛觉减弱。中医辨证为气血虚。

4. 灼热

灼热是由热的病理变化作用于皮肤而引起。多伴有皮损色红、瘙痒。中医辨证为热盛。

3.2　皮肤损害

1. 斑疹　为有明显界限和颜色改变的平于皮肤的皮损。

辨证：红斑为热或血热；紫斑为血瘀或热毒炽盛；白斑为气滞血虚或肝肾阴虚；褐斑为气滞血瘀或为肝肾虚；黑斑为肾虚；继发性色素沉着斑多属气血不和或血瘀。

2. 丘疹　为高出皮肤的小丘形、界限性、坚实性突起。

辨证：红色丘疹为血热，风热；紫色丘疹为血瘀或热毒；肤色丘疹多为气滞或风寒。

3. 水疱　为高出皮肤，含有液体的损害。

辨证：水疱清盈为湿邪浸聚；水疱周围有红晕，或在红斑上起水疱为湿热；水疱内有血性液体为血热；水疱混浊为湿毒。

4. 脓疱　为高出皮肤含有脓液的损害。

辨证：脓疱为热毒。

5. 结节　为位于皮肤或皮下的局限性、实质性损害。

辨证：红色结节为血热，血瘀；肤色结节为瘀滞或痰湿。

6. 风团　为皮肤的暂时性、局限性、水肿性扁平隆起。常骤起骤消，反复发作，消后不留痕迹。

辨证：风团色红为风热，血热；风团色白为风寒，风湿，或血虚受风。

7. 鳞屑　为皮肤积聚或脱落的鳞片状皮屑。

辨证：皮肤病早期出现者为风热；晚期出现者为血虚化燥，肤失荣养；脂性鳞屑为湿盛；干燥性鳞屑为血燥。

8. 糜烂　为水疱、脓疱等皮损的表皮破损形成的湿烂面。愈后不留痕迹。

辨证：糜烂渗液多属湿热；糜烂面渗液淋漓为湿盛；糜烂面有脓液为湿毒。

9. 溃疡　炎性或非炎性损伤造成皮肤或粘膜的深入真皮的局限性组织缺损。

辨证：急性溃疡疮底肉芽鲜红，脓液稠黄，伴红肿热痛为热毒；慢性溃疡疮底肉芽晦暗或淡红，分泌物稀少，久不愈合者为气血虚；疮面肉芽水肿为湿盛。

10. 皲裂　为皮肤上发生的线形裂隙。多见于手掌和足底。

辨证：皲裂为血虚，风燥，寒盛。

11. 苔藓样变　为局限性皮肤肥厚、干燥、粗糙，皮嵴增高，皮纹加深，或有细碎皮屑的损害。

辨证：苔藓样变为血虚，风燥。

12. 瘢痕　为修复溃疡、缺损形成的结缔组织，或原发性新生结缔组织肿块。分为萎缩性瘢痕和肥厚性瘢痕两种。

辨证：瘢痕属血瘀。

4 皮肤病的中医治疗

中医对皮肤病的治疗有悠久的历史和丰富的临床经验，是中国医学宝贵遗产的重要组成部分，她曾对世界皮肤病学做出过可贵的贡献。如大枫子仁治疗麻风，砷剂、汞剂治疗梅毒，硫磺治疗疥疮等都是首创于中国，后传于世界。

皮肤病的中医治疗以辨证论治为基本法则。辨证论治就是在运用四诊了解疾病的全面病情之后，再用中医辨证理论分析出疾病的病理变化和证候，然后再确定治疗法则、选用方剂和运用药物。治外必本诸内，就是说皮肤病虽发于外，但也与体内因素有关。将局部病变与整个机体的状况和环境条件结合起来，全面分析疾病的性质与治疗，这种整体观念是中医治疗学的基本观念。所以整体观念和辨证论治是中医治疗皮肤病的基本观念和基本法则。

皮肤病的治疗分内治法与外治法两种。无论内治或外治，都继承了中医理法方药的理论和成就，它具有与现代医学不同的诊疗特色。

4.1 内治法

皮肤病的内治方法很多，临床应用多以1种方法为主，配合运用其他方法。

1. 疏风清热法　用于风热客于肌肤所致的皮肤病。如风热所致的荨麻疹、玫瑰糠疹等。

方剂举例：消风散（1）。

常用药物：菊花、薄荷、蝉蜕、浮萍、桑叶、牛蒡子、白藓皮、地肤子、生石膏等。

2. 疏风散寒法　用于风寒侵袭肌肤所致的皮肤病。如风寒所致的荨麻疹、皮肤瘙痒症等。

方剂举例：荆防败毒散(2)。

常用药物：荆芥、防风、羌活、独活、麻黄、桂枝、白芷、细辛、苏叶等。

3. 活血祛风法　用于风邪郁久，宿于血分，久治不愈，或伴有血瘀证候的皮肤病。如结节性痒疹、色素性紫癜性苔藓样皮炎等。

方剂举例：四物消风饮(3)。

常用方药：当归、川芎、丹参、鸡血藤、荆芥、防风、全蝎、乌梢蛇、僵蚕等。

4. 养血祛风法　用于血虚风燥或血燥所致的皮肤病。如神经性皮炎、慢性湿疹等。

方剂举例：当归饮子(4)。

常用药物：当归、白芍、生地、熟地、何首乌、火麻仁、鸡血藤、丹参、荆芥、防风、白蒺藜等。

5. 清热解毒法　用于治疗热毒引起的皮肤病。如脓疱疮、丹毒、疖等。

方剂举例：五味消毒饮(5)、黄连解毒汤(6)。

常用药物：金银花、蒲公英、紫地丁、连翘、黄芩、黄连、栀子、黄柏、野菊花、大青叶、板蓝根等。

6. 清热凉血法　用于治疗证属血热的皮肤病。如银屑病、过敏性紫癜等。

方剂举例：犀角地黄汤(7)。

常用药物：生地、赤芍、丹皮、紫草、玄参、白薇、白茅根、地骨皮、生石膏等。

7. 清热利湿法　用于湿热蕴结肌肤引起的皮肤病。如带状疱疹、急性湿疹等。

方剂举例：龙胆泻肝汤(8)、五神汤(9)。

常用药物：龙胆草、栀子、黄芩、黄柏、苦参、茵陈、萆薢、车前子、茯苓、泽泻、木通、防己、赤小豆等。

8. 活血祛瘀法　用于治疗证属血瘀的皮肤病。如结节性红斑、硬皮病、瘢痕疙瘩等。

方剂举例：桃红四物汤（10）。

常用药物：桃仁、红花、赤芍、川芎、丹参、穿山甲、乳香、没药、三棱、莪术、土元、地龙等。

9. 软坚散结法　用于治疗皮肤痰核、疣赘等症。如皮肤结核、寻常疣、痤疮等。

方剂举例：桃红二陈汤（11）。

常用药物：半夏、陈皮、贝母、橘核、夏枯草、山慈姑、生牡蛎、连翘、昆布、海藻等。

10. 补益肝肾法　用于治疗肝肾不足引起的皮肤病。如斑秃、黄褐斑等。

方剂举例：神应养真丹（12）。

常用药物：熟地、何首乌、当归、白芍、萸肉、菟丝子、枸杞子、旱莲草、女贞子等。

4.2　外治法

外治法是根据自觉症状和皮肤损害的具体表现，选用不同的药物和剂型，进行局部治疗的一种方法。外治法在皮肤病的治疗中起着重要的作用，有些皮肤病单独使用外治法即收到满意疗效。现将临床常用剂型、用法及适应症分述如下：

1. 熏洗剂　又称溶液剂。是将单味或复方药物加水煎煮成一定浓度，滤去药渣所得的水溶液。具有清热解毒、祛风止痒、除湿收敛、活血消肿、杀虫除疣等作用。其用法有熏洗疗法和溻渍疗法两种。熏洗疗法即用热溶液先对准患部热熏，待温后浸洗患部，每日1~2次。每次约30分钟，每剂药可连续使用2~3天，每次煮沸10分钟即可使用。浸洗时注意溶液不宜过高。本法适用于慢性瘙痒性皮肤病，如神经性皮炎、慢性湿疹等。溻渍疗法，又称湿敷法，即用消毒纱布6~8层（或毛巾），浸透药液后，稍加拧挤，敷盖于皮损表面，每隔数分钟更换1次，如此连续进行30~60分钟，每日2~3次。临床多用冷湿敷，湿敷液的温度，夏季以室温或略低于室温为宜，冬季以10℃左右为宜。本法适用于急性或亚急性湿疹、皮炎，有明显渗液、红肿之皮损。

熏洗剂单味药可选用：蒲公英、野菊花、马齿苋、苦参、黄柏、生地榆、蛇床子等。复方药物可选用：解毒洗药（13）、止痒洗药（14）、祛风洗药（15）、硝矾洗药（16）等。

2. 散剂　又称粉剂。是将1种或1种以上的中药研制成的极细粉。具有保护皮肤、散热消肿、收敛干燥、杀虫止痒等作用。根据病情需要，可采用直接干撒患处，或用冷开水、醋、麻油等调成糊状涂布患处。渗出多及多毛部位忌用。散剂一般适用于急性、亚急性无渗液或少量渗液皮损。

散剂举例：黄柏散（17）、青蛤散（18）、颠倒散（19）、大黄粉等。

3. 油剂　油剂是将药物放入香油内炸枯去渣制成的药油，或将含油药物烧制出的药油，或药粉与香油、花生油等植物油混合制成。具有清热解毒、消肿止痛、收敛燥湿、护肤生肌等作用。用棉棒或毛笔蘸药外涂患处，每日2~3次。适用于糜烂渗液皮损湿敷间歇期，化脓性皮肤病出现糜烂渗脓者以及慢性皮炎、湿疹皮损。

油剂举例：紫草油（20）、黄连油（21）、黑豆馏油（22）、糠馏油（23）等。

4. 酊剂　将单味或复方中药置于白酒或酒精中浸泡过滤去渣而成。具有解毒、杀虫、活血、止痒等作用。用棉棒或毛笔蘸药直接外涂患处，每日2~3次。适用于局限性、慢性皮炎无破损者，如神经性皮炎、局限性皮肤瘙痒症，以及皮肤霉菌病、斑秃、白癜风等。

酊剂举例：补骨脂酊（补骨脂25克，75%酒精100毫升，混合浸泡一周去渣而成。治疗白癜风、斑秃等）、百部酊（百部25克，75%酒精100毫升，混合浸泡一周去渣而成。治疗神经性皮炎、荨麻疹、头虱等）、复方土槿皮酊（24）等。

5. 醋剂 ——将药物置于食醋内浸泡过滤去渣而成。具有杀虫止痒、软化角质作用。主要用于治疗手足癣、甲癣。患处洗净擦干后置于醋剂中浸泡。每次浸泡15～40分钟，每日2～3次。

醋剂举例：鹅掌风醋浸剂（25）、藿香醋浸剂（26）等。

6. 软膏 将药粉与植物油、动物油，或凡士林、蜂蜡等煎熬或调制而成。具有清热解毒、杀虫止痒、润肌收敛等作用。适用于一切慢性皮肤病具有结痂、皲裂、苔藓样变等皮损，及未溃破的急性感染性皮肤病。外涂患处，每日2次，或将软膏摊于纱布上敷患处，每日1次或隔日1次更换。

软膏举例：润肤膏（27）、黄连膏（28）、金黄膏（29）、大青膏（30）等。

下篇 各 论

1 病毒性皮肤病

1.1 单纯疱疹

单纯疱疹是由单纯疱疹病毒所致的一种急性疱疹性皮肤病。以常发于皮肤粘膜交界处，表现为局限性簇集性水疱为特征。中医以其常发于热病中，故称为热疮。

病因病机

本病的发生是因於发热性疾病、胃肠道功能紊乱、过度疲劳等情况，造成机体抵御能力降低，即正气虚弱，邪毒乘虚侵袭而发病。

临床表现

1. 本病好发于成年人的皮肤与粘膜交界处，以唇周、鼻孔周围、面颊以及外阴部为多发部位。

2. 局部先有灼热瘙痒感，继而出现红斑，红斑上迅速出现簇集性水疱，水疱基底微红，疱液透明或微混浊。可有擦烂、渗液、结痂等损害，愈后常遗有暂时性色素沉着。

3. 若继发感染，可有化脓、疼痛。局部淋巴结常肿大、压痛。

4. 自觉灼热感、瘙痒感，或有微痛。

5. 病程约1～2周，可以自愈，但易复发。

辨证论治

1. 内治法

(1) 湿热熏蒸型

主证：口唇、鼻孔周围或面颊处出现红斑及簇集性水疱。自觉刺痒、灼热。舌质红，苔薄黄，脉多浮数。

治法：清解肺胃湿热。

方药：辛荑清肺饮（31）加减

辛荑、黄芩、栀子、生枇杷叶、知母、百合、杏仁、蔻仁各9克，生石膏、薏苡仁各15克，甘草6克。

(2) 湿热下注型

主证：红斑、水疱群见于外阴部。有灼热、瘙痒感。舌红，苔黄或黄腻，脉象多滑数。

治法：清泻肝胆湿热。

方药：龙胆泻肝汤（8）加减

柴胡、黄芩、栀子、生地、车前子、泽泻、当归、苦参、萆薢各9克，木通、生甘草各6克。

2. 外治法

(1) 黄柏散（17）用茶水调搽患处。

(2) 2%冰片水擦患处。

1.2 带状疱疹

带状疱疹是由病毒感染而发生的一种急性疱疹性皮肤病。以骤然发生密集的水疱群，沿一侧神经分布区呈带状排列，伴有神经痛，愈后极少复发为特征。

本病在中医古籍中称为缠腰火丹。

病因病机

本病多因情志不遂，肝火妄动，而致肝胆火盛；或因饮食不节，脾失健运，而致脾湿内生；或因疾病之后正气虚弱，复受邪毒侵袭而发病。

临床表现

1. 多发生于一侧腰部或胸部，以及头面颈部等处。春秋季较多见。

2. 发病前常有轻度发热、倦怠、纳呆、全身不适，局部皮肤刺痛、瘙痒、灼热感及感觉过敏。亦可突然发病。

3. 初起患部出现片状红斑，继而出现红色丘疹群，迅速变成簇集性水疱，周围有红晕，水疱累累如珠，五七成簇，疱疹之间常有正常皮肤。皮疹沿一侧神经干路呈带状排列。

4. 自觉有疼痛、灼热、刺痒感，但小儿发病疼痛较轻，老年患者疼痛较剧，甚至皮损消退后仍遗有轻重不同的神经痛。

5. 疱疹严重时可呈现血疱和坏死，伴有发热等全身症状。一般疱疹持续数日后可结痂，结痂脱落后遗有淡红斑或色素沉着。

6. 病程2～3周。部分年老体弱患者，皮肤疼痛可持续数周或数月。

辨证论治

1. 内治法

(1) 热盛型

主证：相当于带状疱疹初期。患部有红斑、红色丘疹群，疼痛、灼热、刺痒感，可有烦躁不宁，口苦咽干，舌质红，舌苔黄，脉象弦数。

治法：凉血清热。

方药：凉血清肝汤 (32)

生地、赤芍各15克，丹皮12克，柴胡、川芎、黄芩、栀子、龙胆草、紫草、青皮各9克，金银花、连翘各15克，生甘草6克。

(2) 湿热型

主证：相当于带状疱疹中期。患部皮肤潮红，簇集性水疱，周围有红晕，或溃破渗液。有疼痛及灼热感，可伴有烦躁、口干、舌质红、舌苔黄腻、脉象滑数。

治法：清泻肝胆湿热。

方药：龙胆泻肝汤（8）加减

金银花、连翘各 15 克，生地、车前子、泽泻各 12 克，柴胡、龙胆草、栀子、黄芩、赤芍、元胡各 9 克，木通、生甘草各 6 克。

(3) 瘀滞型

主证：相当于带状疱疹晚期。患部疱疹结痂，遗有淡红褐斑或色素沉着，仍有疼痛。

治法：疏肝活血，通络止痛。

方药：柴胡疏肝汤（33）加减

白芍、赤芍、丹参各 15 克，柴胡、香附、川芎、枳壳、陈皮、元胡、青皮、川楝子各 9 克，生甘草 6 克。

加减：

热盛者可加大青叶、板蓝根，重用黄芩、龙胆草。

胸腰部灼热剧痛者，可重用黄柏、牛膝。

烦躁不安者，可选加珍珠母、生龙骨、生牡蛎、远志、枣仁。

疼痛剧烈者，可选加乳香、没药、郁金、白芷、细辛、川芎。

2. 外治法

(1) 蜈蚣散：蜈蚣 10 克焙干，加冰片 1 克，共研细粉，用水调涂患部。

(2) 大黄黄柏粉：两药等量研细粉，加冰片少许，水调外涂患部。

(3) 鲜马齿苋适量，洗净捣烂成泥外敷患部。

1.3 疣

疣是病毒引起的常见皮肤病，是发生在皮肤浅表的赘生物。临床上可分为寻常疣、扁平疣、传染性软疣、尖锐湿疣四种。

病因病机

由于皮肤气血失和及腠理不密，复感邪毒侵入，致使气血凝滞瘀聚高突，而出现各种形态的疣赘性病变。

临床表现

1. 寻常疣

(1) 好发于青少年手背及头面部皮肤。

(2) 初发为 1~2 个，约绿豆至黄豆大角质增生性丘疹，表面粗糙略硬，呈淡褐色或正常皮色，后期略增大，数目可逐渐增多，顶端呈乳头状或刺状增生。

(3) 一般无自觉症状，慢性过程，可持续数年，能自愈，愈后不留痕迹。

临床上还可见到以下几种异型寻常疣:

(1) 甲周疣　发于甲周，可延及甲下，呈刺状增生，可有裂隙，易继发化脓感染。

(2) 丝状疣　多发于老年、中年人的颈部及眼睑皮肤，柔软细长，呈丝状突起。

(3) 指状疣　好发于头皮部位，常呈多个参差不齐的指状突起。

(4) 跖疣　好发于足底，由于压迫及磨擦，使跖疣呈现与皮面平行的角化斑，表面粗糙，若削除表面角质层，可出现乳白色角质软芯。多单侧发生，数目不定。

2. 扁平疣

(1) 好发于青年人，女性多见。多发生在面部、手背、前臂。

(2) 常突然发现，初呈针头或芝麻粒大，后呈大米粒大扁平丘疹，淡褐色或淡灰色，表面光滑，呈多个散在或密集分布。

(3) 有微痒或无自觉症状，慢性过程，可自愈，也可复发。

3. 传染性软疣

(1) 多见于儿童和青年，好发于躯干和四肢。有轻度传染性。

(2) 初为针头大小丘疹，逐渐变大、增多。约绿豆或黄豆大时，呈半球形隆起，表面光滑，具有蜡样光泽，中央有脐窝，呈灰白色或正常肤色。刺破其表皮，可挤出乳白色物质，称为软疣小体。

(3) 自觉微痒，经过缓慢。

4. 尖锐湿疣

(1) 发于成年人，多发生在外阴、肛周、腋窝、妇女乳房下部。

(2) 初起为数个乳头状丘疹，渐增多增大，融合重迭。呈疣刺状、乳头状、蕈状、菜花状或巨大皮癌状不一。呈暗褐色或灰色，触之易出血，表面湿润，可有糜烂、裂隙、浆液或脓液。常有恶臭。

(3) 早期无自觉症状，晚期可有瘙痒感及压迫感。

辨证论治

1. 内治法

内治法适应于疣体分布广泛者，如扁平疣、传染性软疣、寻常疣。本病在病机、辨证、治则方面有不同见解：有肝虚血燥，筋气不荣则生疣目之说；有血瘀立论，气血凝滞，瘀聚皮肤之说；有邪毒立论，邪毒侵入皮肤，增殖瘀聚之说。故临床辨证有肝虚血燥、血瘀、毒结之分。

(1) 肝虚血燥型

主证：疣体广泛，表面干燥、粗糙、枯萎。

治法：养血润燥，平肝潜镇。

方药：治疣方（经验方）

当归、白芍、灵磁石、紫贝齿、代赭石、生牡蛎各12克，桃仁、红花、山慈姑、地骨皮、黄柏各9克。

(2) 血瘀型

主证：疣体广泛，呈红褐色，坚实。

治法：活血破瘀。

方药：治瘊方（经验方）

熟地、何首乌、杜仲、白芍、赤芍各 12 克，丹皮、桃仁、红花、穿山甲、赤小豆、白术、牛膝各 9 克。

(3) 毒结型

主证：疣体增殖较巨，有渗液或脓液。

治法：解毒散结。

方药：治疣汤

金银花、连翘、蒲公英、大青叶、板蓝根、白藓皮各 12 克，柴胡、桃仁、红花、赤芍、丹皮、紫草各 9 克，夏枯草 15 克。

2. 外治法

(1) 熏洗法

板蓝根 30 克，水煎洗，日 1～2 次。

洗疣方：板蓝根 30 克，紫草、香附、桃仁各 15 克，水煎洗，日 1～2 次。

擦疣方：白藓皮 60 克，明矾 20 克，香附、木贼草各 30 克，加水 1 000 毫升，水煎透，去渣浓缩至 300 毫升，每日用此药水擦患处 3 次，每次 5 分钟。

(2) 外敷法

鸦胆子泥外敷：将鸦胆子用水浸泡后，剥皮取仁捣泥，敷患处，用胶布固定，3～4 日换 1 次。

乌梅粉外敷法：将乌梅研粉加水调膏，敷患处，用胶布固定。

2 细菌性皮肤病

2.1 脓疱疮

脓疱疮是一种浅在性皮肤脓疱病。多在夏秋季发病，好发于儿童，能接触传染和自身接种，易在儿童集体中造成流行。

病因病机

本病多因于小儿机体虚弱，皮肤娇嫩，再加夏秋暑湿及皮肤在尘污汗浸下，易感邪毒而发病。皮肤感受邪毒，邪毒化热，热毒蕴结皮肤而形成脓疱疮之皮肤损害。

临床表现

临床上以寻常型脓疱疮最常见，此外尚有大疱型脓疱疮、新生儿脓疱疮、深脓疱疮。

1. 寻常型脓疱疮

初起为红斑或丘疹，迅速发展成黄豆大水疱，疱周有红晕，约1～2天后变成脓疱。脓疱呈多个散在发生，疱壁薄而紧张，易溃破，破后露出红色糜烂面，脓液溢出，浸淫四散，随处可生。脓液干燥后形成蜡黄色脓痂。自觉瘙痒。重者可伴有发热，淋巴结肿大等。

2. 大疱型脓疱疮

脓疱较大，如蚕豆或更大，疱周红晕不显著。疱壁始紧后松，由于体位关系，脓液常沉积于脓疱下方，呈半月形坠积状。疱破后脓液干燥结痂，痂呈淡黄色，痂脱即愈，愈后遗留暂时性色素沉着。

3. 新生儿脓疱疮

多在出生后不久即发病，患儿一般体质较弱。脓疱约黄豆至胡桃大，壁薄易破，溃破后出现糜烂，结脓痂。本病发病急，传染性强，病情进展迅速，可迅速扩延到全身较大面积。全身症状明显，出现发热、萎靡、吐泻等。如失治可因并发败血症或毒血症而危及生命。

4. 深脓疱疮

多发生在下肢。初起为红斑或为黄豆大硬结，渐成脓疱，周围有红晕，逐渐增大，侵及深层组织，溃后形成溃疡，脓痂较厚，附着牢固，愈后遗有瘢痕自觉疼痛。

辨证论治

1. 内治法

主证：基本皮损为脓疱，疱周有红晕，疱破结脓痂，附近淋巴结肿大，自觉灼热、瘙痒或疼痛，重者伴有发热、烦渴、便干、溲黄等，此属热毒之证。

治法：清热解毒。

方药：黄连解毒汤（6）合五味消毒饮（5）

金银花、蒲公英、紫地丁、野菊花各15克，黄连、黄柏、栀子、黄芩、天葵子各9克。

重症新生儿脓疱疮应配合现代医学疗法。

2. 外治法

一般轻症可仅用外治疗法。

（1）首先剪除脓疱，用解毒洗药（13）或金银花、野菊花、苦参、黄柏各15克，白矾6克，煎汤洗净脓液、脓痂，再用黄柏散（17）或黄连粉撒布疮面，日1次。

（2）黄连6克，黄柏9克，枯矾3克，冰片1克，氧化锌24克，共研细末，加凡士林45克调软膏，外涂患处，日2~3次。

预防与护理

1. 注意清洁卫生，及时治疗各种瘙痒性皮肤病。
2. 发现患儿立即隔离治疗，患儿用过的衣物要消毒。
3. 每次敷药前，先用麻油湿润患处片刻，揩去原药，然后敷新药。

2.2 丹毒

丹毒是溶血性链球菌感染引起的一种皮肤和皮下组织的急性炎症。好发于下肢及颜面，以界限明显的局限性红肿为特征，伴有发热恶寒等全身症状，发病迅速，极少化脓。

病因病机

本病多因血分有热，外感邪毒。或皮肤破损，邪毒侵袭而发病。邪毒化热，热毒蕴结肌肤而出现红肿热痛。发于头面者，多挟风；发于下肢者，多挟湿；热毒炽盛者，可热入营血，引起严重的并发症。

临床表现

1. 发病初起先有发热恶寒，全身不适等全身症状。
2. 患部出现红斑，迅速向周围扩大，表面光亮，颜色鲜红，边界清楚。发生在皮肤疏松部位（口唇、眼睑等）可呈现明显红肿。伴有附近淋巴结肿大。
3. 患部有明显灼热疼痛感。
4. 严重者可出现水疱、大疱、坏死，也可向他处蔓延。
5. 可出现高热烦躁，神昏谵语，恶心呕吐等症状。
6. 反复发作者，患部可继发淋巴性水肿。
7. 发病中可出现白细胞计数增高，血沉增快，抗链球菌溶血素增高。

辨证论治

1. 内治法

（1）热毒挟风型

主证：头面部红肿，发热恶寒，灼热疼痛或有刺痒。

治法：清热解毒，散风消肿。

方药：普济消毒饮（34）加减

板蓝根、金银花、连翘各18克，黄连、黄芩、马勃、牛蒡子、薄荷、僵蚕、柴胡、桔梗各9克,甘草6克。

(2) 热毒挟湿型

主证:小腿局限性红肿,发热恶寒,灼热疼痛。

治法:清热解毒,佐以利湿。

方药:茵陈赤小豆汤(经验方)

金银花、忍冬藤各30克,黄柏、苦参、茵陈、防己、泽泻、丹皮、赤芍、牛膝、苍术各9克,赤小豆、薏苡仁各15克。

(3) 热毒炽盛型

主证:患部红肿,灼热疼痛,高热恶寒,神昏谵语等。

治法:清营凉血解毒。

方药:犀角地黄汤(7)合黄连解毒汤(6)加味

金银花、连翘、生石膏各30克,生地、赤芍、丹皮各15克,黄连、黄芩、黄柏、栀子、知母各9克,犀角6克。

可配合服紫雪丹(35)或安宫牛黄丸(36),每次1粒,每日2次。

2. 外治法

(1) 金黄膏(29)或大青膏(30)外敷患处,每日换1次。

(2) 黄柏散或大黄粉,水调糊状外涂患处,每日2次。

(3) 鲜马齿苋洗净捣烂为泥外敷患处,每日更换2次。

预防与护理

1. 有皮肤破损者,应及时处理,避免感染。

2. 治疗原发病灶,如足癣。

3. 患病期间,应卧床休息,充分饮水。发于下肢者,应抬高患肢。

3 癣

癣是真菌侵犯皮肤、毛发、指（趾）甲而产生的有传染性的皮肤真菌病。常见的有手足癣、体癣、股癣、甲癣、头癣、花斑癣等。中医称手癣为鹅掌风；称足癣为脚湿气；称体癣为圆癣或钱癣；称股癣为阴癣；称甲癣为灰指甲；称头癣为白秃疮或肥疮等；称花斑癣为汗斑或紫白癜风。因癣的发病部位不同，临床表现各异。本病在温热季节及温热地区发病率较高，有传染性。

病因病机

中医认为本病的致病因素是虫（真菌）。虫毒侵入肌肤蕴热生风化燥化湿，在患处即出现由风、湿、热、燥引起的各种临床表现。

3.1 手足癣

临床表现

多见于成年人，儿童很少见。多在夏秋季发病、加重或复发，冬季可减轻。损害一般局限在手掌、足底及趾间。临床一般分为3种类型：

(1) 水疱型 初起掌跖及指趾间发生散在性或簇集性粟粒大小水疱，疱壁较厚，不易破裂，可引起剧烈瘙痒。疱壁破裂后叠起鳞屑，四周继起小水疱，可逐渐扩大，伴有瘙痒。

(2) 糜烂型 多见于趾指间，水疱破后局部潮湿，皮肤浸渍变白，白色腐皮剥脱后，呈现鲜红糜烂面，有渗出。患部瘙痒。多见于手足多汗者。

(3) 鳞屑角化型 水疱已不存在，或偶尔发生。皮肤干燥、肥厚，不断产生鳞屑，进而粗糙甚至皲裂。多发生在掌跖及侧缘，伴有瘙痒，由于皲裂可引起疼痛。

糜烂型易继发细菌感染，引起淋巴管炎，淋巴结炎、小腿丹毒等。

辨证论治

1. 外治法

（1）熏洗剂　可用止痒洗药（14），祛风洗药（15）或硝矾洗药（16）煎汤，温热时熏洗患部。若继发细菌感染再加解毒洗药（13）熏洗。

（2）酊剂　可用复方土槿皮酊（24）外搽患部，日3次。

（3）醋剂　可用藿香醋浸剂（26），或鹅掌风醋浸剂（25）浸泡患部，每日1～2次。

（4）脚气粉（37）干撒患部，或撒于鞋袜内。

2. 内治法

适用于糜烂渗液或合并急性细菌感染者。

（1）湿盛型

主证：患处糜烂渗液，或反复起簇集性水疱。

治法：淡渗利湿，佐以清热祛风。

方药：萆薢渗湿汤（53）加味

白藓皮、滑石、薏苡仁各15克，萆薢、赤苓、泽泻、黄柏、丹皮、苦参各9克，木通、甘草各6克。

（2）湿热型

主证：皮损为水疱、糜烂、渗出，患处轻度红肿。

治法：清热利湿。

方药：茵陈赤小豆汤（经验方，见丹毒）

（3）热毒型

主证：患部渗出，红肿，疼痛，或继发小腿丹毒，腹股沟淋巴结肿大压痛，可伴发热。

治法：清热解毒，佐以利湿。

方药：黄连解毒汤（6）合五神汤（9）加味

金银花、紫地丁各 30 克，黄连、黄柏、黄芩、栀子、苦参、丹皮、茯苓、车前子、牛膝、泽兰叶各 9 克。

3.2 甲癣

临床表现

多由手足癣蔓延而来。初发时仅侵犯少数甲，久则蔓延及多个甲。不治疗常终生不愈。表现为甲远端或全部甲板增厚，表面凹凸不平，患甲不透明，失去光泽，呈灰褐、灰黄或灰白色。甲变松脆，常有残缺或甲变形。一般无不适感。

辨证论治

外治法

1. 可用藿香醋浸剂（26），或鹅掌风醋浸剂（25）浸泡患部。

2. 荆芥、防风、大枫子各 18 克，皂角、红花、地骨皮各 15 克，明矾 12 克，食醋 1 500 毫升，混合浸泡 7 天，过滤去渣，用药液浸泡患部，每日 2～3 次，每次 20～30 分钟，本法也适用于手足癣。

3. 皂角 30 克，白凤仙花（干者）30 克、川椒 15 克、陈白醋 250 毫升，将上 3 种药物分别研成粗末，装瓶内，注入白醋浸泡，7 天后即可使用。用脱脂药棉蘸药适量，敷患处，纱布包扎每 12 小时换 1 次，直至病愈。

在治疗过程中，应常用洁净刀片轻轻削刮变软之患甲。

3.3 体癣、股癣

临床表现

凡发生在面、颈、躯干及四肢的癣称体癣。仅局限于大腿近端内侧，或同时累及生殖器及臀部者称为股癣。表现为圆形或多环形的红斑，边界清楚且隆起，可有散在的丘疹、水疱、鳞屑或结痂，以边缘为著。中央常有自愈倾向，自觉瘙痒。如治疗不当则呈离心性扩大。搔抓日久可呈现湿疹化或苔藓化皮损。

辨证论治

以外治法为主，可选用以下诸方法：

1. 复方土槿皮酊（24）外涂，或皮肤软膏（85）外涂，每日2～3次。

2. 土大黄60克，用75%酒精250毫升浸泡3天，过滤后每日外涂患部2～3次。

3. 硝矾洗药（16）外洗患部，每日2次，每次30分钟。

3.4 头癣

临床表现

头癣为发生于头皮和头发的一种浅在真菌病。主要在儿童中发病，传染性强。头癣在临床上又分为黄癣、白癣、黑点癣3种。

1. 黄癣

（1）初起毛囊周围轻度发炎，有少量鳞屑，形成黄红色小点，逐渐扩大成黄色癣痂，呈圆碟形，有毛发贯穿。癣痂可融合成不整形，可散在分布或遍及全头。

（2）病发干燥而脆，渐呈不均匀脱落，日久毛囊破坏，呈永久性脱发，可遗有萎缩性瘢痕。

（3）头皮瘙痒，有臭味。

（4）慢性经过，至青春期可减轻，但不会自愈。

2. 白癣

（1）初起先出现毛囊性丘疹，覆有灰白色鳞屑，渐扩大成灰白色鳞屑斑，呈单个或多个出现。

（2）病发干枯变脆，失去光泽，近头皮处毛干有灰白色菌鞘，易在距头皮2～4毫米处折断，故病发参差不齐。

（3）自觉瘙痒。

（4）慢性过程，至青春期可自愈，愈后不留瘢痕。继发化脓性感染者，愈后留瘢痕，并在该处出现永久性脱发。

3. 黑点癣

(1) 初起呈散在性局限性红斑，渐发展成圆形白色鳞屑斑，边界清楚。

(2) 病发易在出头皮处折断，形成黑点状。

(3) 自觉瘙痒。慢性经过，愈后遗有小片瘢痕。

辨证论治

1. 外治法

(1) 每周理发 1 次。

(2) 每日用白矾 10 克，或蛇床子 30 克洗头。

(3) 每日早晚各擦 1 次药膏。可选用：

5%硫磺软膏。

雄黄膏（雄黄 30 克，氧化锌 30 克，凡士林 300 克调成软膏）。

一扫光软膏（苦参、黄柏、烟胶各 500 克，枯矾、木鳖肉、大枫子肉、蛇床子、红椒、潮脑、硫磺、白矾、水银、轻粉各 90 克，白砒 15 克，共研细末，熟猪油 1 120 克，化开，入药搅匀即成）。

(4) 每用药 1 周，用雄灰糊溶发 1 次（雄灰糊处方：雄黄与生石灰按 1∶4 比例装入容器，加冷水搅拌均匀，使成稀糊状，放置 1 天后应用）用法：将雄灰糊均匀涂于头皮，20 分钟后洗头，头发即可脱落。此药有溶发作用，不破坏毛囊，故毛发可再生。

以上治疗应连续使用，直至真菌检查确认治愈为止。

3.5 花斑癣

临床表现

1. 好发于成人的胸背部、上肢近端及颈部。常冬轻夏重。

2. 损害为黄豆大小斑点，呈淡白色、黄褐色或灰白色，边界清楚,表面光滑,上覆极细鳞屑。

3. 一般无自觉症状,或有微痒。

4. 慢性过程,可持续多年不愈。

辨证论治

外治法

1. 硫黄醋液。硫磺30克与100毫升醋混合,浸泡一周后外涂患处,每日2～3次。

2. 5～10%硫黄乳剂或复方土槿皮酊(24)外涂,每日2～3次。

3. 密陀僧30克、乌贼骨30克、硫磺15克、川椒15克,共研成极细粉,用时取生姜1块,斜形切断,以断面蘸药粉少许擦患处,擦至皮损为淡红色为度,每日早晚各1次,擦后勿用水洗。一般治疗1～2周可愈。为预防复发,愈后再擦3～6天。

预防

1. 头癣的预防　凡患者用过的帽子、枕套、梳子等生活用品,未经消毒不得使用;理发工具要严格消毒处理;早发现,早治疗,彻底治愈后方可入托、入学。

2. 足癣的预防　保持足部清洁干燥;脚盆、脚布、拖鞋等用品不能互相借用;患者穿过的鞋袜要经常洗刷、曝晒。

(赵纯修)

4 昆虫所致皮肤病

4.1 疥疮

疥疮是由疥虫寄生于人体所致的传染性皮肤病，传染性强，易于在家庭及接触者之间传播流行。中医文献称本病为疥疮、虫疥等。

病因病机

接触疥疮病人，或使用病人衣物，疥虫侵入皮肤所致。

临床表现

1. 有接触疥疮病人或使用疥疮病人用过的衣物史。
2. 本病可发于任何年龄，好发于皮肤较薄而柔软的部位，如指缝、腕屈面、肘窝、脐周、下腹部、股内侧及外生殖器等处。一般不发于头面、掌蹠部。
3. 皮肤损害主要为小丘疹、小水疱及隧道。丘疹多为针头至米粒大小。隧道为本病之特征，系疥虫在表皮内钻行而成之通道，约3～15毫米长，常弯曲，微隆起，呈淡灰色或皮色，其末端常有小水疱形成。阴囊、阴茎、腹股沟、腋窝等处可发生结节性损害。
4. 剧烈瘙痒，以夜间为甚，常影响睡眠。
5. 常因搔抓而产生抓痕、皮肤肥厚、色素沉着和化脓性感染。
6. 刮取新发的水疱疱液进行显微镜检查，可查到疥虫。

辨证论治

1. 外治法

本病一般不需内治，主要靠外用药物杀灭疥虫。

临床常用5～15%硫磺软膏，小儿用5～10%，成人用10～

15%。先用温热水和肥皂洗浴，擦干后搽药，除头面外，自颈部遍及全身，搽药时要稍用力，皮损处多搽，每日早晚各1次，连用3天。在搽药期间不洗澡，不换衣服，第四天再洗浴，换上经过消毒的衣服、被褥。观察1周，如无新皮疹出现，即为痊愈。若未愈，应重复治疗1次。

2. 内治法

如继发化脓性感染时，可用五味消毒饮（5）加减

生地15克，赤芍15克，金银花30克，蒲公英30克，白藓皮30克，野菊花15克，地丁15克，连翘15克，生甘草9克。

护理及预防

1. 治疗中必须注意杀灭所有的疥虫，疥疮才能治愈；疗程间注意换用洁净及消过毒的衣服及被褥，以防复发；换下的衣服、被褥，须煮沸或日晒，或用熨斗烫过，必要时应用药物进行消毒，防止再次接触传染。

2. 为杜绝传染，病人家庭内与集体宿舍中同室居住的人，应予同时治疗。

3. 加强个人卫生及服务行业卫生管理，避免疥疮传播。

4.2 虫咬皮炎

虫咬皮炎是由虫类叮咬或刺螫后，通过毒汁、毒刺、毒毛刺激皮肤引起的炎症性皮肤病。引起该病常见的昆虫有蠓、蚊、蚁、蚤、臭虫、蜂、蝎、刺毛虫、蚂蟥、蜈蚣、蛇等。中医文献称恶虫叮咬或毒虫咬伤。

病因病机

恶虫刺咬，邪毒侵入，郁于肌肤而成。

临床表现

1. 多见于夏秋害虫孳生季节，好发于暴露部位。

2. 皮肤以瘀点、丘疹、风团多见，有时可出现水疱、大疱或脓疱，往往在损害中央见有一针头大的小瘀点（刺吮点），散

在分布或数个成群。蜂、蝎、蜈蚣螯咬后则局部红肿明显，蚂蝗咬伤后则以出血为主。

3. 局部有不同程度的瘙痒、麻木、烧灼或疼痛感，重者可伴有恶寒发热、头晕胸闷、恶心呕吐，甚至抽搐昏迷等全身中毒症状。

辨证论治

1. 外治法

虫咬皮炎，轻者为多，一般仅有局部症状，故以外治为主。

（1）有毒刺进入皮肤者，应小心将其完全拔除。毒毛刺入者可用橡皮膏或狗皮膏（38）粘贴，将其拔出。伤口大或明显者，用吸奶器或火罐吸出毒液。

（2）局部用肥皂水彻底清洗（黄蜂、蜈蚣、蝎螯伤后用醋洗）后，可选用必舒膏（39）、风油精（40）、止痒酊（41），外涂患处。

（3）南通蛇药片（42）适量，用冷开水溶成糊状，涂于伤口周围（中央留出伤口不涂）。

（4）鲜马齿苋适量，捣烂敷患处。

2. 内治法

重者往往伴有全身中毒症状，除进行局部处理外，服用南通蛇药片（42），每日3次，每次10片，同时可服用五味消毒饮（5）合黄连解毒汤（6）加减。

金银花30克，蒲公英30克，野菊花15克，地丁30克，黄芩9克，黄连9克，栀子12克，车前草30克，生甘草9克。

护理及预防

1. 皮炎产生后，切忌搔抓、热水烫洗等不适当刺激。

2. 注意改善环境卫生，昆虫孳生地要喷洒杀虫剂。

3. 夏季要使用蚊帐、蚊香等防护用品。

5 物理性皮肤病

5.1 冻疮

冻疮是发生于寒冷季节的 1 种血瘀性皮肤病。好发于手足、外耳及面部，轻者出现暗紫肿块，重者溃烂成疮。

病因病机

素体阳虚，外寒侵袭，寒凝肌肤，气滞血瘀，发为本病。

临床表现

本病发于寒冷季节，好发于手足、外耳及面部，常对称发生。初起患处出现浮肿性红斑，逐渐变暗紫色，重者暗紫色斑片上发生水疱或大疱，疱破后发生溃烂，自觉肿胀感，遇热后灼热瘙痒，溃破后有疼痛，创面不易愈合，天气转暖时可自愈。

辨证论治

1. 内治法

宜温经散寒、活血通脉，服用当归四逆汤（43）加味

当归 15 克，白芍 15 克，桂枝 15 克，炮姜 9 克，附子 9 克，制川乌 9 克，制草乌 9 克，细辛 3 克，通草 9 克，大枣 5 枚，炙甘草 9 克。

2. 外治法

（1）活血止痛散（44）或干辣椒煎汤烫洗患处，日 1～2 次。亦可用山楂 120 克，煎汤烫洗。

（2）外搽生姜酊、辣椒酊或冻疮膏（45）。

（3）溃烂处可用鲜山楂去核，捣成糊状，外敷患处，用山楂膏外敷亦可。

护理及预防

1. 注意保暖防寒，尤其是已发生冻疮的部位。冷天外出，

要适当添衣、戴口罩、手套，穿宽松适当而保暖的鞋袜，避免长时间受冻。

2. 注意保持手足干燥，对潮湿的口罩、手套、鞋袜，应及时更换或烤干。

5.2 手足皲裂

手足皲裂是发生于手掌、足底部的线形裂隙，为冬季常见的皮肤病。中医文献称为皲裂、皲裂疮。

病因病机

外受风、寒、燥邪，郁于皮肤，气血阻滞，肤失濡养而致。

临床表现

1. 多发于寒冷的冬季，好发于皮肤肥厚而经常摩擦的手指、手掌屈侧、足跟、蹠外侧等处。

2. 初起皮肤干燥、发紧、变硬，以后皮肤变粗糙、肥厚，失去光泽，继之出现深浅不一、长短不等的裂隙。

3. 裂口深者疼痛难忍，可有出血，屈伸不利，甚至影响劳动和生活。

辨证论治

本病一般勿需内治，仅外用药物治疗即可。

1. 活血止痛散（44）煎汤乘热熏洗患处，每日1~2次，每次30分钟;或用地骨皮30克，白矾15克，煎汤熏洗。

2. 外用润肌膏（46）、蛤蜊油（47）、润肤膏（27）等涂搽患处，每日2~4次。

护理及预防

劳动时应注意保温、防寒，避免摩擦，震荡刺激及油垢浸渍，不用碱性过强的肥皂洗手，冬季外涂护肤油脂。

5.3 痱子

痱子是1种发生于夏季高温季节,皮肤出现丘疹的皮肤病。中医文献又称其为热痱、汗疹等。

病因病机
暑湿熏蒸皮肤,闭塞毛窍,汗出不畅所致。

临床表现
1. 本病多发于炎热的夏季。
2. 好发于肥胖小儿及妇女的前额、颈周、胸背、乳房下皱折、肘腘窝、腹股沟等多汗部位。
3. 发病较急,患处出现密集成片的丘疹、丘疱疹,针头大小,周围绕以红晕,触之粗糙有芒刺样感觉,皮疹可成批出现。
4. 自觉瘙痒和灼热。
5. 如果天气转凉爽,皮疹可于数日内自行消退,脱屑而愈。
6. 本病可因搔抓继发感染而成痱毒,发生毛囊炎、脓疱疮和疖肿。

辨证论治
1. 内治法

皮损广泛者可用清暑化湿的清暑汤(48)加减

赤芍9克,白茅根30克,金银花12克,连翘9克,车前草15克,泽泻9克,淡竹叶9克,滑石18克,牛蒡子9克,生甘草3克。

形成痱毒时应清热解毒,可用五味消毒饮(5)加减

生地12克,金银花15克,蒲公英15克,野菊花15克,地丁15克,连翘9克,车前草15克,生甘草9克。

2. 外治法

用韭菜250克或鲜马齿苋250克,煎水洗浴。擦干后撒布六一散(49)、止痒扑粉(50)或痱子粉(51)

护理及预防

1. 发病后患处不宜用热水烫洗，不可用毛巾重擦及搔抓。
2. 居室宜空气流畅，炎热季节应注意通风降温，避免过热。大汗时不要用冷水淋浴。
3. 不要穿衣过多，衣服宜宽大，注意保持衣服的清洁干燥。
4. 常洗浴，婴幼儿浴后可扑痱子粉。

5.4 鸡眼

鸡眼是长期受挤压、摩擦部位发生圆柱状角质增生物，形似鸡眼为特征的皮肤病。中医文献又称肉刺。

病因病机

足底或趾间长期受挤压、摩擦，气血运行不畅，肌肤失养而发生。

临床表现

本病多发于长久站立或行走的男性青年。皮损常见于足跖前中部、踇趾内侧、小趾外侧、趾背、足跟等处，少数可发生于手部。可单发，亦可多发，通常1～2个。皮疹绿豆至豌豆大，色淡黄。初起患处皮肤肥厚，渐成圆锥形的硬结，略隆出皮面，中央有凹陷。纵向挤压时，有明显疼痛。

辨证论治

本病以外治为主。

1. 活血止痛散（44）煎汤乘热熏洗患处。
2. 鸡眼膏（52）贴敷患处。或用适量鸦胆子，去壳取仁捣为泥敷患处，胶布复盖固定，隔日或3日换药1次，直至鸡眼完全脱落。治疗前先用活血止痛散（44）或热水烫洗，洗软患处后用小刀将鸡眼削刮变薄再用药，效果更佳。

护理及预防

1. 注意减少局部挤压、摩擦，鞋靴大小松紧应合适，鞋底要柔软。
2. 足骨畸形者，应尽早矫治。
3. 不滥用强烈腐蚀性药物。
4. 忌用不干净的刀剪修削，以防继发感染。

6 变应性皮肤病

6.1 接触性皮炎

接触性皮炎是皮肤或粘膜接触某种物质后，在接触部位所发生的一种急性浅在性炎症性皮肤病。表现为红斑、肿胀、丘疹、水疱甚至坏死等。有原发性接触性皮炎和变应性接触性皮炎两种类型，而以后者为多见。由于接触物的不同，在中医文献中有不同的病名，如漆疮、粉花疮、膏药风和马桶癣等。

病因病机

先天禀性不耐，皮肤腠理不密，感受外界邪毒，毒热蕴于肌肤而发病。

临床表现

1. 原发性接触性皮炎无潜伏期，立即发病。变应性接触性皮炎有5～21天潜伏期。

2. 皮损的部位与接触部位一致，境界清楚。由于搔抓、衣服摩擦等原因，可在接触部位附近和身体其他部位发病，亦有因高度敏感而泛发全身者。

3. 病轻者表现为红斑、丘疹，并伴有肿胀；病重者可发生水疱、大疱、糜烂、结痂，甚至可发生溃疡和坏死。

4. 自觉不同程度的瘙痒和灼热感，重者可有灼痛感，可伴有发热及全身不适。

5. 本病有自限性，去除病因和经恰当处理后，皮损能很快消退，一般数日至10数日痊愈、反之则使病程迁延变为慢性，患处可呈苔藓样变，而类似慢性湿疹。

辨证论治

1. 内治法

(1) 湿热型

主证：发病急，病程短，局部皮损潮红、肿胀，有丘疹、水疱、糜烂渗出，自觉痛痒，舌质红，苔白或黄腻，脉滑数或缓。

治法：清热除湿。

方药：萆薢渗湿汤 (53) 加减

萆薢15克，泽泻15克，薏苡仁30克，茯苓皮15克，车前草30克，生地15克，丹皮15克，黄芩12克，黄柏12克，木通9克，地肤子30克，生甘草9克。

加减：发热者，加生石膏30克，知母12克。湿重者，加茵陈15克，冬瓜皮15克。痒重者，加白藓皮30克，蝉蜕9克。

中成药：龙胆泻肝丸 (8) 或防风通圣丸 (54)。

(2) 血燥型

主证：病程迁延日久，皮损肥厚、粗糙，表面可有抓痕、血痂，色素沉着或呈苔藓样变化，瘙痒剧烈。舌质淡，苔白，脉沉或缓。

治法：活血润燥，祛风止痒。

方药：当归饮子 (4) 加减

当归15克，生地15克，赤芍15克，白芍15克，丹参15克，何首乌15克，生黄芪24克，苍耳子15克，生甘草9克。

加减：痒甚难眠者，加全蝎9克，乌梢蛇9克，合欢皮15克，炒酸枣仁15克。大便干燥者，加番泻叶6克。

中成药：秦艽丸 (55) 或润肤丸 (56)。

2. 外治法

(1) 急性期可用解毒洗药 (13) 合止痒洗药 (14) 煎汤，候冷后湿敷患处，然后选用黄柏散 (17) 或湿疹散 (57)，撒布或用麻油调涂患处，每日2～3次。

(2) 慢性皮炎可外搽黑豆馏油软膏 (58)，每日2～4次。

护理及预防

1. 追查病因，清除致病物质，并避免再次接触。

2. 避免搔抓、摩擦、热水或肥皂水洗涤及其他不良刺激。
3. 忌食鱼虾等水产品及辛辣刺激性食物。
4. 保持大便通畅。

6.2 湿疹

湿疹是一种常见的过敏性炎症性皮肤病。可见于任何年龄，可泛发全身或局限于某些部位。临床一般分为急性湿疹、亚急性湿疹和慢性湿疹三种类型。

中医文献依据发病部位和临床表现有多种名称。如泛发的称浸淫疮、湿疮；局限的由于发病部位不同而有旋耳疮、四弯风、肾囊风等。

病因病机

禀性不耐，风、湿、热、燥诸邪客于肌肤而成。

急性、亚急性湿疹多因风、湿、热邪客于肌肤，以致血行不畅，营卫失和而发病；慢性湿疹则多为反复发作，日久邪深，伤阴耗血，血虚风燥，皮失所养所致。

临床表现

1. 急性湿疹

(1) 发病急，可发于任何部位，但多见于头面、四肢、会阴部等处。

(2) 皮损呈对称性。

(3) 皮损呈多形性。开始患处皮肤潮红，继而出现丘疹、水疱、糜烂、渗液、痂皮等，皮疹常群集成片，边界不清，常数种皮损同时存在，也可以1~2种疹形为主。

(4) 自觉剧烈瘙痒及灼热。皮疹广泛者可有低热。

(5) 经适当治疗2~3周可愈。但容易反复发作，倾向慢性。

2. 亚急性湿疹

(1) 为介于急性湿疹与慢性湿疹间的阶段，常由于急性湿疹未能及时治疗或治疗不当，以致病情迁延。

(2) 皮损表现较急性湿疹缓和，炎症部分消退，渗液减少，瘙痒减轻，并出现鳞屑、痂皮等皮疹。

3. 慢性湿疹

(1) 多由急性、亚急性湿疹演变而成，也有开始即为慢性的。

(2) 患处皮肤肥厚、粗糙，触之较硬，呈暗红色或褐色，可有鳞屑，或呈苔藓样变。边界较急性期、亚急性期清楚。有时部分皮损可有小片糜烂，少量渗液及痂皮，附近还可有少数丘疹或水疱，发于手足者常有皲裂。

(3) 呈阵发性剧烈瘙痒，遇热及入睡前较著。

(4) 慢性病程可达数日或数年，时轻时重，常反复呈急性或亚急性发作，精神紧张时为甚。

以上3种类型不是固定不变的，可相互转化。总的来说，湿疹有以下4个特点：

(1) 多形性皮损，有渗出倾向。

(2) 皮损发生部位有对称性。

(3) 剧烈瘙痒。

(4) 病程容易趋向慢性，容易反复发作。

辨证论治

1. 内治法

(1) 湿热型

主证：皮损潮红肿胀，糜烂渗液或结痂，有剧烈瘙痒及灼热感，心烦，口渴，舌质红，苔薄白或黄，脉滑或弦数。

治法：清热利湿，祛风止痒。

方药：龙胆泻肝汤（8）加减

龙胆草9克，栀子9克，黄芩12克，生地15克，玄参15克，车前草30克，泽泻15克，木通9克，白鲜皮30克，地肤子30克，蝉蜕9克，生甘草9克。

加减：热盛者，加生石膏30克，白茅根30克。湿盛者，加茯苓皮15克，冬瓜皮15克。痒甚者，加全蝎9克，乌梢蛇9克。大便干者，加生大黄9克（后入）。病发于上部，加升麻9克。病发于下部，加牛膝9克。

中成药：龙胆泻肝丸（8）或防风通圣丸（54）。

(2) 风热型

主证：皮损以红斑、丘疹、结痂、鳞屑为主，红肿减轻，渗出减少，自觉瘙痒，舌质红，苔白，脉滑或滑数。

治法：疏风清热利湿。

方药：消风散（1）加减

牛蒡子9克，生地15克，苦参9克，苍术15克，当归15克，知母12克，生石膏30克，木通9克，地肤子30克，白藓皮15克，蝉蜕9克，生甘草9克。

加减：痒重者，加全蝎9克，乌梢蛇9克。渗液明显者，加泽泻15克，车前草30克。纳呆者，去苦参、木通，加陈皮9克，草蔻9克。发于胸胁、外耳、阴部者，加柴胡12克，龙胆草9克。

中成药：可服龙胆泻肝丸（8）或防风通圣丸（54）。

(3) 血虚风燥型

主证：病程日久，反复发作，出现皮肤肥厚或苔藓样变，阵发性剧烈瘙痒，舌质淡，苔白，脉沉细或缓。

治法：养血润燥，祛风止痒。

方药：当归饮子（4）加减

当归15克，丹参15克，白芍15克，何首乌15克，川芎9克，生黄芪24克，防风15克，白蒺藜15克，苍耳子15克，徐长卿30克，生甘草9克。

加减：皮疹色红，有热象者，加生地15克，白茅根30克。瘙痒重者，加全蝎9克，乌梢蛇9克。

中成药：秦艽丸（55）或润肤丸（56）。

2. 外治法

(1) 糜烂渗液明显时，可选用止痒洗药（14）或燥湿洗药（59），煎汤候冷湿敷患处，每日2～3次，每次30分钟。

(2) 渗液不多时，可选用湿疹散或黄柏散，外扑或用麻油调成糊状外涂患处，每日2～3次。

(3) 皮肤肥厚或苔藓样变时，可用止痒扑粉（50）或祛风洗药（15）煎汤，乘热熏洗患处，每日2～3次，每次30分钟。亦可外搽10—20%黑豆馏油软膏或2%冰片霜。

护理及预防

1. 应尽可能避免搔抓，急性发作时忌用热水烫洗，忌用碱类及肥皂洗擦患处。

2. 忌食诱发和加重湿疹的鱼腥海味、蛋类、牛羊肉、鸡鸭鹅肉与辛辣、酒类等刺激性食物。

3. 注意休息，避免过度疲劳和精神过度紧张。

4. 急性期暂缓预防注射。

5. 注意寻找诱因，减少复发。

6.3 荨麻疹

荨麻疹是1种常见的瘙痒性皮肤病，以皮肤发生风团为主要表现。中医文献称该病为瘾疹、风瘩瘤等。

病因病机

1. 禀性不耐，又食鱼虾等腥荤动风之物。

2. 腠理不密，卫外失固，复感风热、风寒之邪。

3. 饮食失节，肠胃失和，湿热内生，复感风邪。

4. 平素体虚或久病耗伤，气血不足，风邪乘隙侵袭。

临床表现

1. 可发生于任何年龄、四季、男女均可发病。

2. 多突然发生，首先皮肤有痒感，不久或经搔抓后即发生风团，风团形状及大小不一，可相互融合成片，颜色可鲜红、淡红或瓷白。皮损时发时消，发生迅速，消退亦快，消退后不留痕迹，1日内可反复数次，出疹部位不固定，常此起彼伏。重者可泛发全身。

3. 发病时伴有剧烈瘙痒感，也可有灼热或刺痛感。部分急性患者可有发热（一般不超过 38.5℃）、恶心、呕吐、腹痛、腹泻等消化道症状，或有胸闷、喉头阻塞感、呼吸困难等呼吸道症状。

4. 病程不定，急性者多于数日到两周痊愈。若反复发作持续 3 个月以上者，为慢性荨麻疹，可迁延数月至数年，呈连续发作或有缓解期。

辨证论治

1. 内治法

（1）风热型

主证：风团色红，遇热发生或增剧，得冷则减，皮疹灼热，瘙痒剧烈。可伴有口渴、心烦。舌质红，苔薄白或薄黄，脉浮数。

治法：清热祛风利湿。

方药：消风散（1）加减

牛蒡子 9 克，生地 15 克，苦参 9 克，苍术 15 克，当归 15 克，知母 12 克，生石膏 30 克，木通 9 克，地肤子 30 克，白藓皮 15 克，蝉蜕 9 克，大胡麻 15 克，全蝎 9 克，生甘草 9 克。

加减：热重者，加白茅根 30 克，金银花 15 克。难眠者，加合欢皮 15 克，炒枣仁 15 克。口渴者，加玄参 15 克。心烦者，加莲子心 4.5 克。

（2）风寒型

主证：风团（荨麻疹团）色淡红或瓷白，遇冷易发，恶风怕冷，得暖则缓解，冬重夏轻，舌质淡，苔薄白，脉浮缓。

治法：疏风散寒，调和营卫。

方药：麻桂各半汤（60）加味

麻黄9克，桂枝9克，白芍15克，炒杏仁9克，生姜3片，大枣5枚，荆芥9克，防风15克，蛇床子12克，苍耳子15克，炙甘草9克。

加减：体虚自汗者，去麻黄加生黄芪30克。日久反复发作者，加黄芪30克，炒白术30克，全蝎9克，地龙9克。

(3) 胃肠湿热型

主证：发生风团时，伴有脘腹疼痛或恶心呕吐，大便秘结或泄泻，苔黄腻，脉滑数。

治法：疏风解表，通腹泄热。

方药：防风通圣散（54）加减

防风15克，桔梗9克，生石膏30克，滑石18克，大黄9克（后入），芒硝9克，白术15克，白藓皮30克，薄荷9克，连翘12克，黄芩12克，栀子12克，生甘草9克。

加减：腹痛者，加元胡12克，御米壳罂粟壳12克。腹泻者，去大黄、芒硝，加白扁豆花15克，金银花15克。恶心呕吐者，加竹茹9克，代赭石30克。

中成药：防风通圣丸（54）。

(4) 气血两虚型

主证：平素体虚或病久，风团反复发作，劳累及受凉后加重，神疲乏力，面色无华，舌质淡，苔薄白，脉沉细。

治法：养血祛风，益气固表。

方药：当归饮子（4）合玉屏风散（61）加减

当归15克，白芍15克，丹参30克，川芎9克，何首乌15克，荆芥9克，防风15克，生黄芪30克，炒白术15克，徐长卿30克，苍耳子15克，蛇床子12克，炙甘草9克，全蝎9克。

加减：纳呆者，加焦楂9克，鸡内金9克。难眠者，加炒枣仁15克，夜交藤15克。神疲乏力者，加熟附子9克，仙灵脾（淫羊藿）12克。

中成药：选用十全大补丸（62）、玉屏风散（61）、归脾丸（63）。

2. 外治法

（1）皮损广泛者，可用止痒洗药（14）合燥湿洗药（59）共同煎汤洗浴，每日1~2次。

（2）外涂止痒酊（41）、百部酊（见总论外治法）。

（3）止痒粉（64）外扑并揉擦患处。

护理及预防

1. 忌食鱼腥虾蟹等水产品，不饮酒，不吃刺激性食物。因某种食物引起发作时，应注意禁食该食物。

2. 应避免各种刺激性因素，如穿化纤衣物、寒冷、搔抓、精神紧张等。

3. 对花粉过敏者，室内禁放花卉。

6.4　丘疹性荨麻疹

丘疹性荨麻疹是1种好发于儿童的过敏性皮肤病。以发生红色风团样损害，其中心常有小水疱或小丘疹，伴剧烈瘙痒为特征。中医文献称本病为细皮风疹、水疥等。

病因病机

1. 禀性不耐，复受蚊虫叮咬，毒邪内侵，散发肌肤。

2. 饮食失节，湿热内蕴，或食入荤腥类动风助火之品，或外受风邪，风湿热郁于肌肤。

临床表现

1. 好发于学龄前儿童，夏秋季多见。

2. 皮疹好发于躯干及四肢伸侧，散在或群集分布。

3. 皮疹为突然发生的绿豆至花生米大小，圆形或略带纺锤形的红色风团样损害，其长轴多与皮纹一致，触之略硬，边缘可有伪足。皮疹顶端常有小水疱或小丘疹，有的可成为与皮疹等大的水疱，疱液清，周围无红晕。

4. 皮疹常成批出现，新旧皮疹可同时存在。每批皮疹经2～3天至10多天消退，留有暂时性轻度色素沉着。本病可反复发作，迁延数日或数年。

5. 一般无全身症状，自觉剧烈瘙痒，可因搔抓而发生糜烂或感染。

辨证论治

1. 内治法

(1) 风热型

主证：发疹多为风团样斑丘疹或红斑，水疱少见，色泽较红，剧烈瘙痒。舌质红，苔薄黄。

治法：疏风清热

方药：生地方（经验方）

生地9克，白茅根30克，金银花15克，蒲公英15克，地肤子30克，蝉蜕6克，荆芥穗6克，防风9克，赤小豆30克，生甘草9克。

加减：热重者，加生石膏30克，牛蒡子9克。痒甚者，加白藓皮12克，苍耳子9克。

中成药：犀角化毒丸（65）防风通圣丸（54）。

(2) 湿热型

主证：皮疹多发于4肢，有大小不等水疱，疱破后可有糜烂、渗液、痂皮，剧烈瘙痒，舌质红，苔黄腻。

治法：健脾利湿，清热除风。

方药：小儿化湿汤加味（经验方）

苍术9克，陈皮6克，茯苓9克，泽泻9克，炒麦芽9克，滑石15克，地肤子30克，蝉蜕9克，防风9克，生甘草6克。

加减：湿重者，加车前草15克，冬瓜皮9克。热重者，加生地9克，生石膏30克。继发感染者，加金银花15克，连翘9克。

中成药：犀角化毒丸（65）防风通圣丸（54）。

2. 外治法

(1) 皮损无破溃时，可选用风油精 (40)、止痒酊 (41) 等外搽，每日 3～4 次。亦可用喉症丸 (66) 150 粒用食醋 3 毫升浸泡化开，外涂患处，每日 3～4 次。

(2) 皮损有糜烂、渗液或继发感染时，可用黄柏散 (17) 或湿疹散 (57)，用麻油调为糊状，涂擦患处，每日 2～3 次。

护理及预防

1. 尽量减少搔抓，及时外用止痒药物。
2. 注意家庭卫生。采用喷洒药物、挂蚊帐等措施防止蚊虫叮咬，不要让儿童到杂草丛生处玩耍，以防虫咬。
3. 忌食鱼腥发物。

6.5 药物性皮炎

药物性皮炎又称药疹，是药物通过不同途径进入人体，在皮肤粘膜上引起的炎症反应，是药物反应的 1 种表现。中医文献称该病为中药毒。

病因病机

本病由于禀性不耐，药毒内侵，入于营血，外蕴肌肤腠理，内传经络脏腑所致。

临床表现

1. 本病有明确的用药史。
2. 从首次用药到出现皮损有一定的潜伏期，多在 4～20 天以内，重复用药则潜伏期大为缩短，常在 1 天内，也可短至 2 小时以内发病。
3. 皮疹的形态多种多样，色泽鲜艳，分布范围广，且常对称。
4. 自觉瘙痒、灼热感，重型药疹多伴有全身症状。
5. 除少数重型药疹外，一般病程短，停药及适当治疗后，可较快痊愈。

临床上药物性皮炎有以下常见类型：

(1) 荨麻疹型：广泛发生大小不等的风团，较一般荨麻疹色泽红，持续时间较长，自觉瘙痒，并可伴刺痛、触痛。

(2) 猩红热样或麻疹样型：广泛性鲜红色斑或粟粒至豆大丘疹、斑丘疹，密集对称分布，自觉微痒。虽然皮疹明显，但缺乏全身症状，这是与麻疹、猩红热的鉴别要点。

(3) 多形性红斑型：皮疹呈豆大至钱币大水肿性紫红斑，中央色深可有水疱，对称性发生于躯干、4肢、口、眼、唇周、外阴等处也可发生，且常出现糜烂渗液。本型常伴有瘙痒、发热、关节痛、腹痛等。

(4) 固定性红斑型：为较常见类型。皮疹为局限性圆形或椭圆形水肿性鲜红斑或紫红斑，中央可有水疱。眼、口周、肛门、龟头等皮肤粘膜交界处多见，其次为躯干、4肢、红斑消退需1～10天不等，阴部发生糜烂溃疡时病程较长。自觉瘙痒。愈后留有色素沉着，经久不退。下次再用同样药物，仍在原皮损处发病。

(5) 紫癜型：为针头大至豆大或更大的瘀点或瘀斑，平坦或稍隆起，轻者多发生于双下肢。重者可泛发全身。

(6) 剥脱性皮炎型：是1种较严重的药疹。潜伏期20天以上。多突然发病，先出现麻疹样丘疹、斑丘疹，迅速融合呈全身弥漫性潮红，手、足、面部可有水肿、糜烂，然后皮损开始反复剥脱，头发、指（趾）甲亦可脱落。全身有瘙痒、灼热感，常伴有恶寒发热、恶心呕吐等全身症状，病程常超过1个月。

(7) 大疱性表皮松解型：为药疹中最严重性。发病急，持续高烧。皮疹初为鲜红或紫红色、大小不一的斑片，迅速布满全身。然后皮损表面出现皱折，继而出现松弛的大小不一的暗紫色水疱，易破溃糜烂。如合并感染，常引起败血症。本型多数伴有口腔、食道、气管粘膜脱落及肝肾损害。

辨症论治

首先应立即停用致敏或可疑致敏药物,然后按病情缓急与证型不同采用相应治法。

1. 内治法

(1) 风热型

主证:以发疹为主要表现者。皮肤出现红斑、丘疹、风团、伴有瘙痒,轻度发热,口渴,舌质红,苔薄黄,脉浮数。

治法:清热解毒,疏风止痒。

方药:消风散 (1) 加减

生地15克,赤芍15克,苦参9克,金银花30克,大青叶15克,连翘15克,牛蒡子9克,蝉蜕9克,大胡麻15克,生石膏30克,知母12克,生甘草9克。

加减:热重者,加白茅根30克,紫草12克。瘙痒甚者,加白藓皮30克,全蝎9克。大便干者,加生大黄9克(后入)。

中成药:犀羚解毒丸 (67)。

(2) 湿热型

主证:以发疹为主要表现,但兼有红肿、糜烂、渗液,同时伴有瘙痒,舌质红,苔薄白或黄,脉滑数。

治法:清热解毒,祛风除湿。

方药:龙胆泻肝汤 (8) 加减

龙胆草9克,黄芩9克,栀子9克,金银花30克,连翘15克,生地30克,白茅根30克,车前子15克,泽泻15克,木通9克,白藓皮15克,地肤子30克,生甘草9克。

加减:热重加生石膏30克,知母12克。湿重加茯苓皮15克,冬瓜皮15克。瘙痒甚者加全蝎9克,苦参9克。

中成药:龙胆泻肝丸 (8)。

(3) 热毒型

主证:全身弥漫性潮红或皮肤剥脱,或出现广泛紫红斑。大疱、糜烂及合并感染。可伴有高热神昏、烦燥口渴、舌质红绛、苔黄燥、脉洪数。

治法：清热解毒，凉血清营。

方药：犀角地黄汤（7）合黄连解毒汤（6）加减

水牛角30克，生地30克，丹皮15克，赤芍30克，黄连9克，黄芩12克，栀子12克，金银花30克，玄参15克，生石膏30克，知母12克，生甘草9克。

加减：神昏谵语者，加紫雪丹（35）0.9克，分两次服。口干者，加石斛12克，天花粉12克。

中成药：安宫牛黄丸（36）或至宝丹（68）。

(4) 阴虚血燥型

主证：严重药疹期及恢复期，大热已退，皮肤损害好转，干燥有屑，面色无华，倦怠乏力，舌质淡，苔薄白或少苔，脉细数。

治法：滋阴养血，益气疏风。

方药：当归饮子（4）合增液汤（69）加减

当归15克，生地15克，熟地15克，川芎9克，白芍15克，玄参30克，麦冬9克，生黄芪30克，炒白术15克，地肤子30克，白藓皮15克，生甘草9克。

加减：烦热，加沙参15克，莲子心4.5克，石斛15克。痒重，加蝉蜕9克，全蝎9克。

中成药：选用十全大补丸（62）、知柏地黄丸（70）。

2. 外治法

根据皮损的不同，采用不同的外治法，具体治法，可参照湿疹处理。

3. 其他疗法

对于重型药疹，在辨证论治的同时，应采用现代医学疗法，根据病情，可使用激素、抗生素、输液、输血等。

护理及预防

1. 用药应有高度警惕性，应详细询问患者的药物致敏史，严格掌握用药指征，避免滥用药物。

2. 在用药过程中，如出现局部红斑或皮肤瘙痒等过敏症状时，应立即停用可疑药物。

3. 忌用热水烫洗及搔抓皮疹，以防病情加重及继发感染。

4. 注意多饮水，以加速药物排泄。

6.6 过敏性紫癜

过敏性紫癜是1种因过敏反应而发生的皮肤和粘膜出血性疾病。中医文献称该病为葡萄疫、紫癜等。

病因病机

禀性不耐，风湿热外袭或饮食不节，食入禁忌，湿热内生，以致血热内蕴，热伤血络，血溢肌肤而成；或因肝肾阴亏，虚火伤及血络而致；亦有因气虚不摄，脾不统血，血不归经而致者。

临床表现

本病多发于青少年，发病前或有咽喉疼痛，发热恶寒等风热外感病史，因受累部位及表现不同，可分为以下4种类型：

1. 单纯性紫癜：一般仅有皮肤发疹。皮疹好发于下肢，尤其是小腿伸侧，间或发于上肢及躯干部。皮疹常突然发生，为针头至黄豆大小的瘀点或瘀斑，成批反复发作。初起鲜红，数日后转暗紫色，再转为黄褐色，经2～3周消退，无明显全身症状。部分病人可有轻度瘙痒。容易复发。

2. 关节性紫癜：除皮肤发疹外，尚有关节肿痛，尤以膝关节常见，其次为肘、踝关节。皮疹多形性，除发生瘀点、瘀斑外，尚可出现风团、水疱、血疱等，可伴发热、疲倦等全身症状。病程数周及数月，容易反复发作。

3. 腹性紫癜：除多形性皮疹外，尚伴有恶心呕吐，腹痛腹泻，甚至便血等。重者可发生肠套叠，肠坏死，肠穿孔等。可有发热，关节肿痛，疲倦等全身症状。病程约3～4周，常可复发。

4. 肾性紫癜：皮疹亦为多形性。伴有血尿、蛋白尿或管型尿，少数可出现浮肿及少尿等肾炎的症状。

上述分型不是绝对的，患者有时可同时出现两型或两型以上的症状。

辨证论治

1. 内治法

(1) 风热型

主证：皮肤突然发斑，色鲜红或紫红，压之不退色，可有轻度瘙痒或低热，舌质红，苔薄黄，脉浮数。

治法：凉血止血，疏风清热。

方药：犀角地黄汤 (7) 合桑菊饮 (71) 加减

水牛角 30 克，丹皮 15 克，生地炭 15 克，赤芍 15 克，桑叶 9 克，菊花 9 克，金银花炭 9 克，连翘 15 克，藕节炭 9 克，侧柏叶 9 克，薄荷 9 克，生甘草 9 克。

加减：瘙痒明显者，加地肤子 30 克，蝉蜕 9 克。心烦者，加灯芯草 3 克，淡竹叶 9 克。

中成药：选用十灰散 (72)、清瘟败毒丸 (73)、犀羚解毒丸 (67)。

(2) 风湿型

主证：皮疹多形性，瘀斑色红隆起，关节肿胀疼痛，肢体乏力，或有发热，下肢浮肿。舌质红，苔黄或白腻，脉滑数。

治法：凉血清热，祛风除湿。

方药：犀角地黄汤 (7) 合独活寄生汤 (74) 加减

水牛角粉 3 克（冲），生地炭 15 克，丹皮 15 克，赤芍 30 克，独活 12 克，桑寄生 9 克，威灵仙 15 克，秦艽 15 克，防己 15 克，川牛膝 12 克，薏苡仁 30 克，海风藤 15 克，生甘草 9 克。

加减：下肢浮肿者，加茯苓皮 15 克，车前草 30 克。

中成药：消络痛 (75) 或四妙丸 (76)。

(3) 脾胃湿热型

主证：除多形性皮疹外，可有恶心呕吐，腹痛腹泻或便血。舌质红，苔黄腻，脉濡数。

治法：清脾利湿，凉血止血。

方药：清脾除湿饮（77）加减

茯苓15克，炒白术15克，黄芩12克，栀子15克，茵陈15克，生地炭15克，地榆炭15克，泽泻15克，竹叶9克，竹茹9克，厚朴9克，元胡9克，生甘草9克。

加减：呕吐者，加半夏9克，生姜6克。腹泻者，加木香9克，黄连9克。

中成药：防风通圣丸（54）或香连丸（78）。

(4) 肝肾阴虚型

主证：皮疹为多形性，有血尿、蛋白尿、少尿、浮肿等，可伴有低热烦躁，耳鸣目涩，消瘦腰酸，舌红少苔，脉细数。

治法：养阴清热，凉血化斑。

方药：六味地黄汤（79）加减

生地15克，丹皮15克，玄参24克，麦冬9克，赤芍30克，泽泻15克，茯苓12克，山萸肉9克，大蓟12克，小蓟12克，龟板12克，鳖甲12克，生甘草9克。

加减：心烦加淡竹叶6克，灯芯草3克。浮肿加车前子12克，冬瓜皮15克。腰酸加狗脊15克，怀牛膝15克。

中成药：六味地黄丸（79）或知柏地黄丸（70）。

(5) 气不摄血型

主证：病久反复，皮损紫暗，压之不退，伴有面色萎黄，神疲乏力，头晕目眩，食少纳呆，舌淡少苔，脉细弱。

治法：补气摄血，健脾和中。

方药：归脾汤（63）加减

黄芪30克，党参15克，白术15克，茯苓15克，熟地15克，当归15克，血余炭9克，仙鹤草15克，远志9克，木香9克，炒枣仁15克，龙眼肉9克，陈皮9克，炙甘草9克。

加减：关节痛者，加豨莶草 15 克，络石藤 15 克。腹痛者，加元胡 9 克，五灵脂 9 克。血尿，加小蓟 15 克，藕节炭 9 克。
中成药：归脾丸（63）或人参健脾丸（113）。
2. 外治法
可参考湿疹处理。
护理及预防
1. 患病期间，应卧床休息，抬高患肢。
2. 忌食鱼腥海味、牛奶、蛋类、辛辣类动风助火之品。

7 神经功能障碍性皮肤病

7.1 皮肤瘙痒症

皮肤瘙痒症是一种自觉瘙痒而无原发性损害的皮肤病。由于不断搔抓，常有抓痕、血痂、色素沉着及苔藓变等继发损害。本病临床上有泛发性、局限性两种。中医文献称泛发性瘙痒为痒风、风瘙痒等，因局限性瘙痒的部位不同又有阴痒、肛门作痒等名。

病因病机

多因风、寒、湿、热诸邪蕴阻于肌肤，不得疏泄而发；或血虚化燥，血燥生风，肤失濡养而致；阴痒、肛门瘙痒多与肝胆湿热有关。

临床表现

1. 多见于成年人与老年人。
2. 泛发性为全身多部位瘙痒，可同时发作，也可由1处移到另1处，此起彼伏。初期瘙痒较轻微，历时亦短，以后逐渐增剧，瘙痒时间延长；局限性以肛门、女阴、阴囊多见。
3. 瘙痒均成阵发性，多较剧烈，每日发作次数不定，每次持续数分钟至数小时。情绪激动、温度改变、过度疲劳、饮酒及吃辛辣食物，易诱发和加重瘙痒。晚间入睡时，更易发作，常影响睡眠。
4. 皮肤检查无原发疹可见。
5. 由于瘙痒而搔抓，可在皮肤上继发抓痕、血痂及色素沉着，病程长者可出现皮肤肥厚或苔藓样变，以及失眠、精神萎靡、食欲不振等。
6. 该病病程较长，数周、数月及数年不等。

辨证论治

1. 内治法

(1) 风热型

主证：病属新起，全身多处部位作痒或局限于某一部位，遇热加剧，自觉焮热，可有抓痕、血痂，舌质红，苔白或薄黄，脉弦数。

治法：凉血清热，祛风止痒。

方药：白藓皮饮（80）加减

金银花15克，白藓皮30克，当归12克，生地15克，蝉蜕9克，白蒺藜15克，黄芩9克，紫草9克，防风15克，地肤子30克，生甘草9克。

加减：热重者，加生石膏30克。痒重者，加全蝎9克，乌梢蛇9克。难眠者，加合欢皮15克，夜交藤15克。大便干者，加大黄9克（后入）。

中成药：防风通圣丸（54）。

(2) 血虚风燥型

主证：病程日久，皮损干燥、肥厚或呈苔藓样变，阵发性剧烈瘙痒。舌质淡，苔薄白，脉沉细或弦滑。

治法：养血润燥，除风止痒。

方药：当归饮子（4）加减

当归15克，生地15克，熟地15克，白芍15克，川芎9克，何首乌15克，生黄芪30克，炒白术15克，防风15克，苍耳子15克，合欢皮15克，白藓皮15克，生甘草9克。

加减：有热象者，去熟地加生石膏30克，牛蒡子9克。心烦难眠者，加莲子心4.5克，酸枣仁15克。顽固性瘙痒者，加乌梢蛇9克，全蝎9克。中成药：选用养血安神丸（81）、四虫片（82）、秦艽丸（55）。

(3) 肝胆湿热型

主证：阴囊或女阴瘙痒，局部肿胀、潮红、舌质红、苔黄、脉滑数。

治法：清利肝胆湿热，祛风止痒。

方药：龙胆泻肝汤（8）加减

龙胆草9克，柴胡12克，黄芩9克，栀子12克，生地15克，车前草30克，泽泻15克，木通9克，地肤子30克，白藓皮15克，生甘草9克。

加减：痒重加全蝎9克，乌梢蛇9克。伴有糜烂、渗液者，加茯苓皮15克，茵陈15克。

中成药：龙胆泻肝丸（8）。

2. 外治法

（1）可选用止痒洗药（14）、祛风洗药（15）煎汤温洗患处，每日1~2次。

（2）外涂药物选用止痒酊（41），神经性皮炎药水（83），2%冰片霜，黑豆馏油软膏（58）等，每日涂3~4次。

护理及预防

1. 禁用碱性强的肥皂洗浴及热水烫洗。

2. 保持患处清洁，但不要过多洗擦，冬季洗澡不宜太勤，以每周1次为度。尽量避免和减少搔抓。

3. 保持被褥衣物清洁舒适，不宜穿用化纤、毛织衣物。

4. 禁食刺激性食物、饮料、如辣椒、酒、浓茶、咖啡等。忌食鱼虾蟹等水产品。

5. 保持大便通畅。

6. 避免过度劳累和精神紧张。

7.2 神经性皮炎

神经性皮炎是以阵发性瘙痒和皮肤苔藓样变为特征的皮肤病。中医文献记载，因其顽固难治而称为顽癣；又因其状如牛项之皮，厚而且坚，故又称牛皮癣。

病因病机

初起为情志失调，风热之邪外袭肌肤，蕴聚不散所致。日久风热炽盛，耗血伤津，血虚化燥生风，肌肤失养而成。

临床表现

临床上分局限性和泛发性两种，而以局限性多见。

1. 多见于青年人和老年人。

2. 好发于颈后及两侧，其次是肘部伸侧、骶尾部、腘窝、踝部、眼睑等处。

3. 初起皮肤有阵发性瘙痒而无皮肤损害，经搔抓后，逐渐出现成片的扁平圆形或多角形坚实性丘疹，呈正常肤色或淡红、红褐色，日久局部皮肤干燥肥厚，形成皮嵴隆起、皮纹加深的苔藓样变之斑片，呈黄褐、淡褐或正常肤色，边缘清楚，表面光滑，或少量糠状鳞屑，周围可有少量散在的扁平丘疹。可因搔抓而有抓痕、血痂、糜烂渗出甚至化脓性感染。

4. 自觉阵发性剧痒，以夜间为重。泛发性神经性皮炎，常奇痒难忍，须搔抓至局部疼痛为止。

5. 病程慢性，时轻时重，缠绵不愈。

辨证论治

1. 内治法

（1）风热型

主证：红色扁平丘疹群，痒甚，舌质淡，苔薄黄或薄白，脉浮数。

治法：凉血清热，祛风止痒。

方药：白藓皮饮（80）加减

金银花15克，白藓皮30克，生地15克，丹参15克，赤芍15克，蝉蜕9克，黄芩9克，紫草9克，防风15克，地肤子30克，白蒺藜15克，生甘草9克。

加减：痒甚者，加全蝎9克，乌梢蛇9克。难眠者，加合欢皮15克，炒枣仁15克。发于颈部者，加柴胡12克。

中成药：防风通圣丸（54）或丹栀逍遥丸（84）。

(2) 血虚风燥型

主证：病程日久，皮损呈苔藓样变或局限性肥厚，或有脱屑、抓痕、血痂，舌质淡红，苔薄白，脉沉细。

治法：养血润燥，祛风止痒。

方药：当归饮子（4）加减

当归15克，熟地15克，川芎9克，白芍15克，何首乌15克，炙黄芪30克，白蒺藜15克，徐长卿30克，苍耳子15克，全蝎9克，乌梢蛇9克，防风15克，生甘草9克。

加减：心烦难眠者，加莲子心4.5克，炒酸枣仁15克。纳呆腹胀者，加炒麦芽15克，草蔻9克，炒莱菔子15克。皮损红热者，去熟地、白芍，加生地15克，赤芍15克，生石膏30克。

中成药：秦艽丸（55）或润肤丸（56）。

2. 外治法

(1) 风热型可用止痒洗药（14）或祛风洗药（15）煎汤候冷湿敷患处，每日1～2次，每次30分钟。血虚风燥型可用上药煎汤，乘热熏洗患处，每日1～2次，每次30分钟。

(2) 可选用止痒酊（41）、神经性皮炎药水（83）、黑豆馏油软膏（58）、黄升皮肤软膏（85），外涂患处，每日3～4次。

(3) 狗皮膏（38）或伸筋膏（86）加热后，在表面撒布少许樟脑或冰片，外贴患处，每3日换贴一次。

护理及预防

1. 尽量避免各种不良刺激，如搔抓、热水烫洗、衣领摩擦、饮酒、食刺激性食物、外用刺激性强的药物等。

2. 避免过劳和精神紧张，克服急躁情绪，如有神经衰弱者，应同时进行治疗。

(杨东海)

8 红斑类皮肤病

8.1 多形性红斑

多形性红斑是以红斑为主，兼丘疹、水疱等多形性损害的急性炎症性皮肤病。典型红斑，形如猫眼，故在中医文献中有猫眼疮之称。根据发病特点，又称寒疮。

病因病机

总由禀性不耐所致。或因风寒外袭，以致营卫不和，气血凝滞而成；或因风热外感，湿热内蕴，郁于皮肤而成；或因饮食失节，食入禁忌（如药物、鱼、虾、蟹等）而诱发。

临床表现

1. 好发于青壮年男女，以女性较多见。常见于春秋或冬季，也有在夏季发作者。

2. 损害好发于手背、手掌、指缘、足背、足底、颜面、颈旁，亦可见于口腔粘膜及生殖器，少数可累及全身皮肤。常呈对称性分布。

3. 皮疹呈多形性。初起多为红斑，以后可出现风团、丘疹或水疱、糜烂、紫癜等。常数种皮疹同时存在。红斑颜色鲜红，或暗红到紫红，可相互融合。有些红斑边缘呈堤状隆起，中央凹陷。典型者中心部常发生重叠水疱，形如猫眼。发于粘膜的损害，溃后常形成糜烂。

4. 自觉灼热痒痛。一般无全身症状。重者皮损广泛，甚至并发内脏病变，如累及肾脏，可出现蛋白尿、血尿、纳呆、乏力等全身症状。

5. 病程2～3周左右，但愈后易于反复发作。

辨证论治

1. 内治法

(1) 湿热型

主证：斑色鲜红，并见水疱，水疱破后，或累及粘膜者可见糜烂、渗液。自觉灼热痒痛，发热恶寒，心烦口渴，关节酸痛，溲黄便干。苔黄腻，舌质红，脉多滑数。

治法：清热利湿，佐以凉血散风。

方药：萆薢渗湿汤（53）加减

蒲公英 30 克，连翘 12 克，栀子 9 克，黄柏 9 克，萆薢 9 克，薏苡仁 15 克，泽泻 12 克，木通 6 克，车前子 15 克（包煎），生石膏 15 克，生地 15 克，丹皮 9 克，牛蒡子 9 克，浮萍 9 克，水煎服。

加减：便秘者加生大黄 9 克（后入）。关节酸痛者加防己 12 克，秦艽 9 克。

(2) 风寒型

主证：遇寒则发或加重，得暖减轻或渐愈。斑色紫暗，肢端皮温偏低，指趾可肿胀。可伴有畏寒肢冷，腹痛便溏等症。苔薄白，脉濡缓。

治法：疏风散寒，活血化瘀。

方药：当归四逆汤（43）加减

桂枝 9 克，赤芍 9 克，当归 9 克，鸡血藤 15 克，川芎 9 克，丹参 15 克，细辛 3 克，熟附子 6 克，干姜 6 克，羌活 9 克，防风 9 克，甘草 6 克，水煎服。

加减：腹痛者加元胡 9 克，乌药 9 克。便溏者加茯苓 12 克，猪苓 12 克。

2. 外治法

(1) 湿热型：以红斑、丘疹为主者可选用炉甘石洗剂（87）、三石水（88）外涂。有水疱、糜烂、渗液者用燥湿洗药（59）煎水冷湿敷，湿敷间用黄连油（89）外涂。有口腔粘膜病损时可用白菊花、金银花各 15 克，加 500 毫升开水浸泡，取其药液含漱，1 日多次。

(2) 风寒型：2 号洗药 (90) 煎汤熏洗患处，日 2 次，每次 20~40 分钟。

8.2 结节性红斑

本病是 1 种以皮下结节为特征的急性炎症性皮肤病。常侵犯下肢伸侧，春秋多见，好发于青年女性。与中医文献记载的瓜藤缠或湿毒流注相类似。

病因病机

素有蕴湿，郁久化热，湿热蕴结，导致脉络阻塞、气血凝滞而发病；或因脾虚蕴湿不化，兼感寒邪，寒湿凝结，阻滞血脉而致。

临床表现

1. 好发于青年女性，春秋季节多见。

2. 皮损一般对称发生于小腿伸侧，少数亦可发生于小腿屈侧、股部等处。

3. 发病常较突然。发病前或发病时可有轻重不等的畏寒、发热、头痛、咽痛、关节酸痛、食欲不振、神疲乏力等症。

4. 皮疹为直径 1~5 厘米大小的圆形皮下结节，略高起于皮面或隐没于皮下，质地坚实，互不融合，始终不溃。结节颜色初为鲜红，渐变暗红、紫红或黄褐色，中央着色较深。结节数目多寡不一，少则数个，多则数 10 个。自觉灼热疼痛，并有压痛。重者可见下肢浮肿。

5. 病程一般为 6 周左右，但亦有长达数月者。常可反复发作，并在劳累后或月经期容易复发。

辨证论治

1. 内治法

(1) 湿热型

主症：起病急骤，常有头痛、咽痛、关节痛，或有发热。皮疹色红，灼热肿痛。可有口渴、便干、尿黄，舌红苔黄腻，脉滑数。

治法：清热利湿，活血通络。

方药：四妙勇安汤（91）加味

金银花30克，蒲公英30克，连翘15克，地丁15克，栀子9克，黄柏9克，防己9克，玄参30克，丹参15克，赤芍15克，当归12克，川牛膝9克，甘草6克，水煎服。

加减：发热者加生石膏30克，柴胡9克。咽痛者加牛蒡子9克，山豆根9克。关节酸痛者，加威灵仙9克，独活9克。

(2) 寒湿型

主证：结节经久不消，颜色紫暗，4肢不温，关节疼痛，遇寒加重，甚则腿胫浮肿。舌质淡，苔薄白或白腻。脉沉细或迟缓。

治法：温经散寒、除湿通络。

方药：当归四逆汤（43）加减

当归15克，桂枝9克，细辛3克，川牛膝15克，鸡血藤15克，川芎9克，丹参15克，威灵仙9克，茯苓12克，苍术12克，白术9克，木瓜9克，薏苡仁15克，水煎服。

2. 外治法

(1) 湿热型：外敷大青膏（30）或芙蓉膏（92），隔日更换药膏1次。

(2) 寒湿型：活血止痛散（44）煎汤乘热熏洗患处，每日2次，或外敷回阳玉龙膏（93），隔日更换一次。

9 红斑鳞屑性皮肤病

9.1 玫瑰糠疹

玫瑰糠疹是一种常见的急性红斑鳞屑性皮肤病。以好发于躯干，4肢近端，斑色紫红，上覆白屑，斑疹长轴与皮肤一致为特征。本病与中医文献中记载的风热疮相似。

病因病机

本病多因血热内蕴，复感风邪，风热相搏，郁于肌肤，腠理闭塞，阴津灼伤，血燥而成。

临床表现

1. 好发于青年及中年人，以春秋2季多见。皮损多发于躯干与4肢近端，也可泛发于全身皮肤，但不累及头面部。

2. 初起大多在躯干或4肢某处先出现一个红斑，逐渐扩大成圆形或椭圆形，大小如指甲或钱币，周边微隆起，中央较平坦，上覆细碎白色鳞屑，此称母斑。若无瘙痒，常被忽视。约经10天左右，母斑渐转暗淡，并趋向消退，而在其它部位则相继成批出现较母斑小的大小不等的同样皮疹，此称子斑。常对称性散在分布，皮疹长轴与皮肤纹理平行，中心可见细微皱纹，边界清楚，极少融合。

3. 自觉有轻重不等的痒感。大多数无全身症状。部分患者发病初起可伴有低热，头痛，咽痛，心烦口渴，关节酸痛，全身不适。

4. 病程有自限性，一般经4—6周左右可自愈。亦有拖延2—3个月，甚至更多时间才痊愈的。愈后常不再复发。

辨证论治

1. 内治法

凡初起皮疹广泛，鲜艳紫红，自觉灼热瘙痒，并可伴有低热、头痛、咽痛、心烦口渴，小便黄赤。苔薄白或薄黄，舌质红，脉弦滑微数者属血热风盛。

治法：清热凉血，散风止痒。

方药：白藓皮饮（80）加减

金银花 15 克，大青叶 15 克，紫草 9 克，黄芩 9 克，白藓皮 15 克，防风 9 克，蝉蜕 6 克，白蒺藜 12 克，丹皮 12 克，生地 15 克，赤芍 15 克，生石膏 15 克，生甘草 6 克，水煎服。

加减：瘙痒重者，加重白藓皮至 30 克，加苦参 9 克。病久证属血虚风燥者去金银花、大青叶、紫草、黄芩，加当归、鸡血藤、何首乌、丹参各 15 克。

2. 外治

(1) 外涂炉甘石洗剂（87）或 5%硫黄乳剂。

(2) 苦参 30 克，蛇床子 30 克，川椒 12 克，明矾 12 克，加水煎汤约 2000 毫升，待温洗患处，每日 1—2 次，每次 20—30 分钟。

(3) 针刺：取合谷、曲池、大椎、肩髃、肩井、血海、足三里等穴，用泻法，留针 10—15 分钟，每日 1 次。

护理及预防

1. 急性期勿用热水洗浴。避免外用刺激性药物。
2. 忌食辛辣、鱼腥。

9.2 银屑病

银屑病是 1 种常见的红斑鳞屑性皮肤病。与中医文献中记载的白疕、松皮癣等名相似。以在红斑上反复出现多层银白色鳞屑为其皮损特征。男女老幼皆可患病，但以青壮年患者多见。

病因病机

外感风邪，搏于肌肤，郁久化热，以致血热、血燥或血瘀；

或因肝肾亏损，冲任不调，营血不和，脏腑阴阳失调所致。

临床表现

本病临床上可分寻常型、关节型、脓疱型和红皮症型，以寻常型为多见。

1. 寻常型

(1) 皮疹可发于全身各处，但好发于头皮、四肢伸侧及腰骶部。

(2) 皮疹初为米粒至黄豆大小红色丘疹或斑丘疹，以后扩大融合成片，边缘清楚，可呈点滴状、钱币状或地图状，其上覆有多层银白色鳞屑，状如松皮。刮除鳞屑后，可见有半透明的薄膜，称为薄膜现象。再刮之有点状出血，称为露滴现象。发生于头皮部位的皮疹呈暗红色，上覆灰白色厚屑，头发常因鳞屑牵拉而成束状，但不脱发。若侵犯甲部，甲板呈点状小凹陷。

(3) 大多急性发病，病程经过缓慢，易反复发作。发病有明显的季节性，多冬季发病或加剧，夏季自愈或减轻，部分患者亦可相反。病久季节性常不明显。根据皮疹活动情况可将本病分为进行期、静止期和消退期。进行期：新皮疹不断出现，旧皮疹不断扩大，鳞屑增厚，炎症明显，皮疹周围绕以红晕。在此期间常出现同形反应，即在皮肤外伤处或注射针眼处发生银屑病皮疹。静止期：病情保持于静止阶段，无新疹出现，旧疹也不消退。消退期：皮疹变平缩小乃至逐渐消失。消失后常在原皮疹处遗留暂时性色素减退或沉着斑。

(4) 自觉有不同程度瘙痒。

2. 关节型

除具有寻常型皮疹以外，还伴有类风湿性关节炎样症状，如发热、关节肿痛等，这些症状往往与皮疹同时加重或减轻。关节病变多累及指趾小关节，也可侵犯大关节，日久关节僵硬变形、活动受限。

3. 脓疱型

好发于掌跖部,重者可泛发全身。表现为在红斑上出现浅在小脓疱。脓疱泛发者常伴有恶寒发热及关节疼痛等。

4. 红皮症型

多由寻常型转变而来。全身皮肤潮红或紫红,浸润及大量脱屑。仅存在少数片状正常皮肤。可伴有发热,掌跖角化,指趾甲增厚等。

辨证论治

1. 内治法

(1) 血热型

主证:皮疹的发生发展较迅速,且泛发,色红,屑多。瘙痒明显。常有同形反应。可伴有怕热,心烦易怒,咽干口苦,便秘溲黄,苔薄黄,质红或红绛,脉弦数或滑数。

治法:清热凉血,活血祛风。

方药:双花土苓饮(94)加减

土茯苓30克,金银花30克,炒槐米15克,黄芩9克,知母9克,紫草9克,生地15克,赤芍15克,丹皮12克,丹参15克,当归9克,柴胡9克,蝉蜕6克,白藓皮15克,水煎服。

(2) 血燥型

主证:病程较久,皮疹停止发展或有部分消退,皮疹色淡、干燥,鳞屑减少。舌质淡红,苔少或薄白,脉弦细或沉细等。

治法:养血祛风润燥。

方药:养血润肤饮(95)加减

当归15克,白芍9克,赤芍9克,生地15克,熟地15克,鸡血藤30克,玄参15克,何首乌15克,天冬9克,麦冬9克,小胡麻9克,白藓皮9克,白蒺藜9克,僵蚕9克,水煎服。

(3) 血瘀型

主证:皮疹经久不消,色暗红或色素沉着。鳞屑较厚,或呈蛎壳状。有的伴有关节活动不利。舌质紫暗有瘀斑，脉细涩等。

治法：活血化瘀。

方药：桃红四物汤（10）加减

归尾9克，川芎9克，赤芍15克，桃仁9克，红花9克，三棱9克，莪术9克，丹参15克，鸡血藤30克，土元9克，白花蛇舌草15克，水煎服。

(4) 冲任不调型

主证：见于女性患者。皮疹在怀孕时消失或减轻，产后则出现或加重，平素常伴有月经不调，腰酸肢软，头晕耳鸣等。

治法：调摄冲任。

方药：二仙汤（96）合四物汤（97）加减

熟地15克，当归9克，赤芍12克，白芍12克，益母草12克，首乌15克，黄精15克，仙茅9克，仙灵脾15克，菟丝子12克，巴戟天9克，苍耳子9克，水煎服。

(5) 风湿阻络型

主证：本型相当于关节型银屑病。关节肿胀、疼痛，甚至僵硬畸形，活动受限。

治法：散风祛湿，活血通络。

方药：独活寄生汤（74）加减

秦艽9克，防风9克，桑枝30克，独活9克，威灵仙9克，川牛膝9克，当归9克，川芎9克，白芍9克，鸡血藤15克，白藓皮15克，土茯苓15克，甘草6克。

(6) 热毒挟湿型

主证：多见于脓疱型银屑病，或有潮红、糜烂、渗液皮损者。重者可伴有发热口渴，便秘溲黄等全身症状。舌质红，苔黄或黄腻，脉弦滑或滑数。

治法：清热解毒利湿。

方药：龙胆泻肝汤（8）合五味消毒饮（5）加减

龙胆草9克，黄芩9克，黄柏9克，栀子9克，金银花30

克，地丁15克，蒲公英30克，野菊花15克，连翘9克，土茯苓15克，车前子9克（包煎），泽泻9克，木通6克，水煎服。

(7) 火毒炽盛型

主证：相当于红皮症型银屑病。全身皮肤呈现弥漫性潮红或暗红，大量脱屑，皮肤灼热。病久者皮损浸润肥厚。常伴有发热畏寒，心烦口渴，大便秘结，小便短黄等。舌质红绛，苔少或无苔，脉滑数。

治法：凉血清热解毒。

方药：清营汤 (98) 加减

水牛角15克（先煎），生地30克，玄参15克，丹皮9克，赤芍15克，金银花30克，蒲公英15克，连翘15克，黄连6克，生石膏30克，竹叶6克，生甘草6克，水煎服。

中成药：寻常型银屑病可选用消银片 (94)，每次10片，日3次；克银丸 (99)，每次1丸，日3次；防风通圣丸 (54)，每次6克，日3次。

2. 外治法

(1) 病情进展期宜用温和、低浓度药膏，如5%硼酸膏，5%硫磺软膏等。

(2) 静止期可用5—10%硫磺软膏或黑豆馏油软膏 (58)，皮肤软膏 (85) 等。

(3) 皮损广泛者可配合硫化钾浴、温泉浴或中药浴：枯矾120克，小椒120克，野菊花240克，芒硝500克，煎水适量，作全身浴，每次20—60分钟，每日一次。

(4) 石榴皮（研细粉）10克，麻油20毫升，混合调为油膏外涂，每日2次。

10 结缔组织病

10.1 红斑性狼疮

本病属结缔组织病范畴,因其有自身免疫现象,故亦属于自身免疫性疾病。临床上分为盘状红斑狼疮和系统性红斑狼疮。前者主要表现为皮疹,多为慢性局限性,后者除表现皮疹外,同时累及内脏器官,病变一般呈进行性经过。在中医文献中,尚无类似本病的相应病名。根据临床表现,一般认为系统性红斑狼疮近似阳毒发斑、阴阳毒;盘状红斑狼疮类似鬼脸疮、蝴蝶丹等。也有人以证候为辨病的主要依据,凡以关节疼痛为主者,属痹证;以浮肿为主者,属水肿;出现胸腔积液者,属悬饮;出现心肌损害,急性心内膜炎者,属心悸或怔忡;病久,呈现一系列虚劳证候者,属虚劳。由于本病症状错综复杂,变化多端,故很难归属于单一病证。

病因病机

本病多因先天禀赋不足,肝肾亏损,或因七情内伤,劳累过度,以致阴阳不调,气血失和,气滞血瘀,经络阻塞;或因日光曝晒,热毒入里,瘀阻脉络,内伤脏腑,外阻肌肤所致。

临床表现

1. 盘状红斑性狼疮

(1) 皮损好发于面部,尤以鼻梁、鼻旁及双颊为主,常连接成蝴蝶形,亦可累及口唇、外耳、手背、头皮等处,皮损限于下颌以上者为局限型;皮损超过下颌者为播散型。

(2) 典型皮疹为浸润性隆起红斑,边缘清楚,中央萎缩凹陷,状如盘形。初起色泽鲜红,日久转暗红,表面紧附粘着性灰黄或灰白色鳞屑。鳞屑下皮肤可见毛孔扩大,状如筛孔,剥下的鳞屑底面有角质栓,状如钉板。愈后残留萎缩性疤痕,或色素沉着,或色素减退。在头部形成萎缩性秃发斑。粘膜损害多发生在下唇,常因浸渍而呈灰白色糜烂或浅在性溃疡。

(3) 一般无明显全身不适。少数病例可伴有低热,乏力,关节酸痛等症状。局部通常无自觉症状,或有微痒和灼热感。

(4) 病程慢性。少数病例可转变成系统性红斑狼疮。

2. 系统性红斑狼疮

(1) 多发于15~40岁女性。

(2) 皮损常多而广泛,分布对称,好发于暴露部位,如面部、手背,亦可发于躯干。皮损呈多形性。常见的皮损为水肿性红斑或紫红斑。大小形状不一。发于面颊者,可呈蝶形。发于指(趾)末端的损害、多为紫斑、水疱、溃疡。发于口腔粘膜者,常为出血点、糜烂、浅在性溃疡,以及齿龈炎等。其它可表现为类似多形红斑,网状青斑,结节性红斑样皮疹,或见结节、风团、脱发等损害。约15%左右的病人始终无皮损。

(3) 本病常以发热、头痛、关节肌肉酸痛开始,以后可因侵犯不同脏器而出现不同症状。多数为肾脏损害,多表现为肾炎,或为肾病综合征及肾功能衰竭。后期常引起尿毒症和高血压;半数病例有心血管系统的病变,如心包炎、心肌炎、心内膜炎、心脏扩大、心力衰竭等。也有的表现为血栓性静脉炎、血栓闭塞性脉管炎,或雷诺氏现象等;呼吸系统和消化系统也常被累及,表现为慢性咳嗽、胸痛、咯血、呼吸困难等,甚则呼吸衰竭。或有食欲不振、恶心呕吐、腹痛腹泻和便血等症状;约1/3的患者有神经系统受累,出现性情急躁、意识模糊、幻想、痴呆、谵妄、偏瘫、周围神经麻痹等症状;其他可有月经失调,肝脾淋巴结肿大,眼底出血,视网膜病变等。

(4) 实验室检查

a 有不同程度的贫血,红细胞数减少,部分患者血小板减少。

 b 血沉大多加快。

 c 蛋白电泳显示丙种球蛋白增高，白蛋白降低。

 d 周围血液或骨髓中可找到红斑狼疮细胞，急性期阳性率较高。

 e 间接荧光免疫抗核抗体试验大多数可呈阳性反应，以周边型为特异性，偶见核仁型。

 f 部分患者类风湿因子试验阳性。

辨证论治

1. 内治法

（1）气滞血瘀型

主证：多见于盘状红斑性狼疮及以肝损害为主的系统性红斑狼疮。面部等处有暗红斑，或有雷诺氏现象，肝脾肿大，肌肉关节酸痛，胸胁疼痛，脘腹胀满，月经不调等证。舌质暗红，或见瘀斑，苔薄白，脉弦细。

治法：舒肝理气，活血化瘀。

方药：柴胡疏肝汤（33）合通窍活血汤（100）加减。

柴胡9克，赤芍12克，白芍12克，川芎9克，桃仁9克，红花9克，丹参15克，枳壳9克，郁金9克，川楝子9克，陈皮9克，白花蛇舌草15克，水煎服。

中成药：活血祛瘀片（101），每次5片，每日3次。病久阴虚内热者，六味地黄丸（79），每次1～2丸，每日2次。青蒿蜜丸（青蒿研粉，炼蜜为丸），每丸10克，每次1～2丸，每日3次。

（2）热毒炽盛型

主证：相当于系统性红斑狼疮急性期。证见高热，关节肌肉酸痛，烦躁口渴，喜冷饮，溲赤便秘，精神恍惚，甚或神昏谵语、抽搐。皮损为水肿性红斑，亦可出现瘀斑、鼻衄、吐血、便血等出血症状。舌质红或绛，苔黄，脉弦数或洪大。

治法：清热解毒，凉血护阴。

方药：犀角地黄汤（7）或化斑汤（102）加减

水牛角6克（冲服），生地30克，丹皮9克，赤芍15克，栀子12克，生石膏30克，知母9克，金银花15克，连翘9克，玄参15克，麦冬15克，白茅根30克，水煎服。

加减：神昏谵语者，加用安宫牛黄丸（36）1～2粒（化服），或紫雪丹（35）0.9克（冲服）；壮热不退者加羚羊粉0.3～0.6克（冲服）。

(3) 阴虚火旺型

主证：多属系统性红斑狼疮缓解期。壮热已退，转为持续低热，五心烦热，口干唇燥，头昏乏力，耳鸣目眩，腰腿酸软，关节酸痛，盗汗，落发，月经不调。舌质红，苔薄黄或无苔，脉细数。

治法：养阴清热。

方药：知柏地黄汤（70）加减

生地30克，玄参15克，天冬12克，麦冬12克，知母9克，黄柏9克，青蒿9克，地骨皮15克，丹皮9克，茯苓9克，山萸肉12克，旱莲草12克，女贞子12克，水煎服。

(4) 气阴两虚型

主证：多属系统性红斑狼疮缓解期。全身乏力，纳呆，精神萎靡，心悸气短，或有低热，口干不欲饮，大便燥结，舌质红，脉沉细而弱。

治法：益气养阴。

方药：生脉散（103）加味

太子参15克，麦冬15克，五味子9克，南北沙参各15克，玄参30克，石斛15克，生地30克，生黄芪30克，黄精15克，茯苓9克，白术9克，当归9克，丹参15克，水煎服。

(5) 热毒扰心型

主证：见于有心脏病变者。证见心悸怔忡，气短胸闷，自汗不眠，心神不安，面色苍白，四肢逆冷，舌淡苔薄白，脉细弱或见结代。

治法：益气养心、安神。

方药：养心汤（104）加减

太子参 15 克，南北沙参各 15 克，炙黄芪 30 克，当归 9 克，生地 15 克，丹参 15 克，茯神 9 克，炒枣仁 15 克，柏子仁 15 克，五味子 9 克，远志 9 克，珍珠母 30 克，炙甘草 6 克，水煎服。

(6) 脾肾阳虚型

主证：多见于肾脏损害后期。证见面色㿠白，畏寒肢冷，浮肿，乏力，精神萎靡，腰痛腹胀，不思饮食，便溏溲少，或面如满月，肩背肿胖。甚则胸水、腹水，心悸气促，舌质淡而体胖，边有齿印，脉沉细弱。

治法：温阳利水。

方药：金匮肾气丸（105）合二仙汤（96）、参附汤（106）加减。

熟附子 9 克，仙灵脾 15 克，仙茅 10 克，巴戟天 9 克，菟丝子 15 克，生黄芪 15 克，党参 15 克，炒白术 9 克，淮山药 15 克，茯苓 9 克，桂枝 9 克，猪苓 12 克，泽泻 12 克，水煎服。

2. 外治法

(1) 生肌玉红膏（128）外涂患处，每日 2～3 次。

(2) 密陀僧散（107）适量，醋调擦，每日 2～3 次。

3. 其他疗法

急性发作期或重型病例常须配合西医疗法。

护理与预防

1. 避免日光曝晒。

2. 适当增加营养。浮肿时应低盐或无盐饮食。

3. 防止劳累、注意保暖，急性发作期卧床休息。

4. 节制生育。

10.2 硬皮病

硬皮病是一种以皮肤肿胀、硬化,最后发生萎缩为特征的结缔组织病。临床上一般分为局限性与全身性两型。近似于中医文献中记载的皮痹,属痹证范畴。任何年龄均可发病,女多于男。病程缓慢。

病因病机

素体肾阳虚损,营血不足,卫外不固,腠理失密,兼风寒湿邪乘虚侵袭,凝结于经络、肌表、血脉之间,以致营卫不和,气血凝滞,痹塞不通;或外邪由之入侵脏腑,以致脏腑不和,气血凝滞而成。

临床表现

1. 局限性硬皮病

病变仅侵犯皮肤,偶可侵犯其下之肌肉,不累及内脏,预后较好。常见皮损形态有斑状、带状、点状3种。

(1) 斑状硬皮病:最常见。可发生于身体任何部位,损害多寡不定,不对称。初起为轻度水肿性发硬斑片,呈淡红色,边缘清楚。皮损渐扩大,呈圆形、椭圆形或不规则形。中央颜色逐渐变淡,呈黄白色,略凹陷,周围有1细狭淡紫晕,表面皮肤光亮如涂蜡。其下肌肉亦可变硬。病久,皮肤萎缩菲薄,弹性消失,毛细血管扩张,色素沉着与脱失夹杂,轻度脱屑,毛发脱落。一般局部自觉症状不明显,或有紧张不适感。病程缓慢,数年后可自愈。

(2) 点状硬皮病:较少见。多发于颈部和胸部。为多数黄豆大小、集簇性、发硬的小斑点,白色或象牙色,圆形,稍凹陷,周围有淡紫红色晕。日久变萎缩。可与斑状硬皮病同时并发。

(3) 带状或线状硬皮病:皮损与斑状相似,但呈条索状分布。多见于头面、躯干或4肢,常单侧分布。在额部的皮损可由头皮向前后方延伸,日久凹陷,萎缩,色白,毛发脱落,状如刀砍。躯干部皮损常呈半环状围绕躯干分布。四肢皮损常沿肢体长轴排列，偶有呈环状排列者。

2. 系统性硬皮病

病变除侵犯皮肤外，还常累及内脏，预后较差。

(1) 早期症状：发病隐匿，可渐感有倦怠乏力，消瘦，不思饮食，关节疼痛等。肢端动脉痉挛（雷诺氏现象）常为本病的前驱症状。

(2) 皮肤损害：常由4肢远端或面部开始，呈对称性分布，逐渐向近端或全身发展，重者开始即为全身性。病变过程经过浮肿、硬化、萎缩3个时期。浮肿期，皮肤呈现实质性非凹陷性浮肿，皮纹消失，表面光滑，色淡黄或黄白。硬化期，浮肿处逐渐绷紧发硬，表面光滑，呈蜡样光泽，伴有色素沉着或夹杂色素脱失。毛发渐脱，知觉迟钝。萎缩期，皮肤萎缩变薄，皮肤附属器萎缩消失，毛发脱落，出汗障碍，色素加深。皮损僵如皮革，紧贴于骨。

(3) 中晚期病人随侵犯部位不同而出现各种表现：侵犯面部时，呈假面样，面色如土，表情淡漠，开口及眼睑张合均感困难。口唇变薄，口缩小，口周有放射状沟纹，牙齿外露，鼻部尖细如刀削，耳部变薄等特殊面容。侵犯胸腹部时，皮肤坚硬，犹如披甲，呼吸表浅。若侵犯4肢，则关节僵硬，屈伸受限。发生在肢端者，指尖变细，手指僵硬，屈如鹰爪。部分病人可发生指（趾）端溃疡，经久不愈。

(4) 内脏损害：消化道受累，伸舌受限，食道变硬、变狭窄，吞咽困难，恶心呕吐，腹胀，腹泻或便秘等；心脏受累，心肌可产生纤维化，可导致心律不齐，心脏扩大，甚至心力衰竭；肺脏受累，可产生肺纤维化，导致肺活量减少，呼吸困难，继发感染等；肾脏受累，可导致高血压，蛋白尿及尿毒症等。

(5) 病程经过缓慢。全身性进行性者，常因心肾功能衰竭、营养障碍、支气管肺炎等而致死亡。

(6) 实验室检查：贫血；血沉增快；部分病人血清球蛋白升高，类风湿因子阳性，抗核抗体阳性，少数（7%）可找到红斑性狼疮细胞；肾脏损害时则有蛋白尿、血尿、管型等；因皮下、肌肉等软组织有广泛钙盐沉积，故 X 线检查可见点状或片状阴影。

辨证论治

1. 内治法

(1) 气血凝滞型

主证：多见于无全身症状的硬皮病。证见皮肤硬化萎缩，色素加深或色素脱失。或伴有肢端动脉痉挛现象。舌质暗或见瘀斑，脉象可涩滞。

治法：活血祛瘀。

方药：血府逐瘀汤（108）加减

生地 30 克，桃仁 9 克，红花 9 克，当归 15 克，赤芍 15 克，丹参 15 克，川芎 15 克，三棱 9 克，川牛膝 9 克，鸡血藤 30 克，水煎服。

(2) 脾肾阳虚型

主证：多见于系统性硬皮病。证见皮肤硬化，面色㿠白，肢端发绀，形寒肢冷，腰酸乏力，脱发，自汗，阳痿，遗精，纳呆，腹胀，便溏。舌胖有齿印，脉象沉细或迟缓。

治法：健脾益肾，温阳通络。

方药：阳和汤（109）加减

麻黄 6 克，熟地 15 克，鹿角胶 9 克，制附子 9 克，肉桂 9 克，干姜 9 克，白芥子 9 克，黄芪 15 克，威灵仙 12 克，茯苓 9 克，鸡血藤 15 克，甘草 6 克，水煎服。

加减：气虚者加党参 15 克，黄精 15 克。血虚者加当归 15 克，首乌 15 克，阿胶 9 克。便溏者加车前子 15 克（包煎）。

中成药：根据病情可单用或配合使用以下药物。脾肾阳虚者，金匮肾气丸（105），每次 1~2 丸，日 2 次；气血虚者，十全大补丸（62），每次1~2丸，日2次；关节活动受限者，小活络丹（110），每次1~2丸，日2次，或伸筋片（111），每次3片，日3次；气滞血瘀者，活血祛瘀片（101），每次5—10片，每日3次。

2. 外治法

（1）伸筋草30克，透骨草30克，艾叶15克，乳香、没药各6克，煎水适量薰洗患处，每次30分钟，日2次。

（2）回阳玉龙膏（93）用蜂蜜调敷，再以火烘患部。每日1次，每次约20分钟。

10.3 皮肌炎

皮肌炎是1种肌肉及皮肤的非感染性弥漫性炎性病变，属结缔组织病范畴。以皮肤红肿，肌肉疼痛、无力、肿胀、萎缩为主征。本病也可累及内脏，成为全身性的疾病。中医文献尚无相符之病名，但根据临床表现似与肌痹相类似。《素问》记载："病在肌肤，肌肤尽痛，名曰肌痹，伤于寒湿。"本病多见于中年以上女性（与男性比为2∶1），儿童患者年龄常在10岁以下。病程多为慢性经过。

病因病机

禀性不耐，卫气不固，以致风热毒邪或风寒湿邪乘虚入侵肌肤所致。急性者，风热毒邪除蕴阻肌肤外，还常因热毒炽盛而内传脏腑；慢性者，多为风寒湿邪蕴滞肌肤，阻隔经络，致使营卫不和，气血运行不畅。也有风寒湿邪郁久化热而致热毒炽盛者。不论急性、慢性，病久均可耗伤气血，导致气血虚亏。

临床表现

根据临床表现，一般将本病分为急性、慢性两型。急性型：先有短时间（数日）全身不适，尔后突然出现四肢肿胀、疼痛，常伴有高热、头晕、乏力，四肢肌肉对称性疼痛，活动及持物时加重，并有压痛；慢性型：一般为潜伏性，多先有上呼吸道感染，也有因日光暴晒或受寒起病者。初起常表现为面部红斑，疲乏无力，肿胀，肌痛，肢端动脉痉挛现象等。

1. 皮肤症状

初起常于面部，尤其是眼睑部出现水肿性淡紫红色斑，称为紫红眼睑，颇具特征性。水肿为实质性，压之不陷，具有特殊韧感。红肿可渐向颈、胸、肩及4肢伸侧等处扩延，并可相互融合。日久皮损逐渐干燥，出现糠秕状脱屑，或呈轻度皮肤萎缩及色素沉着，兼有点状色素减退和毛细血管扩张，因而具有皮肤异色症之表现。由于肌肉受累部位的皮肤为非凹陷性浮肿，皮肤肥厚、硬化，因而又有硬皮病样改变。毛发，尤其头发亦可脱落、变稀、变细、无光泽。粘膜病变也颇为多见，如红肿、糜烂、溃疡等。

2. 肌肉症状

肌肉症状是本病重要症状之一。受累肌肉一般为多发性，对称性分布，偶为局限性。与皮损或同时出现或先后出现。二者症状严重程度可不一致。以4肢近端肌肉最易受累，其次为肩胛部、颈部、面部、咽部等处。主要感觉症状为肌肉表现严重无力、紧张，自发痛、压痛，活动时疼痛加剧。患者常感觉蹲坐起立和步登台阶困难，步履蹒跚。严重者卧床不起，转辗困难。由于受累肌群不同，临床上可有种种表现，如颈部肌肉受累，头颈难于保持挺立；咽后肌和食道肌受累，可导致吞咽困难；呼吸肌受累，可致发音异常和呼吸困难；心脏受累，常表现为心肌炎，心力衰竭。受累区肌肉早期可显示肿胀，肌力减退，晚期可萎缩、变硬，活动受限，甚至痿废。

3. 全身症状

常有不规则发热、神疲乏力、易于出汗、消瘦、贫血、淋巴结和肝脾肿大、肢端动脉痉挛、类风湿性关节炎样表现等。约20%的患者并发恶性肿瘤。据报道，40岁以上的皮肌炎病人癌并发率高达52.2%。

4. 实验室检查

白细胞增高；血沉加快；24小时尿中肌酸测定量显著增高；肌酐排出量减少；球蛋白升高；血清酶特别是肌酸磷酸激酶、醛缩酶、乳酸脱氢酶、谷-草及谷-丙转氨酶增高；肌原性肌电图以及肌肉活组织检查显示肌炎变化。

辨证论治

1. 内治法

(1) 热毒炽盛型

主证：相当于急性活动期。发病急，面部红斑鲜艳、弥漫，高热、汗出、头晕、口渴、口苦、咽干，肌肉关节酸痛无力。苔黄厚，舌质红绛，脉象洪数。

治法：清热解毒，凉血养阴。

方药：清瘟败毒饮（73）加减

生地30克，丹皮9克，赤芍15克，黄芩9克，黄连6克，栀子9克，连翘9克，板蓝根30克，生石膏30克，知母9克，玄参15克，牛蒡子9克，生甘草6克，水煎服。

加减：热盛高热不退者加羚羊粉0.3～0.6克（冲服）。肿胀明显者加车前子12克（包煎），泽泻15克。关节肌肉痛重者可加秦艽9克，威灵仙9克。

(2) 湿热郁蒸型

主证：多见于急性、亚急性活动期。常有中等度发热或低热，倦怠乏力，胃纳呆滞，脘腹胀满，便秘溲黄，肌肤潮红肿胀、疼痛。苔黄腻，脉濡数。

治法：清热解毒，利湿消肿。

方药：茵陈蒿汤（112）合草薢渗湿汤（53）加减

茵陈15克，栀子9克，生大黄6克（后入），黄柏9克，草薢9克，茯苓12克，薏苡仁30克，车前子9克（包煎），泽泻15克，滑石15克，通草6克，丹皮9克，生甘草6克，水煎服。

加减：纳呆腹胀加焦楂 15 克，枳壳 9 克。低热不退者加银柴胡 9 克，地骨皮 12 克。

(3) 气虚血亏型

主证：多见于慢性期。皮损暗红，或色素沉着，干燥脱屑，肌肤消瘦或有硬化，疲倦乏力，腰膝酸软，畏寒肢冷，或自汗盗汗，咽痛口干，腹胀纳差。舌质淡或质红，苔薄或光剥无苔，边有齿印，脉沉细。

治法：益气养血，活血通络。

方药：十全大补汤（62）加减

黄芪 15 克，党参 12 克，白术 9 克，茯苓 12 克，当归 15 克，熟地 15 克，赤芍 12 克，白芍 12 克，鸡血藤 15 克，丹参 15 克，威灵仙 9 克，炙甘草 6 克，水煎服。

加减：咽喉干痛，舌红苔剥者加生地 15 克，麦冬 12 克，石斛 12 克。形寒肢冷，关节肌肉酸痛，肢端动脉痉挛者可加桂枝 9 克，细辛 3 克，川芎 9 克。自汗盗汗加浮小麦 30 克，五味子 9 克。

中成药：慢性期可选用人参健脾丸（113），十全大补丸（62），金匮肾气丸（105）等，每服 1～2 丸，日 2 次；伸筋片（111），每次服 6 片，日 3 次，小儿酌减。

2. 外治

局部可配合理疗、按摩、针灸等治疗方法，以防止和减轻肌肉萎缩。

3. 其他疗法

急性期可根据病情需要配合西医疗法。

预防与护理

1. 急性期应保持安静，卧床休息。病情缓解后则需适当活动。
2. 避免暴晒与防寒。
3. 应给予营养丰富并易于消化的高蛋白饮食。
4. 避免妊娠，以防止病情恶化或复发。

11 皮肤附属器疾病

11.1 寻常性痤疮

寻常性痤疮是1种青春发育期常见的毛囊皮脂腺疾病。主要发生于颜面及胸背等处。中医文献有痤、粉刺等名。

病因病机

本病多因肺经血热,薰蒸颜面;或饮食不节,过食肥甘厚味,脾胃积热,又感风毒之邪,凝滞而成。

临床表现

1. 多见于青春期男女,男性多于女性。
2. 皮疹好发于颜面、肩周、胸背等皮脂腺较丰富的部位。
3. 初起为粉刺,即针头大小的丘疹,丘疹呈灰白色或肤色的称白头粉刺;丘疹顶端黑色者称黑头粉刺。用手挤压,可挤出乳白色或黄白色脂栓。粉刺继发感染后,发展成粟粒至赤豆大小的红丘疹,有的顶部可发生小脓疱,有的可形成结节、脓肿、囊肿及疤痕等多种形态损害。患者常同时伴有皮脂过度溢出。
4. 一般无自觉症状,较重者可有不同程度的痒痛感觉。
5. 病程经过缓慢。皮疹常此愈彼起,缠绵不断。青春期过后,大都自愈或减轻。

辨证论治

病程轻者可不需治疗或仅用外治法,重者可配合内治。

1. 内治法

(1) 肺胃湿热型

主证:颜面潮红油腻,皮疹以红丘疹和脓疱为主,常伴有不同程度瘙痒或疼痛。可有口臭、喜冷饮、大便干燥等。舌质红,苔黄或黄腻，脉弦滑或滑数。

治法：清泄肺胃湿热，佐以凉血解毒。

方药：枇杷清肺饮（114）加减

枇杷叶9克，桑白皮9克，黄芩9克，黄柏9克，黄连6克，栀子9克，生地15克，丹皮9克，赤芍15克，生石膏15克，茵陈15克，生甘草6克，水煎服。

加减：脓胞明显，热毒炽盛者，可加金银花30克，蒲公英30克，地丁15克，便秘者，加生大黄6克（后入）。皮脂溢出明显者，加薏苡仁30克，生白术12克，车前草30克。

(2) 痰瘀凝结型

主证：反复发作，久治不愈，皮疹以结节、囊肿、疤痕为主。

治法：活血化瘀，消痰软坚。

方药：海藻玉壶汤（115）加减

当归12克，川芎12克，赤芍15克，丹参15克，青皮9克，陈皮9克，半夏9克，浙贝9克，昆布15克，海藻15克，夏枯草15克，连翘12克，水煎服。

中成药：属肺胃湿热型者，可服防风通圣丸（54）或龙胆泻肝丸（8），每次6克，每日2次。痰瘀凝结型者可服散结片（116），每次10片，每日3次。

2. 外治法

颠倒散（19）适量，茶水调成糊状，睡前涂患处，次晨洗净。

护理与预防

1. 经常用温水肥皂洗脸。
2. 禁忌挤压患处。
3. 少食油腻及糖类，忌酒及辣等刺激性饮食，多吃蔬菜、水果，保持消化道通畅。

11.2 酒渣鼻

酒渣鼻系发生在鼻部的慢性皮肤病。因鼻色紫红如酒渣而得名。损害特征为皮肤潮红，伴有丘疹、脓疱及毛细血管扩张。近年来，在酒渣鼻的皮损中，常发现有毛囊虫的存在，因此，也有人提出该病应改名为毛囊虫皮炎。

病因病机

肺经血热内蒸；或嗜酒，热势冲面；或过食辛辣厚味，胃肠积热上薰，复感风寒外束，以致血瘀凝结而成。

临床表现

1. 本病多发于中年人。
2. 皮疹发生于颜面中部，以鼻尖、鼻翼为主，其次为两颊和前额。少数病例只发于两颊和前额，鼻部正常。
3. 按皮疹的进展过程可分为 3 期，但各期并无明显界限。

（1）红斑期：初为暂时性、阵发性红斑，呈弥漫性分布。遇寒风、食用刺激性饮食及精神兴奋时红斑显著。日久红斑持续不退，并有轻度毛细血管扩张，呈树枝状。有的数年后可发展成丘疹期。

（2）丘疹期：在红斑的基础上出现多数散在的粉刺样小丘疹，有的可变成脓疱，尤以鼻尖为甚。皮色由鲜红渐变为紫褐。此期毛细血管扩张明显，呈蛛网状，故又称此期为毛细血管扩张期。可迁延数年，极少数可发展成鼻赘期。

（3）鼻赘期：少数晚期患者，鼻部组织增生变厚，鼻尖部的丘疹发展成结节性肥大，表面凹凸不平，形成鼻赘。

患者多伴有皮脂溢出症，颜面油腻如涂脂。

4. 病程缓慢，一般无明显自觉症状，或有微痒。

辨证论治

1. 内治法

（1）肺胃湿热型

主证：相当于红斑期和丘疹期。皮疹以红斑、丘疹及毛细血管扩张为主，可伴有瘙痒，渴喜冷饮，小便短黄，大便干燥。舌红，苔薄黄或黄腻，脉象滑数。

治法：清热祛湿，凉血活血。

方药：枇杷清肺饮（114）加减

枇杷叶9克，生槐花9克，桑白皮9克，生石膏30克，黄芩9克，黄连6克，栀子9克，丹皮9克，生地15克，赤芍15克，白茅根30克，红花9克，水煎服。

加减：脓疱明显者，加蒲公英30克，野菊花15克。便秘者，加生大黄6克（后入）。

（2）血瘀凝滞型

主证：鼻部呈暗红或紫红色，皮肤肥厚，或见鼻赘，舌质暗或见瘀斑，脉弦或涩滞。

治法：活血化瘀。

方药：通窍活血汤（100）加减

归尾15克，赤芍15克，桃仁9克，红花9克，川芎9克，五灵脂9克，蒲黄9克，桑白皮9克，陈皮9克，白芷9克，老葱白9克，生姜6克。

中成药：血瘀甚者，并服大黄䗪虫丸（117）早晚各1丸。

2. 外治

（1）5～10%硫磺霜外涂，每日2～3次，或颠倒散（19）清水调为稀糊状，睡前涂患处，次晨洗去。

（2）大枫子肉、水银、核桃仁各6克，先把大枫子肉、核桃仁捣成泥后，再加入水银，捣打至不见水银为度。用纱布裹药少许，在患部揉擦，使患处有热感即可，每日擦药4～5次。

护理与预防

1. 饮食宜清淡，避免各种刺激性饮食，如酒、辣椒等。避免过热饮食和油腻等，并保持大便通畅。

2. 避免面部过冷过热刺激。

3. 保持情绪稳定，避免情志过急。

11.3 皮脂溢出症与脂溢性皮炎

皮脂溢出症是以皮脂分泌过多为特征的常见疾病。脂溢性皮炎为在皮脂溢出症的基础上发生的一种慢性皮肤炎症。继发湿疹样变化者有人称为脂溢性湿疹。中医文献称发于头部者为白屑风；发于面部者为面游风。皮脂溢出症和脂溢性皮炎多发于青壮年，也见于初生婴儿。

病因病机

因风热之邪外袭，郁久则耗伤阴血而血虚，血虚则生风化燥，风燥热邪蕴阻肌肤，肌肤失养所致，表现以干性皮损为主；或过食肥甘油腻，辛辣酒类等，肠胃湿热壅滞，复受风邪，内外合邪，蕴阻肌腠而成，表现以湿性皮损为主。

临床表现

1. 皮脂溢出症

（1）青壮年皮脂溢：主要发生于皮脂腺丰富的部位，如头皮、颜面等处。临床上可分为油性皮脂溢和干性皮脂溢两种。油性皮脂溢：皮脂分泌过多，毛发、头皮及面部油腻光亮，颜面以鼻部最为明显，可见毛囊口扩大，易于挤出黄白色脂栓。干性皮脂溢：头皮遍布灰白色细小鳞屑，易于脱落，脱而又生，梳发或搔抓时常飘扬坠落。日久，毛发往往变细变软，稀疏脱落，称脂溢性脱发。

（2）初生婴儿皮脂溢：多见于营养良好，喂养过多脂肪的新生儿。头皮可见黄厚脂性痂皮。面颊部皮肤潮红，并有油腻性鳞屑覆盖。

2. 脂溢性皮炎

（1）好发于头皮、面部、外耳部、腋窝、胸背等皮脂腺丰富部位。常自头部开始向下蔓延，重者泛发全身。

（2）皮疹为略带黄色的红斑或粉红斑片，大小不一，边缘不整。临床上分鳞屑型和结痂型。鳞屑型：皮疹呈斑片状，表面有油腻性鳞屑。痂皮型：油腻性鳞屑及渗液结成黄厚痂，本型以婴儿最多见。

(3) 由于部位不同，其表现不一。头部：主要为边界不清的红斑，油腻性鳞屑与痂皮，搔抓后可发生糜烂、渗液。面部：最常见于鼻翼旁沟、鼻唇与眉弓部，表现为淡红斑，上有油腻性鳞屑。耳部：可见糜烂、黄痂或皲裂。躯干：最常见于胸前与肩胛骨间的皮肤，为圆形或椭圆形，黄红色或淡红色斑片，表面覆有油腻性鳞屑，少数散在，也可多数融合，或倾向于中心痊愈而形成环状或多环状，类似玫瑰糠疹样发疹。皱褶部：常见于腹股沟、腋窝、臀缝、男性阴囊和女性乳房下等处。一般呈黄红色鳞屑斑片，常呈湿疹样糜烂。

(4) 病程缓慢。常伴有不同程度骚痒。患病日久者，皮肤浸润肥厚，呈慢性皮炎改变。

辨证论治

1. 内治法

(1) 湿热型

主证：皮疹潮红，上覆油腻性鳞屑，或见糜烂、渗出、结痂，自觉骚痒。可伴有胸闷、口苦、纳呆。舌质红，苔黄腻，脉滑数。

治法：清热利湿，祛风止痒。

方药：龙胆泻肝汤 (8) 加减

龙胆草9克，黄芩9克，黄柏9克，栀子9克，苦参9克，白藓皮15克，地肤子15克，柴胡9克，厚朴9克，车前子9克（包煎），茵陈15克，泽泻12克，木通6克，水煎服。

(2) 风燥型

主证：证见干性鳞屑，炎症轻微，或见皮肤粗糙、干燥、肥厚，骚痒明显，或伴毛发干枯脱落。舌红苔少，脉弦。

治法：养血祛风润燥。

方药：当归饮子（4）加减

当归 15 克，生地 30 克，何首乌 30 克，川芎 9 克，赤芍 9 克，白芍 9 克，牡丹皮 9 克，玄参 15 克，麦冬 15 克，刺蒺藜 15 克，防风 9 克，侧柏叶 9 克，水煎服。

2. 外治法

（1）燥湿洗药（59）煎水洗患处，或硝矾洗药（16），热水溶解后洗患处。每日 1～2 次，每次 20～30 分钟。

（2）有糜烂、渗出者，可先以燥湿洗药（59）煎水待凉湿敷，湿敷间歇期，黄柏散（17）用麻油调成糊状外涂。

（3）以红斑为主，无糜烂、渗液者，可外涂 5～10%硫磺霜或颠倒散洗剂（硫磺、生大黄各 7.5 克，石灰水 100 毫升混合即成）外搽，每日 2～3 次。

11.4 斑秃

斑秃是一种以头发突然呈斑片状脱落，而脱发处无炎症和自觉症状的皮肤附属器疾病。中医文献称油风。

病因病机

本病多因血虚不能随气濡养皮肤，使腠理不密，玄府不固，毛孔开张，风邪乘隙外袭，风盛血燥，发失所养而致；或因情志不遂，肝气郁结，过分劳累，心气乃伤，气滞血瘀，气血不能上荣毛发所致；又因肝藏血，发为血之余，肾主骨，其荣在发，故肝肾不足亦能导致脱发。

临床表现

1. 本病可发生于任何年龄，但以青壮年居多。

2. 常在过度劳累、睡眠不足或精神受到刺激后发病。

3. 起病突然，常在无意中发觉或被他人发现头发呈斑片状脱落。脱发区呈圆形、椭圆形或不规则形，小如指甲，大若钱币或更大。数目 1 至数个不等。表面平滑，略有光泽，境界清楚。脱发斑有时可长期静止不变，亦可逐渐扩大增多。

4. 严重者可累及全头部，以致头发大部或全部脱落，称"全秃"；若全身毛发包括眉毛、睫毛、胡须、腋毛、阴毛、毳毛均脱落者称"普秃"。

5. 脱发处一般无任何自觉症状。

6. 病程缓慢。可逐渐自愈，亦可反复发作。

辨证论治

1. 内治法

(1) 血虚风燥型

主证：除脱发外，同时伴有头晕、目眩、心烦、失眠、多梦。舌淡，脉细。

治法：养血祛风。

方药：神应养真丹（12）加减

当归15克，白芍12克，熟地黄15克，何首乌30克，川芎9克，红花9克，女贞子12克，菟丝子12克，羌活9克，天麻6克，水煎服。

加减：失眠多梦者，加炒枣仁15克，茯神9克，远志9克。若病程日久，甚至全秃或普秃，兼见腰膝酸软，耳鸣目眩，遗精盗汗，舌淡苔少，脉象细弱者，可加枸杞子15克，桑椹15克，旱莲草15克。

中成药：养血生发片（118），每次10片，每日3次。七宝美髯丹（119），每次1丸，每日3次。

(2) 气滞血瘀型

主证：脱发久治不愈，面色晦暗，可伴头痛，胸胁痛，病变处或有外伤血肿史。舌质暗红或有瘀点，脉象涩滞或弦细。

治法：活血祛瘀。

方药：通窍活血汤（100）加减

当归尾9克，赤芍9克，川芎9克，桃仁9克，红花9克，三棱9克，莪术9克，柴胡9克，郁金9克，姜黄9克，生姜6克，老葱白9克，水煎服。

中成药：活血祛瘀片（101），每次 5～10 片，每日 3 次。
2. 外治
(1) 25%补骨脂酊外涂，每日 3 次。
(2) 鲜姜块用切开面频擦患处。
(3) 梅花针敲打患处，每日 2 次。

III.5 腋臭

腋臭是 1 种以腋下汗出，带有狐狸之腺臭味为特征的皮肤病。故俗称狐臭。根据其发病特点，中医文献中又有腋气、体气等名。如清代《外科大成·腋气》记载腋气，俗名狐臭，受秉于未形之初，腋内有窍，浊气由此而出，诸药鲜能根除。

病因病机

本病多由父母遗传所致；或湿热内郁，浊气随汗从毛孔外溢而成。现代医学认为，腋臭之臭味是由于大汗腺分泌物经细菌分解后所产生。

临床表现

1. 多见于青年男女，但以女性更为多见，家族中或有同样患者。
2. 多发于腋窝部，重者亦可发于乳晕、脐、前后阴、腹股沟等大汗腺分布区。
3. 腋下易于汗出，并带有臭气。患部可见棕纹毛孔。因汗液色黄，内衣易于受染。夏季多汗时尤甚。轻者在无汗时几乎无臭气。始发于青春期，老年后逐渐减轻或消失。

辨证论治

一般不需内治。发病部位多，汗出粘腻，色黄，臭气较剧，或伴腹胀纳呆，大便不调，小便黄赤，苔黄腻，脉滑数者，为湿热内郁，浊气外溢，可配合内治。

治法：清热利湿，芳香化浊。

方药：甘露消毒丹（120）加减

藿香 9 克，薄荷 9 克，白蔻仁 9 克，菖蒲 12 克，黄芩 9 克，连翘 9 克，土茯苓 15 克，苍术 9 克，茵陈 15 克，滑石 1.5 克，木通 6 克，泽泻 9 克，水煎服。

2. 外治法

(1) 用密陀僧散（107）或枯矾粉搽患处，每日数次。

(2) 枯矾 30 克，蛤蜊壳粉 15 克，樟脑 15 克，共研细末外搽，早晚各 1 次。

护理与预防

1. 保持患处清洁干燥，做到勤洗澡、勤更衣，常用香皂、温水洗涤。

2. 忌食辛辣等刺激较强的饮食，最好戒除烟酒。

12 色素性皮肤病

12.1 白癜风

白癜风是1种以皮肤出现无自觉症状的白斑，斑内毛发亦可变白为特征的皮肤病。中医文献称白癜、白驳风等。如《诸病源候论·白癜候》记载："白癜者，面及颈项身体皮肉色白，与肉色不同，亦不痒痛，谓之白癜。此亦是风邪搏于皮肤，血气不和所生也。"

病因病机

情志内伤，肝气郁结，气机不畅，或因肾阴虚，复感风邪，风邪搏于皮肤，致令气血不和，或气滞血瘀，血不滋养肌肤而成。

临床表现

1. 任何年龄均可发生，但好发于青年，亦可见于儿童。

2. 全身各部均可发生，但以面部、颈部、手背等局限发病者为多。可对称亦可单侧发生，有时可呈节段性或带状分布。

3. 皮肤损害为边界清楚、大小不等的圆形、椷圆形或不规则形的白色斑片。周围色素常较深。表面平滑，斑内毛发变白或正常。数目不定，单发或多发，可相互融合成大片。

4. 一般无自觉症状，少数在病情进展期局部可有微痒。露出部经日晒后发红并有灼痛刺痒感。

5. 皮疹发展有时进展快，有时历久静止不变，病程缓慢。少数患者，尤其早期儿童患者可自愈。

辨证论治

1. 内治法

治法：祛风，养血，活血，滋肾。

方药：白驳片（121）加减

防风 9 克，白蒺藜 30 克，浮萍 15 克，川芎 9 克，赤芍 9 克，红花 9 克，当归 9 克，鸡血藤 15 克，补骨脂 9 克，黑豆皮 15 克，陈皮 9 克，水煎服。

中成药：白驳片（121）或豨莶丸（122），每次 1～2 丸，每日 2 次；复方蒺藜片（123），每次 10 片，每日 3 次。

2. 外治法

(1) 密陀僧散（107）适量醋调搽患处，每日 3 次。

(2) 25%补骨脂酊搽患处，每日 3 次。

12.2 黄褐斑

黄褐斑是 1 种面部色素增生性皮肤病。俗称蝴蝶斑。本病与中医文献中记载的面尘、黧黑斑等相似。

病因病机

忧思抑郁、肝气郁结，气滞血瘀于颜面；或饮食不节，以致脾胃湿热薰蒸于面；或因肾阴不足，虚火上炎，郁结不散，阻于皮肤而致。

临床表现

1. 多发于妇女，但少数未婚女青年及男子亦可罹患。也有继发于肝病、结核病或其他慢性病者。

2. 皮损发生于面颊、额部、鼻部及口周围，常对称分布。

3. 皮损呈黄褐色至暗褐色，边界明显或模糊不清。斑片大小不一，表面光滑，有时可互相融合成蝴蝶状。日晒加重，故春夏斑色加深。

4. 病程缓慢。少数可自行消退。局部无自觉症状。

辨证论治

1. 内治法

(1) 肝郁血瘀型

主证：多见于更年期、肝脏病或有生殖系统疾患的妇女。除面部对称性褐斑外，常伴有性情急躁或忧思抑郁，胸胁胀满，月经不调等。舌苔薄白，或见舌质有瘀斑，脉弦。

治法：疏肝理气，活血化瘀。

方药：逍遥散（124）加减

柴胡12克，当归12克，赤芍9克，白芍9克，白术9克，茯苓9克，青皮9克，陈皮9克，香附9克，丹参15克，红花9克，薄荷6克，水煎服。

中成药：逍遥丸（124），每次6克，每日2次。

(2) 脾胃湿热型

主证：斑色黄褐而鲜明，可伴有纳呆，腹胀，口渴，口臭，大便不调，小便黄赤。苔黄腻，脉滑数。

治法：清热渗湿。

方药：清肌渗湿汤（125）加减

苍术9克，白术9克，厚朴9克，陈皮9克，柴克9克，木通6克，泽泻9克，白芷9克，升麻9克，栀子9克，黄连6克，黄芩9克，水煎服。

加减：便秘者加生大黄6克（后入）。

中成药：三黄丸（126），每次4.5克，每日2次。

(3) 虚火上炎型

主证：斑色黄而晦暗，或兼有结核病等慢性疾患，可伴有低热，盗汗，五心烦热，腰膝酸软，失眠多梦等。舌红苔黄，脉细数。

治法：滋阴降火。

方药：知柏地黄汤（70）加减

生地15克，熟地15克，玄参15克，丹皮9克，地骨皮9克，赤芍15克，山药15克，山萸肉12克，泽泻9克，茯苓9克，黄柏9克，知母9克，水煎服。

中成药：六味地黄丸（79）或知柏地黄丸（70），每次1～2

丸，日2次。

2. 外治法

(1) 白附子、白芷、滑石各250克，共研细末，早晚洗脸后涂患处。

(2) 青嫩柿树叶晒干，研细末，取30克，与白凡士林30克，调成膏，每天睡前涂患处，次晨洗净。

12.3 雀斑

根据面部有散在芝麻大小斑点，如雀卵之色，故名雀斑。本病亦名夏日斑。好发于颜面、颈部及手背等处，表现为黄褐色或暗褐色斑点。有遗传倾向。

病因病机

禀赋不足，肾水不能荣华于面，浮火结滞形成；或浮火郁于细小脉络之中，复受风邪侵袭，风火之邪相结而致。

临床表现

1. 男女均可发生，但以青春期后的女性为多见，一般多从儿童期开始发病，至青春期明显增多，成人后停止发展。

2. 皮损以颜面、颈部、手背为多见，亦可见于胸部及4肢伸侧，多对称发生。

3. 为粟粒至芝麻大小褐色或暗褐色斑点，境界明显，与肤面相平，密集或稀疏分布，从不融合。夏季日晒后数目增多，颜色变深。冬季则数目减少，颜色变浅。

4. 无任何自觉症状。

辨证论治

1. 内治法

治法：滋阴降火。

方药：知柏地黄汤（70）加减

生地150克，熟地150克，山萸肉60克，丹皮50克，泽泻50克，茯苓60克，山药90克，玄参90克，白薇60克，白附子 40 克，共为蜜丸，每丸重 10 克，早晚各 1 丸。

中成药：六味地黄丸（79）或知柏地黄丸（70）每次 1～2 丸，每日 2 次。

2. 外治法

（1）黑丑 30 克，研极细粉，每晚睡前取少许，用少量鸡蛋清调成糊状涂患处，次晨温水洗净，连用 5～7 周。

（2）时珍正容散（127）水调成糊状，睡前涂，次晨洗去。

护理与预防

春夏季节应避免暴晒，外出宜戴宽缘帽防护。

（杜锡贤）

THE ENGLISH–CHINESE ENCYCLOPEDIA OF PRACTICAL TCM
(Booklist)
英汉实用中医药大全
(书目)

VOLUME	TITLE	书名
1	ESSENTIALS OF TRADITIONAL CHINESE MEDICINE	中医学基础
2	THE CHINESE MATERIA MEDICA	中药学
3	PHARMACOLOGY OF TRADITIONAL CHINESE MEDICAL FORMULAE	方剂学
4	SIMPLE AND PROVEN PRESCRIPTION	单验方
5	COMMONLY USED CHINESE PATENTMEDICINES	常用中成药
6	THERAPY OF ACUPUNCTURE AND MOXIBUSTION	针灸疗法
7	*TUINA* THERAPY	推拿疗法
8	MEDICAL *QIGONG*	医学气功
9	MAINTAINING YOUR HEALTH	自我保健
10	INTERNAL MEDICINE	内科学

11	SURGERY	外科学
12	GYNECOLOGY	妇科学
13	PEDIATRICS	儿科学
14	ORTHOPEDICS	骨伤科学
15	PROCTOLOGY	肛门直肠病学
16	DERMATOLOGY	皮肤病学
17	OPHTHALMOLOGY	眼科学
18	OTORHINOLARYNGOLOGY	耳鼻喉科学
19	EMERGENTOLOGY	急症学
20	NURSING	护理
21	CLINICAL DIALOGUE	临床会话

(京) 112号

The English-Chinese
Encyclopedia of Practical TCM
Chief Editor   Xu Xiangcai

16
DERMATOLOGY

English Chief Editor   Li Lei
Chinese Chief Editor   Zhao Chunxiu

英汉实用中医药大全
主编　徐象才

16

皮 肤 病 学

中文　　英文

主编　赵纯修　李　磊

*

高等教育出版社出版
高等教育出版社激光照排技术部排版
新华书店总店北京科技发行所发行
国防工业出版社印刷厂印装

*

开本 850×1168 1/32　印张 13.75 字数 350 000
1991年10月第1版　1991年10月第1次印刷
印数 0001—5 175
ISBN 7-04-003670-3/R·14
定价 8.10 元